SMART! Sports Medicine Assessment and Review Textbook

{Miller: *SMART! Sports Medicine Assessment and Review,* ed. 1 (ISBN: 978-1-4377-0286-6)}

Erratum to Chapter 4, Elbow

Figure Citations:

P. 52, Fig. 4-4 was originally cited in O'Driscoll SW, Morrey BF, Jaloszynski R, An KN, 1992: Origin of the medial ulnar collateral ligament. J Hand Surg 17-A: 164-168, not Morrey (2009) as stated in the figure legend.

P. 56, Fig. 4-14 was originally cited in Smith AM, O'Driscoll SW, 2005. Diagnosing medial elbow pain in throwers. J Musculoskeletal Med 22, 305-316.

P. 62, Fig. 4-20 was originally cited in O'Driscoll SW, Lawton RI, Smith AM, 2005. The "moving valgus stress test" for medial collateral ligament tears of the elbow. Am J Sports Med 33, 231-239.

P. 65, Fig. 4-28 was originally cited in Smith AM, O'Driscoll SW, 2005. Diagnosing medial elbow pain in throwers. J Musculoskeletal Med 22, 305-316.

P. 71, Fig. 4-34 was originally cited in Antuna SA, O'Driscoll SW, 2001. Snapping plicae associated with radiocapitellar chondromalacia. Arthroscopy 17, 491-495, not O'Driscoll SW, Morrey BF, Korinek S, An KN: Elbow subluxation and dislocation. A spectrum of instability. Clin Orthop Relat Res 1992; 280:186-197.

Missing Reference:

The following reference should be included in the list of References and Resources:

O'Driscoll SW, 2008. Valgus extension overload and plica. In: Levine WN, Athlete's Elbow. American Academy of Orthopaedic Surgeons, Rosemont, IL, pp. 71-83.

SMART! Sports Medicine Assessment and Review Textbook

First Edition

Mark D. Miller, MD
S. Ward Casscells Professor of Orthopaedic Surgery
Head, Division of Sports Medicine
University of Virginia
Charlottesville, Virginia;
Adjunct Clinical Professor and Team Physician
James Madison University
Harrisonburg, Virginia

Associate Editor-in-Chief
Jennifer A. Hart, MPAS, PA-C
Physician Assistant
Department of Orthopaedic Surgery
University of Virginia
Charlottesville, Virginia;
Adjunct Clinical Assistant Professor
Physician Assistant Program
James Madison University
Harrisonburg, Virginia

SAUNDERS
ELSEVIER

SAUNDERS
ELSEVIER

1600 John F. Kennedy Blvd.
Ste 1800
Philadelphia, PA 19103-2899

SMART! SPORTS MEDICINE ASSESSMENT AND REVIEW TEXTBOOK ISBN: 978-1-4377-0286-6

Notice

Knowledge and best practice in this field are constantly changing. As new research and experience broaden our knowledge, changes in practice, treatment and drug therapy may become necessary or appropriate. Readers are advised to check the most current information provided (i) on procedures featured or (ii) by the manufacturer of each product to be administered, to verify the recommended dose or formula, the method and duration of administration, and contraindications. It is the responsibility of the practitioner, relying on their own experience and knowledge of the patient, to make diagnoses, to determine dosages and the best treatment for each individual patient, and to take all appropriate safety precautions. To the fullest extent of the law, neither the Publisher nor the Authors assumes any liability for any injury and/or damage to persons or property arising out of or related to any use of the material contained in this book.

The Publisher

Library of Congress Cataloging-in-Publication Data
SMART! : sports medicine assessment and review textbook / [edited by] Mark D. Miller ; associate editor-in-chief, Jennifer A. Hart. – 1st ed.
p. ; cm.
Other title: Sports medicine assessment and review textbook
Includes bibliographical references.
ISBN 978-1-4377-0286-6
1. Sports medicine–Examinations–Study guides. 2. Orthopedic surgery–Examinations–Study guides. I. Miller, Mark D. II. Hart, Jennifer A. (Jennifer Adele), 1974- III. Title: Sports medicine assessment and review textbook.
[DNLM: 1. Athletic Injuries–diagnosis. 2. Athletic Injuries–therapy. 3. Sports Medicine–methods. QT 261 S636 2011]
RC1213.S63 2011
617.1′027–dc22

2010015054

Acquisitions Editor: Daniel Pepper
Developmental Editor: Julie Goolsby
Publishing Services Manager: Hemamalini Rajendrababu
Project Manager: Sukanthi Sukumar
Design Direction: Louis Forgione

Cover art permissions:
Center: Adapted from Tria AJ, Lein KS: An Illustrated Guide to the Knee, p 13. NY, Churchill Livingstone, 1992.
Right: From Miller MD: Review of Orthopaedics, 5th Edition, p 275. Philadelphia, Saunders, 2008.

Printed in the United States of America

Last digit is the print number: 9 8 7 6 5 4 3 2 1

Contents

Preface

Review of Sports Medicine and Arthroscopy, which was a subspecialty version of the "best-selling" text *Review of Orthopaedics* (now in its fifth edition), was a very well received book; however, we never got the nod for a third edition. With the advent of Subspecialty Certification in Sports Medicine and increasing interest, we decided it was time to develop a new Sports Medicine text—complete with questions and answers. This is a book that will be helpful for medical students and residents who are doing rotations in Orthopaedic Sports Medicine, attending physicians preparing for the Subspecialty Exam, ancillary personnel, and anyone, really, who has an interest in our subspecialty.

We have attempted to organize the information provided in these pages in a way that will make this a useful tool as both a review textbook and study aide. We have invited renowned experts in the field to contribute to this book to ensure that the information is both up-to-date and inclusive of the most commonly tested themes. Questions and answers are provided in addition to the standard text format to add another layer to this study tool.

Dedication

This book is written for and dedicated to our past teachers who helped us in our own careers, our current colleagues with whom we work across the country in the field of sports medicine, and our future students who are embarking on their own careers in this subspecialty.

Mark D. Miller, MD
Jennifer A. Hart, MPAS, PA-C

Contributors

Brian D. Busconi, MD
Chief and Fellowship Director of Sports Medicine and Arthroscopy
Department of Orthopaedics
Umass Memorial Medical Center
Worcester, Massachusetts
Hip, Pelvis, and Thigh

Angelo R. Dacus
Assistant Professor
Department of Orthopaedic Surgery
University of Virginia
Charlottesville, Virginia
Wrist and Hand

Kathryn A. Dorweiler, MS, PA-C
Spine Physician Assistant
The Steadman Clinic
Frisco, Colorado
Head and Spine

Jason L. Dragoo, MD
Assistant Professor
Department of Orthopaedic Surgery
Stanford University
Palo Alto, California
Shoulder

Sanjitpal S. Gill, MD
Adjunct Assistant Professor
Department of Bioengineering
Clemson University
Clemson, South Carolina;
Orthopaedic Spine Surgeon
The Steadman Clinic
Vail, Colorado
Head and Spine

S. Raymond Golish, MD, PhD
Clinical Instructor
Department of Orthopaedic Surgery
Stanford University
Palo Alto, California
Shoulder

F. Winston Gwathmey Jr., MD
Resident Physician
Department of Orthopaedic Surgery
University of Virginia
Charlottesville, Virginia
Shoulder

Jennifer A. Hart, MPAS, PA-C
Physician Assistant
Department of Orthopaedic Surgery
University of Virginia
Charlottesville, Virginia;
Adjunct Clinical Assistant Professor
Physician Assistant Program
James Madison University
Harrisonburg, Virginia
The Team Physician and General Care of the Athlete
Medical Issues in the Athlete

Joseph M. Hart, PhD, ATC
Assistant Professor
Department of Orthopaedic Surgery
Department of Human Services-Kinesiology
University of Virginia
Charlottesville, Virginia
Sports Medicine Research and Statistics

John V. Ingari, MD
Assistant Professor of Surgery
Department of Surgery
Uniformed Services University of the Health Sciences
Bethesda, Maryland;
Chief, Hand Surgery Division
WellSpan Orthopaedics
York Hospital
York, Pennsylvania
Wrist and Hand

David A. Joos, MD
Resident
Department of Orthopaedic Surgery
University of Michigan Hospitals
Ann Arbor, Michigan
Ankle and Foot

Anish R. Kadakia, MD
Assistant Professor
Department of Orthopaedic Surgery
University of Michigan
Ann Arbor, Michigan
Ankle and Foot

Robert M. Masella, MD
Orthopaedic Surgery Fellow in Sports Medicine
Department of Orthopaedic Surgery
University of Massachusetts Medical School
Worcester, Massachusetts;
Hackettstown Regional Medical Center
Department of Orthopaedic Surgery;
Skylands Orthopaedics
Hackettstown, New Jersey;
Morristown Memorial Hospital
Department of Orthopaedic Surgery
Morristown, New Jersey
Hip, Pelvis, and Thigh

Mark D. Miller, MD
S. Ward Casscells Professor of Orthopaedic Surgery
Head, Division of Sports Medicine
University of Virginia
Charlottesville, Virginia;
Adjunct Clinical Professor and Team Physician
James Madison University
Harrisonburg, Virginia
Shoulder
Knee

Luke S. Oh, MD
Instructor in Orthopaedic Surgery
Department of Orthopaedic Surgery
Harvard Medical School;
Orthopaedic Surgeon
Department of Orthopaedic Surgery
Massachusetts General Hospital
Boston, Massachusetts
Elbow

CHAPTER 1

The Team Physician and General Care of the Athlete

Jennifer A. Hart

Team Physician Responsibilities

General Considerations

- The team physician is generally considered the "captain of the ship" and is ultimately responsible for the medical care and overall wellness of the athletes.
- The team physician must be a Medical Doctor (MD) or a Doctor of Osteopathy (DO) who has experience and training in dealing with injuries and medical conditions involving athletes.
- Although the team physician may have specialized training in any area of medicine, most team physicians are trained in primary care medicine and orthopaedics.

Communication and Delegation of Responsibilities

- The team physician is the leader of the medical team, which includes the athletic trainers, specialist providers, nutritionists, psychologists, coaches, athletes, and parents of minor children athletes.
- Communication among members of the medical team is of paramount importance, and the team physician is responsible for ensuring that adequate communication systems are in place.
- Certain activities of patient care may be delegated to other members of the team, including maintaining equipment, performing initial injury assessments, and managing day-to-day supervision of care.
- Dispensing of prescription medications is the sole responsibility of the team physician and may *not* be delegated.

Athlete Safety

- The team physician is responsible for the overall safety of the athletes in his/her care.
- Regular review of available equipment, training room layout, practice and game playing areas, and locker rooms may be necessary to ensure that there are no obvious problem areas regarding athlete safety.
- A regular restocking of the team physician bag is usually necessary to ensure that all necessary supplies are available on the field (Table 1–1).
- The team physician should be aware of injury prevention programs and should ensure that they are utilized when appropriate.
- With the growing risk of communicable diseases such as methicillin-resistant *Staphylococcus aureus* (MRSA) in the athletic population, the team physician should ensure that proper hand-washing technique and equipment cleaning are performed.

Medical Clearance for Participation

- Although the team physician does not personally have to perform each pre-participation physical examination for all of the athletes under his/her care, he/she is ultimately responsible for ensuring that each athlete is medically cleared for participation.
- The team physician should make the final decision regarding an athlete's return-to-play status after injury or illness.

Table 1–1 The Team Physician Medical Bag

Medications	Anesthetic (lidocaine, bupivacaine [Marcaine]) Topical antibiotic Oral antibiotics (cephalexin, trimethoprim-sulfamethoxazole [Bactrim], erythromycin) Glucose tablets/gel Povidone-iodine (Betadine), alcohol Ophthalmic drops Acetaminophen, nonsteroidal anti-inflammatory drugs (NSAIDs) Albuterol inhaler Epinephrine Emergency cardiac drugs (epinephrine, atropine, lidocaine, sodium bicarbonate)
Diagnostic equipment	Stethoscope Sphygmomanometer Thermometer Otoscope/ophthalmoscope Penlight Reflex hammer
Splints/supports	Elastic bandage (Ace) wraps Aluminum finger splints Stockinette Under-cast padding (Webril) Fiber-glass splint material Sling
Emergency supplies	Endotracheal tubes Laryngoscope (straight and curved blades) Syringes, various sizes (3, 5, 20 cc) Scalpel blades Bolt cutter (for removing face masks) Mouth barrier Intravenous access kit
Suturing supplies	Suture kit (forceps, small scissors, needle driver, sterile drape) Suture removal kit (forceps, small scissors) Suture (3-0, 4-0, 5-0 nylon and 2-0, 3-0, 4-0 polyglactin [Vicryl]) Sterile and nonsterile gloves Gauze (2×2-inch, 4×4-inch) Roller gauze Adhesive bandages (Band-Aids) Tape Scalpel handle and blades (Nos. 15, 10, 11) Sterile basin Bottles of saline Syringes (10- and 60-mL) Needles (16-, 18-, 22-, 25-gauge)

Event Coverage

- It is not feasible for the team physician to personally attend every practice and game of every team at the school for which he/she covers, so some discretion is necessary to plan a schedule for coverage.
  - Generally it is believed that impact sports, such as football, hockey, and lacrosse, require the physical presence of the team physician at each game.
  - Contact sports, such as basketball, soccer, and wrestling, have a high risk of collision resulting in serious injury and should be adequately covered.
- An emergency care plan should be established and coordinated with the athletic trainers, coaches, and emergency medical services (EMS) team.
- It is generally recommended that coverage consist of one physician and four paramedics for every 250 participants. Similarly, it is recommended to have one physician and one or two paramedics on site for every 10,000 spectators.

Emergency Management and Preparedness

- Emergency procedures should be practiced regularly.
- Again, remember to coordinate the care plan with EMS.
- Be sure to maintain and ensure access to emergency medical equipment, such as an automatic external defibrillator (AED), airway management equipment, and a spine board.
- On-field evaluation of athletic injuries must be carefully planned and coordinated among the involved medical team members:
  - First, assess any additional danger to the athlete or caretakers by remaining at the site.
  - Determine responsiveness of the athlete and proceed with checking airway, breathing, and circulation (ABCs).
  - If shoulder pads and helmet are in place, they should remain as they are while the patient is assessed and the spine stabilized, if necessary.
  - Airway access may be obtained by removal of the face mask only in sports involving such equipment.
  - Chest access may be obtained by cutting the shoulder pad string while keeping the equipment in place otherwise.

Illness and Injury Treatment

- The team physician is ultimately responsible for the evaluation and management of athletic illness and injury.
- If the physician is not readily available for on-field evaluation, this task is usually delegated to the athletic trainer covering the team.
- In these cases communication with the team physician may be necessary, and his/her direct involvement may be obtained as needed.
- Timely and appropriate referral to emergency care providers and specialists should be obtained when necessary.
- Treatment decisions and return-to-play recommendations made by specialist providers should be reviewed by the team physician to ensure that the athlete may safely be returned to sports participation.

Team Physician Responsibilities Questions

1. Which of the following statement is the most true regarding the team physician?
   A. The team physician is responsible for the health of the entire sports team and should designate the care of individual athletes to other members of the health team.
   B. The team physician must be an MD.
   C. The team physician is responsible only for the care of musculoskeletal injuries.
   D. The team physician must personally perform each pre-participation physical examination.
   E. The team physician is ultimately responsible for ensuring that athletes are medically able to participate in sports both at the beginning of the season and after injury.

2. A football player takes a hit during a game and remains motionless on the field. Which of the following is the most appropriate first step in managing this athlete?
   A. Remove the helmet.
   B. Stabilize the cervical spine and immediately place the athlete on a spine board.
   C. Assess the airway.
   D. Assess the circulation.
   E. Transport the athlete for cervical spine x-rays.

3. A football player is being evaluated for a possible cervical spine injury. Which of the following describes the most appropriate order for removing the helmet and shoulder pads?
   A. They should be removed together as a unit as soon as possible.
   B. The helmet should be removed first.
   C. The shoulder pads should be removed first.
   D. They should remain in place if at all possible.
   E. The helmet should be removed only if there is concern over the airway, but the shoulder pads should be left in place.

4. The team physician is responsible for dispensing prescription medications to the athletes. When is the one time that he/she may designate this job to one of the athletic trainers?
   A. If the athlete has taken this medication in the past and has had no reaction.
   B. If the athlete is currently taking this medication and simply needs to have it refilled.
   C. If the medication is a common low-dose antibiotic or anti-inflammatory drug.
   D. There is no situation in which this task may be delegated.
   E. If the physician is taking care of an emergency with an athlete and is not readily available to refill the naproxen that another athlete wants to get before heading to class.

■

The Pre-participation Physical Examination

- The primary purpose of the pre-participation physical examination is to screen athletes for potentially life-threatening illness and to identify conditions that may predispose them to injury through sports participation.
- The pre-participation physical examination also has additional benefits to both the athlete and the sports medicine team:
  - Allows one-on-one time between the physician and the athlete.
  - Provides a forum for the athlete to discuss any potential concerns.
  - Assesses the general health and well-being of each athlete.
  - Allows discussion of techniques for injury prevention.
  - Fulfills legal requirements and, often, the requirements of the athlete's insurance company.
  - Establishes the practice of good record keeping.
  - Provides information to populate the team database.

Parts of the Pre-participation Physical Examination

❑ History
- The history should include a complete list of current and past illnesses and injuries, prior treatments of these conditions, and the presence of any lingering signs or symptoms associated with these problems.
- All current medications, both prescription and over-the-counter, should be reviewed and carefully recorded. In addition, the athlete should be questioned about the use of any supplements or performance-enhancing drugs, which may have implications for his/her care.
- Allergies should be documented along with the reported reaction.
- The past medical history should include a prior surgical history.
- A careful review of systems should include a review of any prior syncopal episodes, chest pain, shortness of breath, frequent or recurrent infections, chronic pain, and gastrointestinal complaints.
- A family history should be taken, which should include cardiovascular disease such as Marfan syndrome, long QT syndrome, sudden cardiac death, and hypertrophic cardiomyopathy. Athletes should also be questioned about a family history of diabetes mellitus.
- Make a note of cases of only a solitary remaining organ in a paired-organ system (e.g., single kidney, legal blindness in one eye).

- ❑ Physical Examination
  - Height, weight, and body mass index (BMI) should be measured and recorded.
  - Vital signs should be recorded with special attention to resting heart rate and blood pressure.
  - Visual acuity along with pupil size and tracking should be evaluated.
  - A thorough cardiac examination should identify and describe any murmurs or arrhythmias.
  - A lung examination should evaluate for wheezing, which could signify the presence of asthma.
  - The abdomen should be evaluated for tenderness, masses, and hepatosplenomegaly.
  - A genital examination is indicated in male athletes to identify cases of undescended testis, testicular masses, and hernia.
  - A musculoskeletal screening examination should at the least evaluate each joint for range of motion and ligamentous instability. A screening for the presence of a scoliotic curve should also be performed. A more focused orthopaedic exam should be performed on any area in which there is a present or past history of pain or injury.
  - A neurologic examination should include a brief sensory and motor examination. For participants in high-risk (i.e., collision) sports, some centers perform pre-season neurocognitive testing to serve as a baseline in the event of a head injury during the season.
- ❑ Additional Tests
  - The use of additional testing, such as electrocardiogram (ECG) and echocardiogram for the detection of cardiac abnormalities, is controversial. Although these tests are generally performed as part of the routine examination in many European countries, they have not as yet become part of the recommended routine sports participation examination in the United States.
- ❑ Assessment and Final Plan
  - The assessment and final plan after the pre-participation physical examination may include any of the following recommendations:
    - Cleared without restriction.
    - Cleared with further evaluation recommended (e.g., spine consultation for scoliosis evaluation).
    - Cleared with restrictions (i.e., collision sports, overhead lifting).
    - Not cleared for participation.
- ❑ Condition Requiring Limitation of Sports Participation
  - Solitary kidney:
    - Athletes with a solitary kidney may participate in contact sports only after a careful explanation of the risk involved.
    - If there is any detectable abnormality in the remaining kidney, participation in contact and collision sports should be restricted.

Pre-participation Physical Examination Questions

1. The purpose of a pre-participation physical examination is:
A. A general annual health examination ("well-child check").
B. To identify athletes with medical conditions and exclude them from activity.
C. To identify those at risk of heart disease and exclude them from activity.
D. To identify conditions that may predispose the athlete to further injury or harm.

2. A soccer player answers on a pre-participated screening sheet that he has donated a kidney to his sister. What should you do about allowing this athlete to participate in his sport?
A. Allow full participation after carefully discussing the risk of injury to the remaining healthy kidney.
B. Allow full participation because his decision to be a donor has nothing to do with his sport.
C. Allow full participation but take the athletic trainer aside and ask him/her to pad the athlete's flank prior to practice and games.
D. Inform the athlete that he is unable to participate in soccer any longer.

■

Return-to-Play Issues

- Generally speaking, the decision to return an injured or ill athlete to play depends on two things:
  - The safety of the injured/ill athlete with return to play.
  - The safety of the other athletes with the injured/ill athlete's return to play.
- In some cases, further treatment or testing may be necessary to determine whether return to play would be safe.
- Some medical conditions have specific aspects that must be considered in the decision to allow an athlete return to play. Some are discussed here, and others are discussed throughout this chapter.

Bleeding

- An athlete may return to play when the bleeding has stopped, the site is covered, and any contaminated clothes have been changed.

Infection

- The athlete may return to play once there is no more fever or active sign of the infection (e.g., diarrhea, vomiting).

Brachial Plexus Injuries ("Burners"/ "Stingers")

- The athlete may return to play when the symptoms of a "burner" or "stinger" fully resolve and strength is fully returned.

Head Injury

- Refer to Chapter 9 for more details.
- Decisions about return to play after a head injury must be made on a case-by-case basis.
- For minor cases, athletes may return to play that day only if:
  - There is no loss of consciousness
  - *All* symptoms *fully* resolve within 15 minutes.
- The general recommendation is that the athlete be completely symptom-free for a minimum of 7 days before return to play is allowed.

Return-to-Play Questions

1. An athlete has been diagnosed with a viral upper respiratory infection and is generally improving but has a lingering fever. What is the primary reason that he/she should not be returned to play until the fever resolves?
   A. The athlete may have undiagnosed mononucleosis with an enlarged spleen.
   B. The athlete is at risk of making his/her own condition worse or infecting other participants.
   C. The athlete has missed too much practice to be in the proper condition for playing.
   D. The athlete should finish a course of antibiotics before returning to play.
2. A high school football player is hit on the head during a play and comes off the field complaining of headache and dizziness. You evaluate him on the sideline. Which of the following findings would prevent the player's returning to play the same day?
   A. Brief loss of consciousness (less than 30 seconds).
   B. Headache that resolves after 10 minutes.
   C. Dizziness that resolves after 5 minutes.
   D. Difficulty concentrating for 5 minutes.
   E. Prior similar injury in 6th grade, also of short duration.
3. A basketball player falls into the bleachers during practice and gets a laceration on his/her side. A few days later during a game, he/she notices that the area has started bleeding and has soaked through his/her shirt. What must happen before the athlete can return to play?
   A. The injury must be disclosed to the other team.
   B. The athlete must undergo HIV testing.
   C. The area must be thoroughly cleaned and a fresh dressing applied.
   D. The area must fully heal so that there is no further risk of bleeding.
   E. The area must be thoroughly cleaned, a fresh dressing must be applied, and the shirt must be changed.

Legal and Ethical Considerations

- The legal and ethical aspects of sports medicine often seem to be interconnected but in reality involve two distinct sets of obligations:
  - *Legal obligations* are those that refer to enforceable rules established by society (laws).
  - *Ethical obligations* are those moral considerations that are deemed to be appropriate but are not necessarily enforceable.
- There are very few, if any, formal guidelines as to the appropriate ethical behavior of an individual team physician.
- Perhaps the best overall statement to define appropriate ethical consideration in this area is that all decisions of the team physician should be in the best interest of the athlete in question.
- The team physician should adhere to the normal ethical considerations of any physician in practice, but this issue can be complicated by some of the relationships unique to this particular practice of medicine:
  - The team physician–athlete relationship is the most similar to the traditional physician-patient relationship.
  - The team physician, however, has additional responsibilities to the team as a whole, which includes the coaching staff. This relationship adds another element of depth to the decision-making process regarding athlete care and, especially, return to play.
- Privacy can be a difficult area in sports medicine because many highly successful athletes are at the forefront of media attention.
  - Athletes have the same rights to privacy as any other patient under the care of a physician regardless of level of competition.
  - The evaluation of athletes itself can make certain privacy issues difficult because it is often performed on the field, on the sideline, or in the training room with various other people present.
  - The U.S. Health Information Portability and Accountability Act (HIPAA) was designed to apply to the traditional patient-physician relationship and does not fully address many of the more unusual aspects of the sports medicine physician–athlete relationship.
  - A good rule of thumb for the team physician is to concentrate on good communication with the direct sports medicine team but to avoid communicating information outside that circle, especially to the media.

Legal and Ethical Considerations Questions

1. Which of the following statements is true regarding an athlete's right to privacy in regard to health matters?
   A. Release of information about a high school athlete's injuries may be allowed only with written permission of the athlete and coach.
   B. All athletes have the same rights of confidentiality as any other patient.
   C. All athletes have the same rights of confidentiality unless they are being paid to perform (i.e., professional level of play).
   D. Anyone directly involved with the career of an athlete has the right to full knowledge of injuries and treatment, including the coach, family, physical therapist, agent, and press.
   E. A team physician may not discuss the care of an athlete with a specialist to whom the athlete has been referred without the written consent of the athlete.

2. The most important consideration of the team physician in the care of a professional athlete is:
   A. Returning the athlete to play as quickly as possible regardless of the injury or illness.
   B. Use of modalities and anesthetic injections as frequently as necessary to allow the athlete to be pain-free enough to continue playing.
   C. Disclosing concerns such as the HIV positivity of the athlete to protect the rest of the team.
   D. Returning the athlete to activity only when the athlete's condition is fully restored and further injury is not being risked, regardless of the potential loss of playing time.
   E. Holding any injured athlete out of play until full evaluation can be performed, including mandatory radiographs.

Resources

TEAM PHYSICIAN RESPONSIBILITIES

Fu, F.H., Tjoumakaris, F.P., Buoncristiani, A., 2007. Building a sports medicine team. Clin. Sports Med. 26, 173–180.

Herring, S.A., Bergfeld, J., Boyd, J., et al., 2001. Sideline preparedness for the team physician: A consensus statement. Sports Med. Update 6–11.

Huff, P., 1998. Drug distribution in the training room. Clin. Sports Med. 17, 211–228.

Konin, J.G., 2007. Communication: The key to the game. Clin. Sports Med. 26, 137–148.

Kuster, T., Knitter, D., Navitskis, L., 2007. Accessibility of the team physician. Clin. Sports Med. 26, 149–160.

Ray, R.L., Feld, F.X., 1989. The team physician's medical bag. Clin. Sports Med. 8, 139–146.

Steiner, M.E., Quigley, D.B., Wang, F., et al., 2000. Team physician consensus statement. Am. J. Sports Med. 28, 440–442.

Steiner, M.E., Quigley, D., Wang, F., et al., 2005. Team physician in college athletics. Am. J. Sports Med. 30, 1545–1551.

THE PRE-PARTICIPATION PHYSICAL EXAMINATION

Armsey, T.D., Hosey, R.G., 2004. Medical aspects of sports: Epidemiology of injuries, preparticipation physical examination, and drugs in sports. Clin. Sports Med. 23, 255–279.

Glover, D.W., Maron, B.J., Matheson, G.O., 1999. The preparticipation physical examination: Steps toward consensus and uniformity. Phys. Sports Med. 27, 29–34.

Gomez, J.E., 2003. Paired organ loss. In: DeLee, J.C., Drez Jr., D., Miller, M.D. (Eds.), DeLee & Drez's Orthopaedic Sports Medicine: Principles and Practice, second ed. Saunders Elsevier, Philadelphia, pp. 264–271.

Grafe, M.W., Paul, G.R., Foster, T.E., 1997. The preparticipation sports examination for high school and athletics. Clin. Sports Med. 16, 569.

Koester, M.C., Amundson, C.L., 2008. Preparticipation screening of high school athletes: Are recommendations enough? Phys. Sports Med. 32, 35–38.

Moeller, J.L., 1996. Contraindications to athletic participation: Spinal, systemic, dermatologic, paired-organ, and other issues. Phys. Sports Med. 24, 57.

RETURN-TO-PLAY ISSUES

Madden, C.C., Walsh, W.M., Mellion, M.B., 2003. The team physician: The preparticipation physical examination and on-field emergencies. In: DeLee, J.C., Drez Jr., D., Miller, M.D. (Eds.), DeLee & Drez's Orthopaedic Sports Medicine: Principles and Practice, second ed. Saunders Elsevier, Philadelphia, pp. 737–748.

Miller, M.D., Arciero, R.A., Cooper, D.E., et al., 2009. Doc, when can he go back in the game? Instr. Course Lect. 58, 437–443.

Putukian, M., 1998. Return to play: Making the tough decisions. Phys. Sports Med. 26, 25–27.

LEGAL AND ETHICAL CONSIDERATIONS

Bernstein, J., Perlis, C., Bartolozzi, A.R., 2000. Ethics in sports medicine. Clin. Orthop. 378, 50–60.

Johnson, R., 2004. The unique ethics of sports medicine. Clin. Sports Med. 23, 175–182.

Tucker, A.M., 2004. Ethics and the professional team physician. Clin. Sports Med. 2, 227–241.

CHAPTER 2

Medical Issues in the Athlete

JENNIFER A. HART

Cardiovascular Issues in the Athlete

The Athlete's Heart

- *Athletic heart syndrome* refers to normal changes of the anatomy and physiology of the heart that result from long-term athletic conditioning.
- These changes occur secondary to an increase in stroke volume and cardiac output.
- Increased vagal tone results in lower resting heart rate.
- Enlargement of the chamber and the left ventricular wall are common characteristics associated with the athletic heart syndrome.
- Common changes seen on the electrocardiogram (ECG) include sinus bradycardia, ST segment changes, T wave changes, and increased QRS intervals.
- The most common change on the echocardiogram is an increased left ventricular wall thickness; however, a thickness greater than 16 mm may indicate other pathology, such as hypertrophic cardiomyopathy.
- Athletic heart syndrome does not predispose the athlete to sudden cardiac death.

Hypertrophic Cardiomyopathy

- Hypertrophic cardiomyopathy (HCM) is the most common genetic cardiac abnormality. It is an autosomal dominant trait with various mutations.
- In the athletic population, HCM is found most frequently in African Americans, who account for 55% of reported cases.
- Symptoms do not always occur, and in some individuals, the first sign of the presence of HCM is sudden cardiac death. If symptoms do occur, they most commonly include exertional chest pain and/or syncopal episodes.
- The physical examination may be normal, but at times a systolic ejection murmur that increases with Valsalva maneuvers may be detected.
- ECG changes are common in cases of HCM and include the presence of Q waves and the inversion of T waves.
- The echocardiogram shows changes distinctive for HCM:
  - Left ventricular wall thickness greater than 16 mm.
  - Ventricular septum–to–free wall thickness ratio greater than 1.3:1.
  - No dilatation of the ventricular cavity (as is seen with athletic heart syndrome).
- Patients who have factors associated with high risk for sudden death related to HCM should be withheld from athletic activity, and an implantable defibrillator or medication treatment may be indicated. These risk factors include:
  - Syncopal episode in the past.
  - Family history of sudden cardiac death.
  - Symptomatic ventricular tachycardia (VT) changes on Holter monitoring.
  - Genotype.
  - Left ventricular wall thickness of greater than 19 mm.

Sudden Cardiac Death

- *Sudden cardiac death* (SCD) is defined as a sudden unexpected heart-related death within 1 hour of symptom onset in a patient with no known preexisting fatal pathology.
- The estimated incidence of SCD in high school and college athletes is 1:200,000, although the reported incidence in older runners is much higher (1:15,000).

- The most common cause of SCD in the young athletic population is hypertrophic cardiomyopathy; coronary artery disease is a more common causative factor in older athletes.

Commotio Cordis

- *Commotio cordis* is defined as a sudden cardiac death that occurs secondary to blunt trauma to the chest, even from a seemingly low-impact blow.
- The timing and location of impact seems to be the key. Impact directly over the left ventricle just before the T-wave peak seems to be the event that triggers the ventricular fibrillation that can lead to death.
- Commotio cordis occurs most frequently in the very young athlete (mean age 13 years) with an anatomically and physiologically normal heart.
- It is most common in sports that involve some type of projectile (e.g., baseball, hockey, lacrosse).
- Chest protectors should be strongly encouraged in high-risk sports, although even they fail to prevent all cases of commotio cordis.
- Treatment involves early defibrillation, although outcomes even with this early intervention are extremely poor.

Wolff-Parkinson-White Syndrome

- Wolff-Parkinson-White syndrome (WPW) involves accessory pathways of conduction between the atria and ventricles that can lead to tachyarrhythmias.
- Many patients with WPW are asymptomatic but an occasional patient presents with syncopal episodes and/or palpitations.
- Diagnosis is made by visualization of the classic delta waves on ECG (Fig. 2–1).
- Sudden cardiac death can occur as a result of the tachyarrhythmia if atrial impulses exceed 240 beats per minute.
- Treatment usually includes medications to control the tachycardia, but definitive management usually involves radiofrequency ablation of the accessory pathway.

Marfan Syndrome

- Marfan syndrome is a genetic disorder with 85% autosomal dominant inheritance with variable expression.
- Signs and symptoms, which appear in adolescence and early adulthood, involve changes in the musculoskeletal, cardiovascular, and ocular systems.
- Major criteria for diagnosis:
  - Four of the following eight musculoskeletal changes:
    - Arm span greater than height
    - Reduced upper segment–to–lower segment ratio
    - Arachnodactyly
    - Scoliosis
    - Pectus carinatum
    - Pectus excavatum
    - Limited elbow extension
    - Pes planus
  - At least one of the following cardiovascular changes:
    - Ascending aorta dilatation with or without associated aortic regurgitation
    - Aortic dissection (ascending aorta)
  - Ectopic lens (diagnosed by slit-lamp examination)
  - Lumbosacral dural ectasia (diagnosed on magnetic resonance imaging [MRI] or computed tomography [CT])
- Minor criteria for diagnosis:
  - Joint hypermobility
  - High arched palate
  - Facial changes
- ECG should be performed in individuals in whom Marfan syndrome is suspected; it may show changes secondary to chronic aortic regurgitation.
- Echocardiography is the "gold standard" for diagnosing aortic dilatation or dissection. The echocardiogram should be repeated at 6-month intervals to monitor the ascending aorta.
- All athletes with Marfan syndrome should be withheld from *contact* sports.

Long QT Syndrome

- Long QT syndrome is a genetic disorder that affects the potassium and sodium channels, leading to elongation of the QT interval on ECG.
- This elongation of the QT interval can lead to torsades de pointes, ventricular fibrillation, and sudden cardiac death.

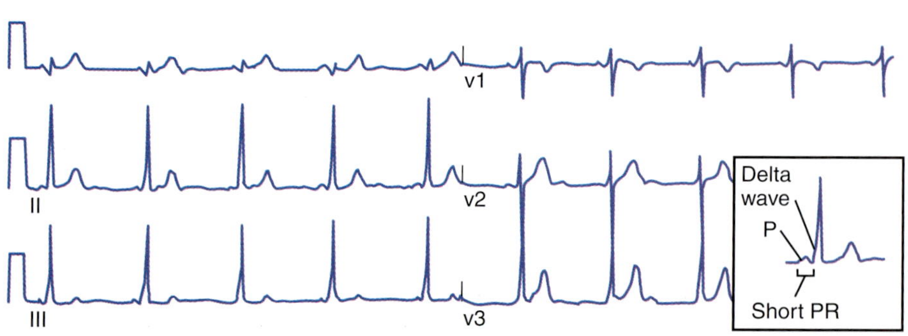

Figure 2–1 ECG appearance of Wolff-Parkinson-White syndrome. *(From Leclerc KM: Risk assessment and management of nonorthopaedic conditions. In DeLee JC, Drez Jr D, Miller MD [eds]: DeLee & Drez's Orthopaedic Sports Medicine: Principles and Practice, 2nd ed. Philadelphia, Saunders Elsevier, 2003, p 282.)*

- Athletes diagnosed with long QT syndrome should be withheld from competitive sports.
- Treatment includes the administration of beta blockers to control the heart rate and restriction on the use of medications that can contribute to a long QT interval.
- Patients with suspected anorexia nervosa should be aggressively treated, because this condition is associated with lengthening of the QT interval as well.

Blood Pressure

- Hypertension is common in the general population and therefore may be one of the most commonly seen cardiovascular problems in athletes.
- Blood pressure elevates normally with exercise but excessive elevation (>250 mmHg systolic) with exercise may require medication treatment.
- Regular endurance exercise can also lead to a reduction in BP (up to 25 mmHg systolic and up to 15 mmHg diastolic).
- Athletes with BP abnormalities should be routinely monitored. Assessing ventricular wall thickness is important as well because LUH with elevated BP may require avoiding heavy resistance exercise.

Cardiovascular Issues Questions

1. A college soccer player without any known medical history is running down the field when she suddenly clutches her chest and falls to the ground. She is unconscious when the athletic trainer arrives at her side. CPR is immediately initiated. What is the most likely etiology?

A. Commotio cordis.
B. Anaphylaxis.
C. Wolff Parkinson-White syndrome.
D. Hypertrophic cardiomyopathy.
E. Athletic heart syndrome.

2. A young baseball player in another part of the state is reported to have died when he was struck in the chest with a ball during the game. The parents of the team in your town are very concerned and want to have a meeting with you to discuss what happened and how they can prevent it. Which of the following statements is correct?

A. That athlete likely had a congenital heart defect, and as long as the children on this team have no known history of heart disorder, they are not at risk for a similar injury.
B. Commotio cordis can be easily prevented by wearing well-fitting chest protectors.
C. You have purchased an automatic electronic defibrillator (AED) to keep at the field, and with immediate recognition and treatment, the survival rates for this condition are extremely high.
D. Commotio cordis occurs as a result of blunt trauma to the chest overlying the heart at a crucial moment in the cardiac cycle and is not related to any known underlying heart disease.
E. Baseball is the only sport that has been associated with commotio cordis.

3. Which of the following findings in an athlete with known hypertension might cause you to recommend restricting heavy exercise?

A. A blood pressure of 140/90 mm Hg 30 minutes after exercise.
B. A positive smoking history.
C. A family history of coronary artery disease.
D. Weight loss of more than 30 pounds in the past 6 weeks.
E. The finding of left ventricular hypertrophy on echocardiogram.

Pulmonary Issues in the Athlete

Exercise-Induced Asthma

- Exercise-induced asthma (EIA) occurs in 12% to 15% of the population in general but at higher rates in patients with environmental allergies (40%) and chronic asthma (50%–80%).
- EIA also has a high association with cold weather sports, such as cross-country skiing.
- EIA is characterized by reversible airway reactivity, inflammation, and cytokine release.
- Symptoms include wheezing, cough, shortness of breath, and chest tightness associated with athletic activity.
- The physical examination may be normal when the athlete is not exhibiting symptoms but may demonstrate wheezing and prolonged expiratory phase after exercise.
- Spirometry demonstrates airflow obstruction that is reversible with the administration of bronchodilators.
- An exercise challenge test may be necessary when normal spirometry fails to confirm the presence of EIA.
- Treatment includes avoiding exposure to known symptom triggers, such as cool, dry air, as well as proper conditioning techniques.
- In some cases, it may be necessary for the athlete to eliminate participation in sports known to increase the risk of EIA, such as running, cross-country skiing, ice sports, rugby, and soccer.
- Pharmacologic treatment usually begins with the introduction of short-acting beta-agonists, which are effective in the vast majority of cases.
- Cromolyn sodium and nedocromil are also effective medical treatments.
- Occasionally, inhaled corticosteroids are necessary for severe "attacks."

Pneumothorax

- Traumatic Pneumothorax
  - Pneumothorax is most commonly associated with trauma, specifically fracture of the ribs, scapula, or clavicle.
  - A tension pneumothorax may develop if there is a steady progressive collection of air leading to mechanical obstruction. A tension pneumothorax may develop rapidly or more slowly and is associated with respiratory distress and eventual hypotension. It should be considered a medical emergency.
  - The athlete with pneumothorax most commonly presents with pleuritic chest pain and dyspnea.
  - The physical examination shows decreased breath sounds on the affected side, resonance to percussion, tachypnea, and tachycardia.
  - The diagnosis is confirmed with chest radiographs (Fig. 2–2).
  - Treatment depends on the severity of the pneumothorax:
    - If less than 15% to 20% of the lung is involved, the athlete may be monitored in an emergency room for several hours with a follow-up chest radiograph the next day.
    - Lesions involving more than 20% of the lung should be treated with a chest tube to decompress (remove the air from) the pleural space.
- Spontaneous Pneumothorax
  - Spontaneous pneumothorax is more common in males than females at a ratio of 6:1, with the most sports-related cases occurring with running, weight training, scuba diving, basketball, and bungee jumping.
  - Spontaneous pneumothorax can be defined as primary or secondary:
    - *Primary pneumothorax* is defined as the rupture of subpleural blebs in patients with no prior diagnosis of lung disorder. It is commonly associated with a very tall and thin body and has been associated with a positive smoking history. Recurrence rates are high in this group, being reported as up to 50%.
    - *Secondary pneumothorax* occurs in patients who do have a previously diagnosed lung disorder, such as asthma, cystic fibrosis, tuberculosis, or chronic obstructive pulmonary disease (COPD). It is also more common in older athletes.

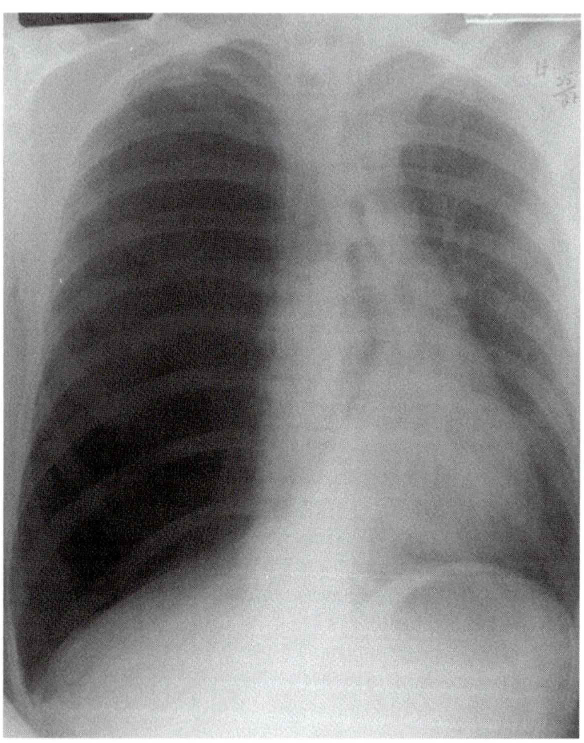

Figure 2–2 Anteroposterior radiograph of the chest showing a right-sided pneumothorax with a left-sided shift of the mediastinum. *(From Mistry DJ, Kramer CM: Imaging of cardiopulmonary diseases. Clin Sports Med 2003;22:197–212.)*

Pulmonary Issues Questions

1. A 17-year-old high school lacrosse player presents after practice with chest tightness, shortness of breath, and audible wheezing on examination. What is the next step to establish a diagnosis?
A. ECG.
B. Echocardiogram.
C. Bronchoscopy.
D. Pulmonary function test.
E. Pulse oximeter.

2. A high school athlete continues to exhibit symptoms that you believe are related to exercise-induced asthma despite the fact that pulmonary function test results are normal. What is your next step to establishing the correct diagnosis?
A. Refer the athlete to a cardiologist to evaluate for hypertrophic cardiomyopathy.
B. Suggest repeating the pulmonary function tests with an exercise challenge component.
C. Start a trial of theophylline.
D. Order a chest radiograph to evaluate for underlying pneumonia.
E. Refer the athlete to a gastroenterologist to evaluate for gastrointestinal reflux, which is commonly mistaken for exercise-induced asthma.

Environmental Illness

Heat Illness

- Mild Heat Illness
  - The most common form of mild heat illness consists of heat cramps and heat edema.
    - Heat edema is characterized by general fatigue, headache, and swelling in the extremities.
    - Heat cramps involve muscular pain and cramping after exercise, with muscle contractions continuing even with cessation of activity.

- In cases of mild heat illness, the core temperature usually remains normal.
- Treatment consists of oral rehydration and cooling.

❑ Heat Exhaustion
- Heat exhaustion is the most commonly encountered heat illness for which athletes seek medical help.
- It most commonly manifests as muscle weakness, confusion, headache, and nausea and/or vomiting.
- Heat exhaustion is characterized by a core temperature of less than 104° F.

❑ Heat Stroke
- Heat stroke is a more advanced condition that occurs when the core temperature exceeds 105° F.
- It is characterized by a progressive deterioration in mental status, tachycardia, tachypnea, and hypotension.

❑ Prevention of Heat Illness
- Prevention of heat illness is extremely important and includes:
  - A training program that acclimatizes the athletes to the heat.
  - Avoiding excessive exercise in extreme temperature conditions, with the general recommendation being to avoid activity if the wet bulb reading is greater than 82° F.
  - Emphasizing rehydration during exercise.
  - Children are more at risk for development of heat illness than adults because children's greater surface area to body mass ratio absorbs more heat from the environment.

❑ Treatment
- Treatment of heat illness begins with a rapid determination of the severity of the condition, including assessment of rectal temperature.
- Cooling must begin immediately with any combination of the following methods:
  - Placing the athlete in a cooling tub.
  - Placing the athlete in front of cooling fans.
  - Pouring water over the athlete.
  - Placing ice bags on the athlete's neck, groin, and axillae.
  - Covering the athlete's body with cold towels.
- In all cases of moderate or severe heat illness, the rectal temperature and vital signs should be closely monitored. Emergency transport is indicated if improvement does not occur rapidly after initiation of appropriate cooling measures.
- Further medical evaluation is required for all cases of severe heat illness to evaluate for any complications, such as electrolyte abnormalities, rhabdomyolysis, and multisystem organ failure.

Cold-Related Illnesses and Injuries

❑ Hypothermia
- Hypothermia is defined as a core temperature that drops below 95° F.
- Shivering is one of the early signs of hypothermia. It rapidly increases in severity but ceases when the core temperature drops below 90° F.
- Other signs and symptoms of hypothermia are mental status changes, lethargy, clumsiness, and slurred speech.
- Rewarming the body is the key to treatment of this condition:
  - Move the athlete to a warmer environment.
  - Replace any wet clothing with dry clothing and blankets.
  - Use external heating devices if available (e.g., warm bottles, heating pads).
  - Encourage the athlete to drink warm fluids if able.
  - In severe cases, begin an intravenous infusion of warmed normal saline solution and transport the athlete to an emergency facility.

❑ Cold-Related Skin Injury
- Injuries to the skin may range from mild (frostnip) to moderate (superficial frostbite) or severe (deep frostbite).
  - *Frostnip* involves constriction of the superficial veins without freezing of the tissue and may be treated by direct warming of area with direct body heat.
  - *Frostbite* involves freezing and possible eventual necrosis of the tissue and is rated as moderate to severe according to the depth of penetration.
- Treatment involves rapid rewarming of the affected tissue, with the most successful method consisting of immersion in a warm water bath (102°–108° F).

Altitude Sickness

- Altitude sickness occurs when an athlete performs in a high-altitude environment without appropriate acclimatization.
- Acute mountain sickness (AMS) is commonly seen in mountain climbers who ascend too quickly.
  - AMS is generally mild and manifests as fatigue, headache, and some mild nausea.
  - It usually resolves with rest and a period of acclimatization.
  - Severe forms of AMS may be seen in extreme conditions and can lead to pulmonary or cerebral edema both of which require immediate descent because they are both potentially life-threatening conditions.

Environmental Illness Questions

1. Which of the following statements is true regarding heat illness in children?

A. Children need electrolyte replacement more than simple water rehydration during activity than adults.

B. Children and adults have equal risks for development of heat illness.

C. Children are more at risk for development of heat illness than adults because children's greater surface area to body mass ratio absorbs more heat from the environment.
D. Children are less at risk for development of heat illness than adults because of children's ability to sweat more efficiently.
E. Children are less at risk for development of heat illness than adults because children's greater body surface area allows them to dissipate heat more rapidly.

2. You are an event physician for the Boston Marathon. It is a particularly warm day, and several of the runners have crossed the finish line with mild signs and symptoms of heat illness. While you are helping distribute water and briefly evaluating them, you notice one runner off to the side who is lying on the ground, conscious but clearly disoriented. She is not sweating and does not respond to your questions. What should your immediate next step be?
A. Measure her temperature orally.
B. Hand her a cup of water and instruct her to drink it as quickly as possible.
C. Because a cooling tub is not immediately available, begin placing ice bags on her axillae, groin, and neck.
D. Begin fanning her with your program and yell for help.
E. Place both of her hands in the cups of the cold water that you have been distributing.

3. You are helping provide medical coverage for a national cross-country skiing team when a hiker stumbles up to your group, claiming to have been lost in the woods for the past 2 days. He is specifically complaining about pain in his right hand. You notice that he is not wearing gloves, and upon examining the hand, you find that the index and middle fingers are white and have diminished sensation. What should your next step be?
A. Immediately refer him to the local emergency room for a surgical consultation.
B. Bring him into the medical cabin to sit by the heater to warm his hand.
C. Rub the fingers slowly until sensation returns.
D. Immerse his hand in a warm water bath.
E. Wrap the hand in layers of pre-warmed gauze and reapply his glove.

■

Infections

Common Cold and Influenza

- Athletes are prone to common viral illnesses owing to their high level of energy expenditure during exercise and their close contact with teammates.
- Athletes who become infected with these common viruses should be managed with symptomatic treatment and monitored for improvement.
- Antibiotics should be administered to an athlete with a cold or flu only if there is strong concern about secondary bacterial infection (e.g., sinusitis, pneumonia, otitis media).
- There should be a strong emphasis on basic hygiene, with special attention to hand washing, to limit exposure of the other athletes.

Gastroenteritis

- Cases of gastroenteritis are most commonly viral in etiology.
- Treatment is generally conservative, consisting of rehydration as the disease is self-limited.
- Athletic participation should be delayed if there is any evidence of dehydration, which greatly increases the risk of heat illness.

Infectious Mononucleosis

- Symptoms of mononucleosis ("mono") include fever, sore throat, fatigue, headache, and nausea.
- The physical examination usually demonstrates an exudative pharyngitis, enlargement of the lymph nodes around the neck, and splenomegaly (50% of cases). A rash may also be present.
- Definitive diagnosis is made by positive results of antibody tests (monospot tests), but results may be negative early in the course of the disease.
- Treatment is symptomatic and largely focuses on rest.
- Contact and collision sports are avoided for 4 weeks to minimize the risk of splenic rupture.
  - The complication of splenic rupture is most common within the first 21 days of the illness, so all athletic activity should be restricted during this period.
  - Full recovery from mononucleosis is expected usually around 4 to 6 weeks, and return to play may be allowed when symptoms resolve and no splenomegaly is detected.

Meningitis

- Viral meningitis is the most common form of meningitis, with most cases being caused by enteroviruses.
- Signs and symptoms include fever, neck stiffness, altered mental status, headache, fatigue, and, occasionally, seizures.
- The classic physical examination findings for meningitis are the presence of Kernig and Brudzinski signs.
  - A positive Kernig's sign is indicated by pain with flexing the hip to 90° and then extending the knee.
  - A positive Brudzinski's sign is indicated by flexion of the hip and knees when the neck is passively flexed.

- Definitive diagnosis is made with a lumbar puncture.
- Treatment should be tailored to the causative organism and should begin immediately upon confirmation of the diagnosis.

Human Immunodeficiency Virus Infection

- To date there have been no cases of human immunodeficiency virus (HIV) transmission related to routine sport contact.
- Because of this fact, there are no mandatory testing policies in place, and disclosure of HIV status is up to the individual infected athlete.
- Regular exercise has been associated with clinical improvement and increased short-term survival rates for HIV-positive patients.
- Strenuous exercise should be avoided if the CD4 (CD4-positive T lymphocyte) count drops below 200 (cells per mm^3 of blood), although mild to moderate exercise may still be encouraged in patients with such a CD4 level.

Infection Questions

1. A soccer player who has been diagnosed with infectious mononucleosis wants to return to practice. When would this be most appropriate?
   A. It has been 2 weeks since diagnosis and he says that he feels well enough to at least return to running during practice.
   B. It has been 3 weeks since diagnosis and he feels well but is still having intermittent fevers.
   C. It has been 3½ weeks since diagnosis, he is asymptomatic, and his physical examination is normal.
   D. It has been 5 weeks since diagnosis, he is asymptomatic, but physical examination shows he still has an enlarged spleen.

2. Which of the following is true regarding an athlete who is HIV-positive?
   A. HIV transmission is commonly reported with athletic participation so great care must be taken in sports that involve direct contact.
   B. HIV screening is mandatory for all NCAA athletes.
   C. Strenuous activity must be avoided in patients with HIV because of the documented detrimental effects of exercise on the immune system.
   D. An athlete should avoid strenuous exercise if his/her CD4 count is less than 200 but may participate in less strenuous activity.

Dermatologic Conditions

Impetigo

- Classic impetigo is characterized by a honey-colored crusted area on an erythematous base. Vesicles or pustules may or may not be present.
- The primary causative agent is *Staphylococcus aureus*, with methicillin-resistant *S. aureus* (MRSA) becoming increasingly more common. *Streptococcus* can also be associated with impetigo.
- Folliculitis is generally considered an associated condition, also caused primarily by *S. aureus*, that affects the hair follicles. It most commonly occurs in areas of shaving.
- The treatment for localized areas of impetigo is topical application of mupirocin (Bactroban), although more extensive skin involvement may require a course of oral antibiotics.
- An abscess requires local incision and drainage (I&D) and culture.
- A high index of suspicion for MRSA should be maintained in athletes with impetigo, and treatment with trimethoprim-sulfamethoxazole or clindamycin should be initiated in these cases.
- National Collegiate Athletic Association (NCAA) guidelines regarding return to play with a bacterial skin infection indicate that:
  - There must be no new lesions in the past 48 hours.
  - All lesions must be free of drainage.
  - A minimum of 72 hours of antibiotic treatment must be completed.

Methicillin-Resistant *Staphylococcus aureus*

- MRSA has become an increasingly common infection seen in training rooms; it is spread by direct skin contact and by contact with contaminated equipment.
- The most common manifestation is a skin pustule on an erythematous base (Fig. 2–3).
- Treatment is with trimethoprim-sulfamethoxazole (Bactrim) and rifampin.

Herpes Simplex

- Herpes simplex virus (HSV) infection is common in "skin-to-skin" sports such as wrestling.

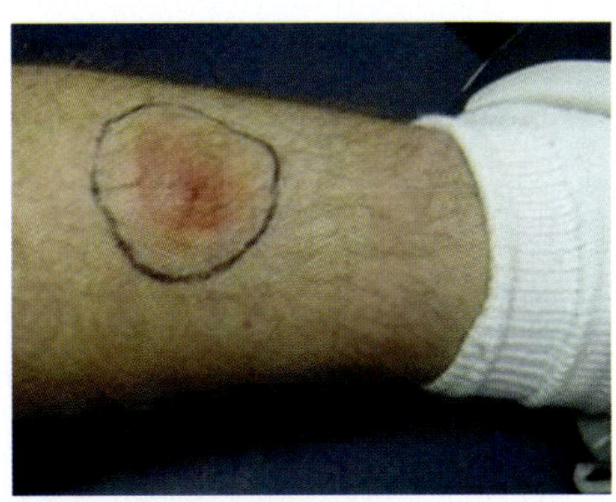

Figure 2–3 Methicillin-resistance *Staphylococcus aureus* (MRSA) lesion on the leg of an athlete 24 hours later.

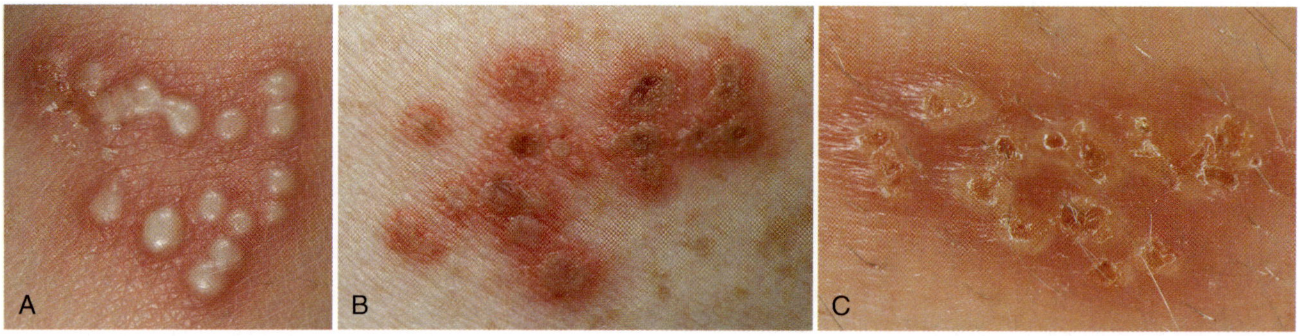

Figure 2–4 Herpes simplex. **A,** Early appearance consists of vesicles on an erythematous base. **B,** Lesions become umbilicated. **C,** Crusts form as lesions begin to heal. *(From Habif TP: Clinical Dermatology: A Color Guide to Diagnosis and Therapy, 4th ed. Philadelphia, Mosby, 2004, p 346.)*

- HSV types 1 and 2 can produce lesions at any place on the body and are spread via direct contact with lesion secretions, saliva, or mucous membranes.
- The diagnosis is usually made from the clinical appearance (Fig. 2–4), but Tzanck staining can be useful to confirm the diagnosis in questionable cases.
- Because of the highly contagious nature of the herpes virus, athletes must be completely clear of disease before return to sport is allowed.
- Antivirals such as valacyclovir, famciclovir, and acyclovir are effective.
  - For primary disease, the treatment course should be extended to 10 days.
  - For recurrent cases, 5 to 7 days of treatment is usually sufficient.
- NCAA guidelines are in place to determine when an athlete with HSV may safely return to sport after treatment:
  - No new lesions for 72 hours.
  - All lesions must be healed over.
  - Antiviral treatment must be ongoing for a minimum of 120 hours.

Molluscum Contagiosum

- Similar to herpes, molluscum contagiosum is commonly seen in "skin-to-skin" sports such as wrestling.
- The clinical appearance is that of small flesh-colored, dome-shaped lesions (Fig. 2–5).
- Treatment is typically via local curettage or the use of topical irritants to stimulate the immune system.

Tinea

- Many forms: corporis, pedis, cruris, capitis.
- Like some other infections already described, tinea is common in close contact sports such as wrestling.
- The classic appearance of tinea is a red scaly border with a center that is slightly lighter in color (Fig. 2–6).
- Topical treatment is indicated only for single or very localized cases; multiple lesions respond more effectively to oral antifungals (e.g., ketoconazole, fluconazole).

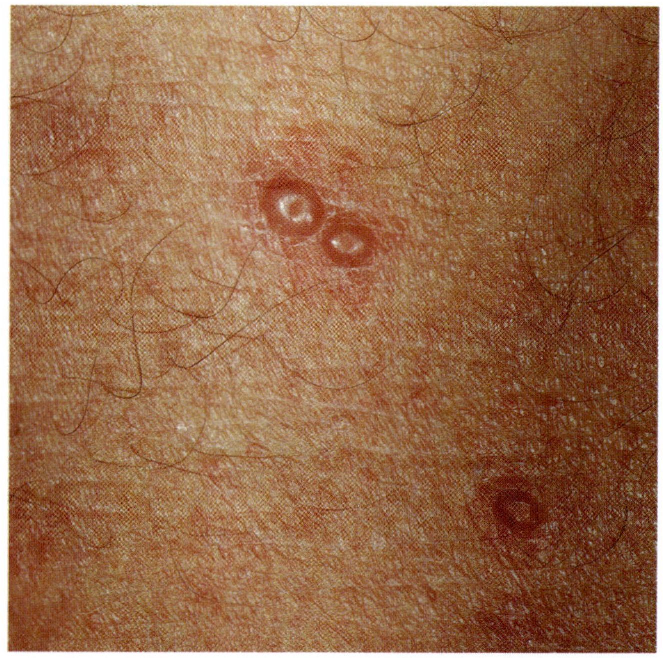

Figure 2–5 Molluscum contagiosum appears as small flesh-colored, dome-shaped lesions. *(From Habif TP: Clinical Dermatology: A Color Guide to Diagnosis and Therapy, 4th ed. Philadelphia, Mosby, 2004, p 344.)*

- NCAA guidelines state that treatment must be ongoing for a minimum of 72 hours and that all areas must be covered with an occlusive dressing before an athlete with tinea may return to sport.

Dermatology Questions

1. An athlete has an area of impetigo on the arm that you have been following in the training room. No new lesions have formed, and there is no active drainage. You have started oral antibiotics in the form of amoxicillin–clavulanic acid. How long must the athlete be taking this medication before you allow him to return to sport?
A. 24 hours.
B. 36 hours.
C. 48 hours.
D. 72 hours.
E. 7 days.

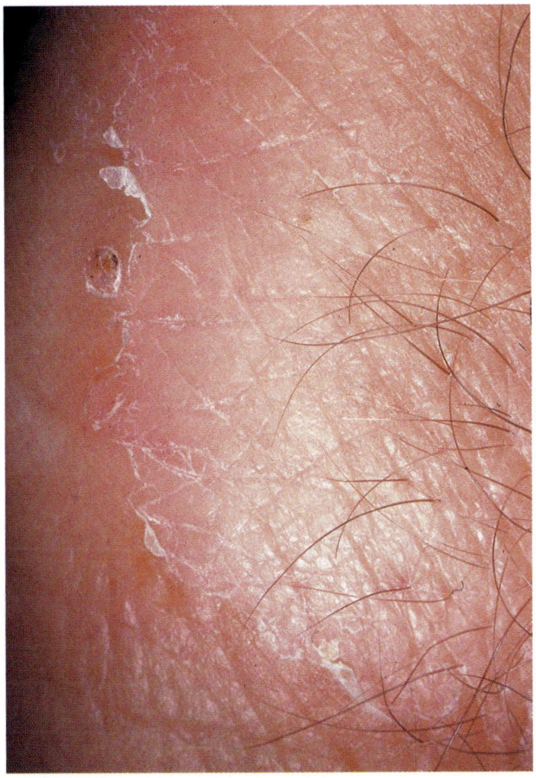

Figure 2–6 The classic appearance of tinea is a rash with a red scaly border and a center that is lighter in color. *(From Habif TP: Clinical Dermatology: A Color Guide to Diagnosis and Therapy, 4th ed. Philadelphia, Mosby, 2004, p 413.)*

2. How long must a college wrestler be free from development of new herpetic lesions before returning to competition, according to the NCAA?
   A. 24 hours.
   B. 36 hours.
   C. 48 hours.
   D. 72 hours.
   E. 7 days

■

Nonmusculoskeletal Injuries in the Athlete

Eye Injuries

- Eye injuries occur most commonly in basketball, baseball, and softball, although many other sports are also associated with a high risk of eye injury, including racquetball, martial arts, and rugby.
- Many of the reported eye injuries can be prevented with the use of proper eye protection.
- It is important to evaluate all eye injuries immediately by means of a close visual inspection; inspection of the pupils for size, shape, and reactivity to light; and testing of extraocular muscle function.
- Appropriate referral should be made to an ophthalmologist for further testing and treatment whenever there is:
  - Persistent loss of visual acuity or blurred vision.
  - Severe pain.
  - Symptoms suggestive of retinal detachment (i.e., cloudy focus of vision or loss of visual field).
  - Foreign body presence.
  - Significant periorbital swelling.
  - Alterations in pupil size or shape.
  - Hyphema.
  - Laceration around the eye, especially involving the lid.

❑ Hyphema
- A hyphema involves bleeding into the anterior chamber of the eye that is usually a result of blunt trauma (Fig. 2–7).
- Initial management should include covering the eye with a patch.
- The presence of a hyphema is an indication for ophthalmologic referral.

Ear Injuries

❑ Otitis Externa ("Swimmer's Ear")
- Otitis externa results when the pH changes in the ear canal as cerumen is lost through frequent or prolonged submersion in water.
- The most common causative organisms are *S. aureus, Pseudomonas aeruginosa,* and *Aspergillus.*
- Treatment includes topical antibiotic and/or antifungal drops.
- If the edema in the canal is severe, the use of corticosteroid agents is helpful. These often must be introduced with a wick to allow maximum penetration of the medication.

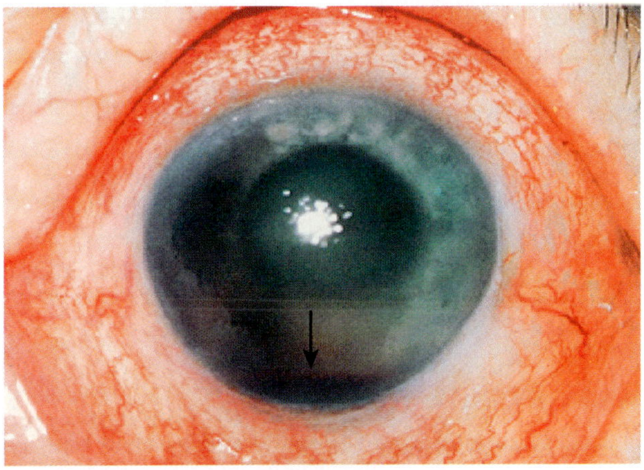

Figure 2–7 Traumatic hyphema. *(From Leclerc KM: Risk assessment and management of nonorthopaedic conditions. In DeLee JC, Drez Jr D, Miller MD [eds]: DeLee & Drez's Orthopaedic Sports Medicine: Principles and Practice, 2nd ed. Philadelphia, Saunders Elsevier, 2002, p 266.)*

❑ Acute Otitis Media
- Acute otitis media can develop secondary to any upper respiratory infection and is associated with the same pattern of acute-onset pain that is common in children with this condition.
- Diagnosis is made by visualization of an erythematous and immobile tympanic membrane on otoscopic examination.
- The most common causative organisms are *S. pneumoniae, Haemophilus influenzae,* and *Moraxella catarrhalis.*
- Treatment includes antihistamines and antibiotics as appropriate.

❑ Perichondrial Hematoma ("Cauliflower Ear")
- Perichondrial hematoma, which is caused by direct trauma to the auricle, occurs most frequently in wrestlers.
- Treatment involves aspirating the hematoma and applying a compressive dressing.

Injuries Involving the Teeth

- Luxation of a tooth or teeth should be treated with repositioning and referral to a dentist.
- Avulsions of a tooth or teeth should be treated with reimplantation as soon as possible.

Blunt Abdominal Trauma

- The concern with blunt abdominal trauma is laceration of a solid organ, injuries to the spleen and kidney being the most common.
- The abdominal examination is the key to the initial evaluation because findings such as tachycardia and hypotension occur later.
- Splenic rupture often requires surgical intervention and may manifest initially as left upper quadrant abdominal pain and a rigid abdomen.
- Trauma to the kidney may manifest as flank pain and hematuria. Most of these injuries are intracapsular and do not require surgical intervention.
- Abdominal ultrasonography of the area of concern is helpful for a quick evaluation.
- CT with use of an intravenous contrast agent is also a reliable method of evaluating the solid organs.

Testicular Injury

- Reports of serious testicular injury are most common in rugby and baseball but may be associated with other sports that involve kicking, such as soccer, football, and martial arts.
- Injuries requiring orchiectomy are rare in the literature.

Nonmusculoskeletal Injury Questions

1. A lacrosse player is hit in the eye with a ball during a game and is complaining of pain but has no change in vision. There is blood in the anterior chamber of the eye. This is best managed by:
A. Covering the eye and returning the athlete to the game.
B. Covering the eye and scheduling a clinic appointment the next morning with a local ophthalmologist.
C. Administration of antibiotic drops and allowing the athlete to return to play.
D. Administration of antibiotic drops, covering the eye, and removing the athlete from play for the day.
E. Immediately transporting the athlete to the local emergency room.

2. A player collides with another player during a rainy soccer game, and his tooth gets knocked completely out and falls onto the field. What is the most appropriate action?
A. Throw away the tooth.
B. Rinse the tooth and scrub it vigorously with a soft brush.
C. Wrap the tooth in dry sterile gauze and send it home with the athlete, instructing him to make an appointment with his dentist.
D. Gently rinse the tooth while holding it by the crown, and replace it in the socket immediately.
E. Instruct the athlete to hold the tooth under his tongue, and transport him to the local emergency room after the game.

■

Supplements and Stimulants

Anabolic Steroids

- The testosterone derivatives known as anabolic steroids have been used as performance-enhancing drugs because of their documented effectiveness in increasing muscle mass and strength.
- Anabolic steroids have a broad side-effect potential, including liver dysfunction, cardiomyopathy, and testicular atrophy.
- Careful testing has greatly reduced the use of these medications, but they are still widely encountered as abused drugs in sports.

Prohormones

- Prohormones such as dehydroepiandrosterone (DHEA) and androstenedione are also derivatives of testosterone that have been used to increase muscle function, although their effects are not well documented.

Creatine

- Creatine has gained popularity as a performance-enhancing drug because it has been shown to increase the muscle phosphocreatine concentration in some people.
- Creatine has been generally realized to have its biggest role in short bursts of exercise, such as seen in weight lifting, but does not seem to have a specific positive effect on aerobic activity.
- Athletes who use creatine are at risk of dehydration and should be carefully monitored for it.

Hormones and Growth Factors

- Human growth hormone (HGH) and insulin-like growth factor I (IGF-I) are both genetically engineered hormones that have found their way into the performance-enhancing drug category. Both of these agents are known to increase muscle mass and shorten muscle recovery time.
- Synthetic erythropoietin has been used to improve aerobic endurance by increasing the oxygen-carrying capacity via a greater number of available red blood cells.
- "Blood doping" involves an autologous transfusion and has similar effects on aerobic endurance.

Supplement Questions

1. Which of the following statements is true regarding creatine?
   A. It is banned by the NCAA.
   B. It can cause dehydration.
   C. It can cause elevation in testosterone levels.
   D. It is most useful during endurance activities.
2. Which of the following substances work to increase the oxygen carrying ability of the blood?
   A. Anabolic steroids
   B. Creatine
   C. Growth hormones
   D. Testosterone
   E. Synthetic erythropoietin

Nutrition and Eating Disorders

Nutrition in Athletes

- Caloric requirements for athletes vary depending on age, gender, size, and activity demands:
  - Female athletes generally require 1600 to 3000 kcal/day.
  - Male athletes typically require 2500 to 6000 kcal/day.
- Dietary sources of energy come primarily from carbohydrates (CHO), protein, and fat.
- CHO is the primary source of energy and should account for 65% of the total daily intake.
  - CHO provides 4 kcal/g of energy, making it the ideal source for high-energy activity.
  - Complex carbohydrates should be the primary source, whereas simple sugars such as those found in sports drinks can be a supplemental source, especially after high-energy activity.
- Protein should account for 10% to 15% of the total daily intake.
  - Protein similarly can provide 4 kcal/g of energy but is the last fuel source called upon during exercise.
  - Slightly higher levels of protein are needed for strength training, but there is no evidence that supplemental protein beyond normal dietary intake is necessary or beneficial.
- Fats should account for 20% to 35% of the total daily intake.
  - Fats can be a significant source of energy during submaximal exercise and should not be excessively restricted from the diet.
  - The dietary emphasis should be on essential fatty acids and unsaturated fats with avoidance of excessive amounts of unsaturated fats and trans-isomer fatty acids (trans fats).

Special Dietary Considerations in Athletes

- Vegetarian athletes must be careful to include a variety of plant proteins in their diets to maintain appropriate energy sources for exercise and may require vitamin supplementation if there is concern about vitamin deficiency.
- Female athletes, especially those suspected of having signs or symptoms consistent with the female athlete triad (disordered eating, amenorrhea, osteoporosis) may require additional supplementation of iron and/or calcium.
  - Screening for iron deficiency anemia by monitoring hemoglobin and serum ferritin levels may be necessary if there is concern.
  - Normal calcium intake should be monitored, and supplemental calcium should be provided if the dietary intake is not meeting the suggested levels:
    - Adolescent athletes: 1300 mg/day.
    - Athletes age 19–50 years: 1000 mg/day.
    - Female athlete triad: 1500 mg/day.
    - Post-menopausal athletes: 1500 mg/day.

Fluid and Dehydration

- Appropriate fluid intake is necessary to maintain maximum performance levels and to prevent dehydration and heat illness.

- The presence or absence of thirst is not a reliable indicator of fluid need; athletes should be instructed to rehydrate frequently during the course of exercise, especially during endurance tasks.
- Early signs of dehydration include thirst and decreased performance level, and later signs include flushing of the skin, nausea, vomiting, and tachycardia.
- Orthostatic vital signs should be assessed if dehydration is suspected, and fluid replacement should begin immediately.
- It can be helpful to weigh the athlete before and after exercise and to suggest a replacement strategy of 24 fluid ounces for each pound of weight lost during exercise.

Hyponatremia

- The signs and symptoms of hyponatremia can be similar to those of dehydration, leading to mismanagement of the former condition.
- Risk factors for development of exercise-related hyponatremia include warm weather, female gender, and the use of nonsteroidal anti-inflammatory medications.
- Rehydration with hypotonic fluids can exacerbate the condition, and electrolyte solutions are often recommended in affected patients.
- The use of hypertonic intravenous solutions should be reserved for severe cases.

Disordered Eating

- Eating disorders are first and foremost manifestations of mental illness rather than true nutritional problems.
- The primary underlying problem in anyone with an eating disorder is a distorted body image.
- Athletes may feel that maintaining a low body weight will increase performance ability.
- Athletes are more commonly affected by disordered eating than the general population.
- Females are much more commonly affected than males, although there has been an increase in the number of males diagnosed with some type of disordered eating.
- Associated disorders, such as depression, generalized anxiety disorder, obsessive-compulsive disorder, and substance abuse problems, are commonly found in patients with eating disorders.

❑ Anorexia Nervosa

- *Anorexia nervosa* is defined as a mental health disorder involving weight loss that leads to a total body weight of less than 85% of normal for age and height.
- The hallmark of anorexia is fear of weight gain in an already thin individual.
- Anorexia can be difficult to diagnose in an athletic population, in which being thin and fit is considered normal.
- Athletes affected by anorexia may exhibit only restrictive behavior (excessive dieting) or episodes of binging and purging.

❑ Bulimia Nervosa

- Bulimia nervosa is similar to anorexia nervosa, in that it also is a type of mental illness that involves a distorted body image.
- Bulimia is characterized by the use of abnormal methods to prevent weight gain, such as fasting, binging/purging, using medication such as laxatives or diuretics, and exercising excessively.
- Bulimia has two characteristic subtypes, purging and nonpurging.

Nutrition and Eating Disorders Questions

1. Which of the following is the single most important source of energy for physical exercise?
A. Carbohydrate.
B. Fat.
C. Protein.
D. Micronutrients.
E. All should be consumed in equal proportions.

2. While you are covering a marathon, one of the female runners crosses the finish line and immediately collapses. She is responsive, and after examining her, you suspect mild to moderate hyponatremia. What is your best first step in treating this condition?
A. Ask her to immediately start drinking as much water as she can tolerate.
B. Give her a sports drink.
C. Immediately establish an IV line and start a hypertonic saline solution.
D. Immediately establish an IV line and start a hypotonic solution.
E. Immediately transport her to the nearest hospital.

The Female Athlete

Menstrual Abnormalities

❑ Amenorrhea

- Amenorrhea may be primary or secondary and may be caused by excessive training, failure to maintain a normal body mass, or stress.
- *Primary amenorrhea* is defined as a delay of menarche beyond the age of 16 years.
- *Secondary amenorrhea* is defined as the cessation of menses for at least 3 consecutive months.
- Treatment of amenorrhea should focus on correcting the underlying problem (i.e., instructing on proper nutrition to normalize body fat percentage) and, occasionally, the use of hormonal supplements if other measures fail.

- Heavy menses may also be a problem for some athletes. Although not specifically affected or caused by exercise, it can lead to an iron deficiency anemia which can cause fatigue and negatively affect performance.

❑ The Female Athlete Triad

- The *female athlete triad* is a term that has been coined to describe a characteristic grouping of disorders that may be seen in some female athletes:
  - Disordered eating.
  - Amenorrhea.
  - Osteoporosis.
- When any one of these elements is suspected, the athlete should be carefully screened for the presence of the other two problems.
- A multidisciplinary approach to evaluation and treatment of the female athlete triad is usually necessary to help prevent some common associated problems, such as development of stress fractures (Fig. 2–8).

The Female Athlete Questions

1. A 16-year-old female cross-country runner presents with symptoms consistent with a metatarsal stress fracture. The prior season she was treated for a contralateral tibial stress fracture. What history points are the most important to obtain in this situation?
A. New prescription medications.
B. The type of shoes that she is wearing to train.
C. Menstrual history and symptoms of disordered eating.
D. Daily calcium intake.
E. Sexual history.

2. A 21-year-old female college soccer player presents to the clinic complaining of increased fatigue that is making it difficult for her to complete her practice sessions. Which test is the most likely to reveal the cause of her fatigue?
A. CBC.
B. Mono screen.
C. TSH.
D. Beta-hCG.
E. Sodium.

Other Special Populations

Down Syndrome

- Exercise has many benefits for Down syndrome patients but careful screening is important to allow safe participation.
- Athletes with Down syndrome should be evaluated for cervical instability by means of standard flexion and extension radiographs prior to sports participation.
  - Radiographically, atlantoaxial instability in this group is defined as an atlas-dens interval greater than 5 mm.

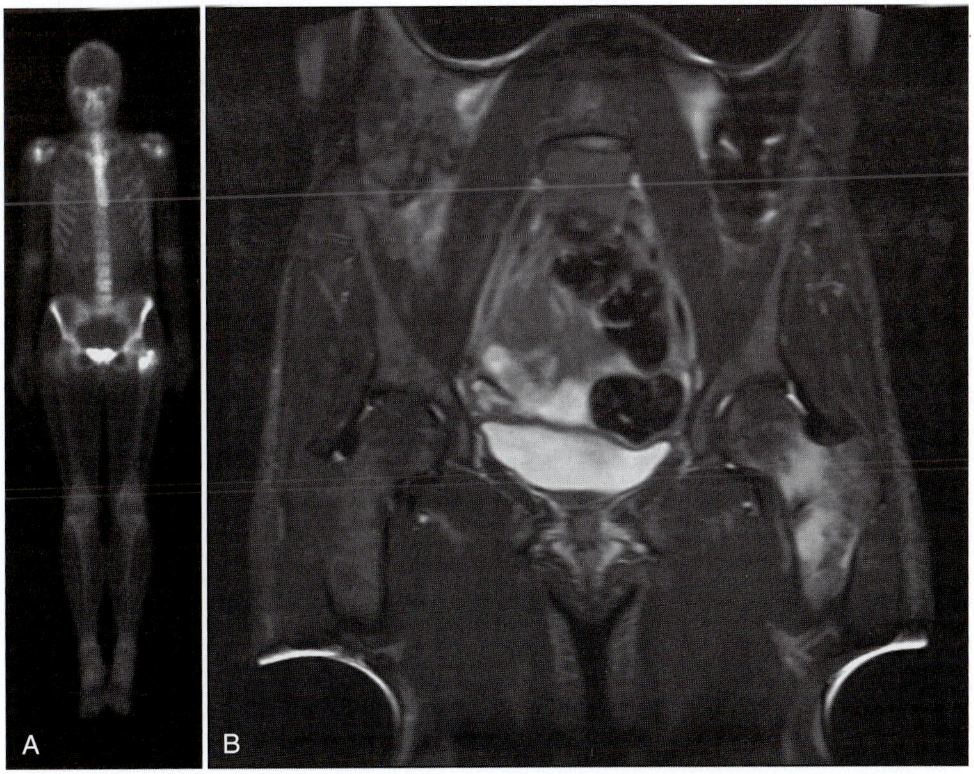

Figure 2–8 A, Bone scan depicting a femoral neck stress fracture in a female runner with classic female athlete triad. B, Magnetic resonance imaging appearance of the same stress fracture.

  - Other spine anomalies are commonly present in addition to the atlantoaxial instability, but the patient is often asymptomatic.
  - All activities that risk loading of the head and neck (e.g., diving, gymnastics, football, skiing) should be avoided if such instability is detected.
- A thorough cardiac history and physical examination are especially important in this population because Down syndrome is associated with an increased risk of cardiac abnormalities of up to 45%.
- Other concerns in athletes with Down syndrome include excess ligamentous laxity, which can predispose to conditions such as patellar instability, shoulder instability, and spinal deformity.

The Diabetic Athlete

- Physical activity should be encouraged in diabetic patients because it has been associated with improved glucose control and long-term outcomes.
- Good glucose control is necessary for diabetic athletes and should be routinely monitored with regular blood glucose and hemoglobin A_{1c} ($HgbA_{1c}$) measurements.
- The biggest risk to diabetic athletes is the development of hypoglycemia up to 24 hours after exercise as a result of the increased glucose uptake by muscles during exercise.
- The team physician's medical bag should contain some form of glucagon for rapid ingestion in case of hypoglycemia.

Special Populations Questions

1. A boy with Down syndrome presents for a pre-participation physical examination for sports. Flexion and extension cervical radiographs taken as per routine show an atlantoaxial interval of 8 mm. What recommendations should you give this patient regarding sport participation?
A. Allow full sports participation.
B. Restrict activity only until MRI is performed to ensure that there is no other abnormality in the spine.
C. Recommend the use of a brace during sports participation.
D. Restrict participation only in sports that produce pain.
E. Restrict participation in all sports that risk head/neck injury.

2. On the pre-participation physical form, one of your athletes answers that he has diabetes mellitus and takes insulin. What is your responsibility to prevent complications relating to athletic activity in this patient?
A. Restrict him from contact and collision sports.
B. Restrict him from all activity unless his screening log shows consistently normal glucose levels.
C. Monitor his glucose levels periodically, especially for 24 hours after exercise, and keep glucagon available in the medical bag.
D. Instruct him to double his insulin dose before activity.
E. Measure his $HgbA_{1c}$ level monthly.

Resources

CARDIOVASCULAR ISSUES

Alpert, J.S., Pape, L.A., Ward, A., Rippe, J.M., 1989. Athletic heart syndrome. Phys. Sports Med. 27, 103–107.
Basilico, F.C., 1999. Cardiovascular disease in athletes. Am. J. Sports Med. 27, 108–121.
Corrado, D., Basso, C., Pavei, A., et al., 2006. Trends in sudden cardiovascular death in young competitive athletes after implementation of a preparticipation screening program. JAMA 296, 1593–1601.
Corrado, D., Basso, C., Schiavon, M., Thiene, G., 1998. Screening for hypertrophic cardiomyopathy in young athletes. N. Engl. J. Med. 339, 364–369.
Corrado, D., Basso, C., Thiene, G., 2001. Sudden cardiac death in young people with apparently normal heart. Cardiovasc. Res. 50, 399–408.
Drezner, J.A., Courson, R.W., Roberts, W.O., et al., 2007. Inter-association Task Force recommendations on emergency preparedness and management of sudden cardiac arrest in high school and college athletic programs: A consensus statement. J. Athl. Train. 42, 143–158.
Epstein, S.E., Maron, B.J., 1986. Sudden death and the competitive athlete: Perspectives on preparticipation screening studies. J. Am. Coll. Cardiol. 7, 220–230.
Fagard, R., 2003. Athlete's heart. Heart 89, 1455–1461.
Haq, C.L., 1998. Sudden death due to low-energy chest-wall impact (commotio cordis). N. Engl. J. Med. 338, 1805–1811.
Kapetanopoulos, A., Kluger, J., Maron, B.J., Thompson, P.D., 2006. The congenital long QT syndrome and implications for young athletes. Med. Sci. Sports Exerc. 38, 816–825.
Link, M.S., 1999. Commotio cordis: Sudden death due to chest wall impact in sports. Heart 81, 109–110.
Maron, B.J., Epstein, S.E., Roberts, W.C., 1986. Causes of sudden death in competitive athletes. J. Am. Coll. Cardiol. 7, 204–214.
Maron, B.J., Zipes, D.P., 2005. Introduction: Eligibility recommendations for competitive athletes with cardiovascular abnormalities—general considerations. J. Am. Coll. Cardiol. 45, 1318–1321.
Mukerji, B., Alpert, M.A., Mukerji, V., 1989. Cardiovascular changes in athletes. Am. Fam. Physician 40, 169–175.
Thompson, P.D., Levine, B.D., 2006. Protecting athletes from sudden cardiac death. JAMA 296, 1648–1650.

PULMONARY ISSUES

Baumann, M.H., Strange, C., Heffner, J.E., et al., 2001. Management of spontaneous pneumothorax: An American College of Chest Physicians Delphi consensus statement. Chest 119, 590–602.
Holzer, K., Brukner, P., 2004. Screening of athletes for exercise-induced bronchoconstriction. Clin. J. Sport Med. 14, 134–138.
Parsons, J.P., Mastronarde, J.G., 2005. Exercise-induced bronchoconstriction in athletes. Chest 128, 3966–3974.
Putukian, M., 2004. Pneumothorax and pneumomediastinum. Clin. Sports Med. 23, 443–454, x.
Randolph, C., 1997. Exercise-induced asthma: Update on pathophysiology, clinical diagnosis, and treatment. Curr. Probl. Pediatr. 27, 53–77.
Rundell, K.W., Im, J., Mayers, L.B., et al., 2001. Self-reported symptoms and exercise-induced asthma in the elite athlete. Med. Sci. Sports Exerc. 33, 208–213.
Rundell, K.W., Jenkinson, D.M., 2002. Exercise-induced bronchospasm in the elite athlete. Sports Med. 32, 583–600.
Storms, W.W., 1999. Exercise-induced asthma: Diagnosis and treatment for the recreational or elite athlete. Med. Sci. Sports Exerc. 31 (Suppl.), S33–S38.
Storms, W.W., 2003. Review of exercise-induced asthma. Med. Sci. Sports Exerc. 35, 1464–1470.
Storms, W.W., 2005. Asthma associated with exercise. Immunol. Allergy Clin. North Am. 25, 31–43.

ENVIRONMENTAL ILLNESS

American College of Sports Medicine; Armstrong, L.E., Casa, D.J., Millard-Stafford, M., et al., 2007. American College of Sports Medicine position stand: Exertional heat illness during training and competition. Med. Sci. Sports Exerc. 39, 556–572.
American College of Sports Medicine; Armstrong, L.E., Epstein, Y., Greenleaf, J. E., et al., 1996. American College of Sports Medicine position stand: Heat and cold illnesses during distance running. Med. Sci. Sports Exerc. 28, i–x.
American College of Sports Medicine; Sawka, M.N., Burke, L.M., Eichner, E.R., et al., 2007. American College of Sports Medicine position stand: Exercise and fluid replacement. Med. Sci. Sports Exerc. 39, 377–390.
Bergeron, M.F., McKeag, D.B., Casa, D.J., et al., 2005. Youth football: Heat stress and injury risk. Med. Sci. Sports Exerc. 37, 1421–1430.
Binkley, H.M., Beckett, J., Casa, D.J., et al., 2002. National Athletic Trainers' Association Position Statement: Exertional heat illnesses. J. Athl. Train. 37, 329–343.
Casa, D.J., Armstrong, L.E., Hillman, S.K., et al., 2000. National Athletic Trainers' Association Position Statement: Fluid replacement for athletes. J. Athl. Train. 35, 212–224.
Convertino, V.A., Armstrong, L.E., Coyle, E.F., et al., 1996. American College of Sports Medicine position stand: Exercise and fluid replacement. Med. Sci. Sports Exerc. 28, i–vii.
Coris, E.E., Ramirez, A.M., Van Durme, D.J., 2004. Heat illness in athletes: The dangerous combination of heat, humidity and exercise. Sports Med. 34, 9–16.
Kenefick, R.W., O'Moore, K.M., Mahood, N.V., Castellani, J.W., 2006. Rapid IV versus oral rehydration: Responses to subsequent exercise heat stress. Med. Sci. Sports Exerc. 38, 2125–2131.
Larsen, T., Kumar, S., Grimmer, K., et al., 2007. A systematic review of guidelines for the prevention of heat illness in community-based sports participants and officials. J. Sci. Med. Sport 10, 11–26.

INFECTIONS

Goodman, R.A., Thacker, S.B., Solomon, S.L., et al., 1994. Infectious disease in competitive sports. JAMA 271, 862–867.
MacKnight, J.M., 2002. Infectious mononucleosis in the athlete: Ensuring a safe return to sport. Phys. Sports Med. 30, 27–41.
Maki, D.G., Reich, R.M., 1982. Infectious mononucleosis in the athlete: Diagnosis, complications, and management. Am. J. Sports Med. 10, 162–173.
Putukian, M., O'Connor, F.G., Stricker, P., et al., 2008. Mononucleosis and athletic participation: An evidence-based subject review. Clin. J. Sport Med. 18, 309–315.
Stringer, W., 1999. HIV and aerobic exercise: Current recommendations. Sports Med. 28, 389–395.

DERMATOLOGIC CONDITIONS

Adams, B.B., 2002. Dermatologic disorders of the athlete. Sports Med. 32, 309–321.
Adams, B.B., 2004. New strategies for the diagnosis, treatment, and prevention of herpes simplex in contact sports. Curr. Sports Med. Rep. 3, 277–283.
Dienst, W.L., Dightman, L., Dworkin, M.S., et al., 1997. Pinning down skin infection: Diagnosis, treatment, and prevention in wrestlers. Phys. Sports Med. 25, 45.

NONMUSCULOSKELETAL INJURIES: INJURIES TO THE EYE, EAR, AND TEETH

Easterbrook, M., 1988. Eye protection in racquet sports. Clin. Sports Med. 7, 253–266.
Easterbrook, M., 1988. Ocular injuries in racquet sports. Int. Ophthalmol. Clin. 28, 232–237.
Gomez, J.E., 2003. Paired organ loss. In: DeLee, J.C., Drez Jr., D., Miller, M.D. (Eds.), DeLee & Drez's Orthopaedic Sports Medicine: Principles and Practice, second ed. Philadelphia, Saunders Elsevier, pp. 264–271.
Heimmel, M.R., Murphy, M.A., 2008. Ocular injuries in basketball and baseball: What are the risks and how can we prevent them? Curr. Sports Med. Rep. 7, 284–288.
Kerr, L., 1983. Dental problems in athletes. Clin. Sports Med. 2, 115–122.
Lee, D., Sperling, N., 1996. Initial management of auricular trauma. Am. Fam. Physician 53, 2339–2344.
Rannelli, D.N., 2005. Dental injuries in sports. Curr. Sports Med. Rep. 4, 12–17.

SUPPLEMENTS AND STIMULANTS

Gilliam, J.D., Hohzorn, C., Martin, D., Trimble, M.H., 2000. Effect of oral creatine supplementation on isokinetic torque production. Med. Sci. Sports Exerc. 32, 993–996.
Haupt, H.A., 1993. Anabolic steroids and growth hormone. Am. J. Sports Med. 21, 468–474.
Perlmutter, G., Lowenthal, D.T., 1985. Use of anabolic steroids by athletes. Am. Fam. Physician 32, 208–210.
Sawka, M.N., Young, A.J., Muza, S.R., et al., 1987. Erythrocyte reinfusion and maximal aerobic power: An examination of modifying factors. JAMA 257, 1496–1499.
Stricker, P.R., 1998. Other ergogenic agents. Clin. Sports Med. 17, 283–297.
Terjung, R.L., Clarkson, P., Eichner, E.R., et al., 2000. American College of Sports Medicine Roundtable: The physiological and health effects of oral creatine supplementation. Med. Sci. Sports Exerc. 32, 06–717.

NUTRITION AND EATING DISORDERS

Hew, T.D., Chorley, J.N., Cianca, J.C., Divine, J.G., 2003. The incidence, risk factors, and clinical manifestations of hyponatremia in marathon runners. Clin. J. Sport Med. 13, 41–47.
Murray, B., Eichner, E.R., 2004. Hyponatremia of exercise. Curr. Sports Med. Rep. 3, 117–118.
Noakes, T.D., 2002. Hyponatremia in distance athletes: Fluid and sodium balance during exercise. Curr. Sports Med. Rep. 1, 197–207.
Sundgot-Borgen, J., 1993. Prevalence of eating disorders in elite female athletes. Int. J. Sport Nutr. 3, 29–40.

THE FEMALE ATHLETE

Barrow, G.W., Saha, S., 1988. Menstrual irregularity and stress fractures in collegiate female distance runners. Am. J. Sports Med. 16, 209–216.
Beals, K.A., Meyer, N.L., 2007. Female athlete triad update. Clin. Sports Med. 26, 69–89.
Clapp 3rd, J.F., 2000. Exercise during pregnancy: A clinical update. Clin. Sports Med. 19, 273–286.
Frankovich, R.J., Lebrun, C.M., 2000. Menstrual cycle, contraception, and performance. Clin. Sports Med. 19, 251–271.
Gidwani, G.P., 1999. Amenorrhea in the athlete. Adolesc. Med. 10, 275–290, vii.
Otis, C.L., Drinkwater, B., Johnson, M., et al., 1997. American College of Sports Medicine position stand: The female athlete triad. Med. Sci. Sports Exerc. 29, i–ix.
Putukian, M., 1998. The female athlete triad. Clin. Sports Med. 17, 675–696, v.
Sanborn, C.F., Horea, M., Siemers, B.J., Dieringer, K.I., 2000. Disordered eating and the female athlete triad. Clin. Sports Med. 19, 199–213.
Teitz, C.C., Hu, S.S., Arendt, E.A., 1997. The female athlete: Evaluation and treatment of sports-related problems. J. Am. Acad. Orthop. Surg. 5, 87–96.

OTHER SPECIAL POPULATIONS

Lisle, D.K., Trojian, T.H., 2006. Managing the athlete with type I diabetes. Curr. Sports Med. Rep. 5, 93–98.
Nemeth, B.A., Allen, D.B., 2003. Diabetes mellitus. In: DeLee, J.C., Drez Jr., D., Miller, M.D. (Eds.), DeLee & Drez's Orthopaedic Sports Medicine: Principles and Practice, second ed. Saunders Elsevier, Philadelphia, pp. 297–317.
Tassone, J.C., Duey-Holtz, A., 2008. Spine concerns in the Special Olympian with Down syndrome. Sports Med. Arthrosc. 16, 55–60.

CHAPTER 3

Shoulder

S. Raymond Golish, Jason L. Dragoo, F. Winston Gwathmey and Mark D. Miller

Anatomy

Bones

- Proximal Humerus
  - Hemispherical head and articular surface, about 45 mm in diameter.
  - Greater and lesser tuberosities are insertions of rotator cuff.
  - The long head of the biceps brachii (LHBB) tendon runs through the bicipital groove that separates the tuberosities.
  - Head is retroverted 35 degrees relative to transepicondylar axis of the elbow and inclined 130 degrees relative to shaft.
- Scapula
  - Triangular bone with multiple fossae for rotator cuff muscles.
  - Coracoid process is the origin/insertion of multiple tendons/ligaments (pectoralis minor, short head of biceps, coracobrachialis).
  - Glenoid is retroverted an average of 5 degrees relative to spine of scapula (best assessed on axillary view) but may vary from 7 degrees of retroversion to 10 degrees of anteversion.
  - Os acromiale is an unfused ossification center of acromion, occurring in 3% of the population, in 60% of whom it is bilateral. Of pre-, meso-, meta-, and basi-acromion, the most common is the meso-acromion.
- Clavicle
  - Sigmoid-shaped bone that acts as strut from sternum (axial skeleton) to scapula (appendicular skeleton).
  - Acromioclavicular (AC) and sternoclavicular (SC) joints have stout ligaments to support the strut.
  - First bone to ossify and last bone to fuse, with medial physis closing in early 20's.
  - Widest at its medial articulation with the sternum.
  - Curves superiorly and posteriorly and tapers in diameter as it approaches its lateral articulation with the acromion.

Joints

- Glenohumeral Joint
  - Ball-and-socket (spheroidal joint) that compromises stability for increased range of motion.
  - Most commonly dislocated joint in the body.
  - Glenoid radius of curvature is larger than that of humeral head.
  - Nonconforming articulation contributes to instability if soft tissue stabilizers are compromised.
  - Has multiple static and dynamic soft tissue stabilizers (see sections on ligaments and biomechanics), which are compromised in injury.
  - Normal glenoid fossa is pear shaped and surrounded by cartilaginous labrum, a critical structure for stability (see sections on biomechanics and instability).
- Acromioclavicular Joint
  - Gliding synovial joint with articular disc.
  - Helps suspend shoulder from thorax as part of clavicular strut.
  - Stout ligaments posteriorly and superiorly aid in stability.
- Sternoclavicular Joint
  - Gliding synovial joint with articular disc like AC joint.
  - SC joint is only bony articulation of shoulder with thorax.
  - Stout ligaments, especially posterior SC ligament, may be disrupted in dislocations.
  - Less than 50% of the medial clavicle articulates with the manubrium and first rib.
  - More angular and rotational motion occurs at the SC joint than at the AC joint.

❑ Scapulothoracic Joint
- A gliding fasciomuscular complex in the absence of a true joint.
- Allows scapulothoracic motion in concert with glenohumeral motion for mobility of shoulder girdle. The normal ratio of glenohumeral motion to scapulothoracic motion is 2:1.

Ligaments

❑ Glenohumeral Ligaments
- Capsular thickenings that are static stabilizers of shoulder (Table 3–1) (Figure 3–1).

Inferior Glenohumeral Ligament (Anterior Band)
- Limits anterior/inferior translation in external rotation and abduction (45–90 degrees of elevation).
- Is injured in classic anterior shoulder dislocation.
- Inferior glenohumeral ligament (IGHL) posterior band is injured in posterior dislocation and prevents translation in internal rotation.

Middle Glenohumeral Ligament
- Limits anterior/posterior translation in 45 degrees of abduction and external rotation.
- Anatomically variable along with anterior labrum (1 to 3 o'clock), resulting in numerous capsulolabral normal variants (Buford complex: a cord-like middle glenohumeral [MGH] ligament inserting onto superior labrum with an absence of anterior labrum [1 to 3 o'clock]).

Superior Glenohumeral Ligament
- Limits inferior translation and external rotation in adduction.
- Acts with coracohumeral ligament to form a pulley for the LHBB tendon.

❑ Other Ligaments (Figure 3–2)

Coracoclavicular Ligaments
- Conoid ligament is more medial, and trapezoid is more lateral.
- Prevents inferior displacement of acromion relative to clavicle (appears as superior displacement of the clavicle).
- Injured in type III AC dislocations but also in type IIb distal third clavicle fractures.

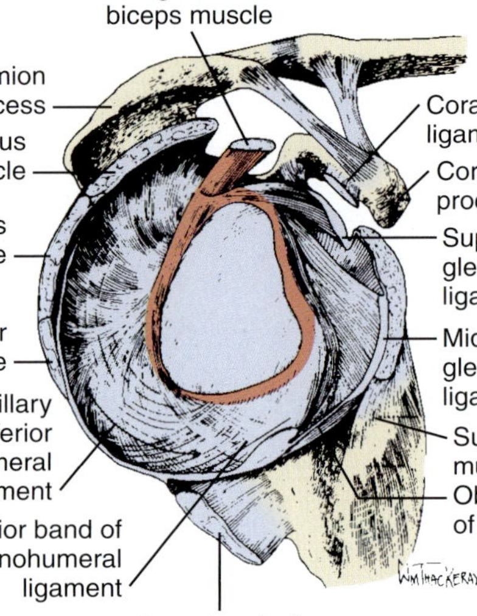

Figure 3–1 Important ligaments of the shoulder. *(From Turkel SH, Panio MW, Marshall JL, et al: Stabilizing mechanisms preventing anterior dislocation of the glenohumeral joint. J Bone Joint Surg [Am] 1981;63:1208-1217.)*

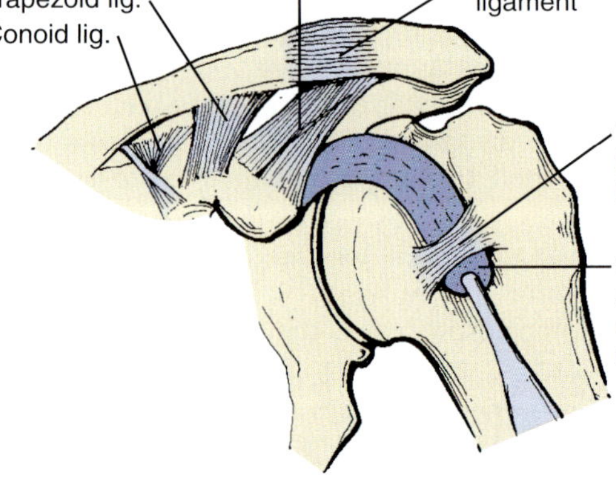

Figure 3–2 Acromioclavicular joint anatomy. *(From Tibone J, Patek R, Jobe FW, et al: Functional anatomy, biomechanics, and kinesiology: The shoulder. In Delee JC, Drez D Jr [eds]: Orthopaedic Sports Medicine: Principles and Practice. Philadelphia, WB Saunders, 1994, p 465.)*

Table 3–1 Glenohumeral Ligaments

Structure	Arm Position	Resists
Superior glenohumeral ligament/ coracohumeral ligament	Adduction	Inferior translation/external rotation
	Forward flexion/abduction/internal rotation	Posterior translation
Middle glenohumeral ligament	Adduction/external rotation	External rotation
	45-degree abduction/external rotation	Anterior/posterior translation
Inferior glenohumeral ligament	45- to 90-degree glenohumeral elevation	Primary restraint to anterior/posterior/inferior glenohumeral translation

From Miller M: Review of Orthopaedics: Expert Consult: Online and Print, 5th ed. Philadelphia, Saunders, 2008.

Coracohumeral and Transverse Humeral Ligament

- Coracohumeral ligament acts with superior glenohumeral ligament (SGHL) to limit inferior translation and external rotation in adduction.
- Transverse humeral ligament, generally thought to be an extension of the subscapularis tendon, stabilizes LHBB tendon in the bicipital groove. It may be compromised in subscapularis tendon ruptures, leading to painful subluxation of the tendon.

Coracoacromial Ligament

- May aid in prevention of anterior/superior displacement of humeral head relative to glenoid.
- Has been implicated in subacromial impingement and may require release during subacromial decompression.
- Release is controversial because an intact ligament may stabilize anterior/superior migration in rotator cuff arthropathy.

❑ Acromioclavicular and Sternoclavicular Ligaments

- AC ligament is capsular thickening that prevents anterior/posterior translation (especially posterior and superior capsule).
- Is injured in AC separations.
- Portion of ligament is retained in arthroscopic distal clavicle resection to preserve stabilizing function.
- SC ligament is a complex of posterior SC, anterior SC, costoclavicular, and interclavicular portions.
- The functions of the ligaments are complex. The posterior SC ligament helps prevent posterior dislocation. The costoclavicular ligament helps prevent anterior dislocation.

Biomechanics

- Glenohumeral joint and shoulder girdle compromise stability for increased range of motion.
- Stability is mediated by static and dynamic stabilizers of the glenohumeral joint, although their relative importance in various positions, activities, and injured conditions is incompletely understood.
- Injury to stabilizers may result in symptomatic instability. The classic example is anterior/inferior labral tear (Bankart lesion) and capsular injury with or without a glenoid rim fracture (bony Bankart lesion) after anterior shoulder dislocation. This may result in repeat low energy dislocations and subjective instability with sports and activities of daily living (ADLs).
- The understanding of surgical biomechanics has been greatly improved, especially in the area of rotator cuff repair. Concepts such as the suspension bridge analogy of the cuff, the coronal and axial plane force couples of the cuff, and the deadman angle of suture anchor placement have improved the management of complex cuff pathology (Burkhart et al, 2006).

Static Stabilizers

❑ Glenoid Labrum

- Critical cartilaginous ring structure that adds stability to glenohumeral (GH) articulation by acting as a chock block and deepening the glenoid fossa.
- Labral injury results in instability in many cases.

❑ Glenohumeral Conformity

- Conformity confers stability to a ball-and-socket joint.
- The bony GH joint is partially nonconforming. The labrum increases effective conformity.
- Injury to glenoid rim (bony Bankart lesion or other fractures) compromises conformity and may require surgical repair.
- Glenoid and humeral version act in complex way to contribute to motion-stability tradeoff.

❑ Capsuloligamentous Structures

- Anterior and posterior capsule can be torn or stretched during instability events.
- Capsule may be imbricated or included in other soft tissue procedures such as Bankart repair.
- The glenohumeral ligaments are capsular thickenings that are extremely important in stability and instability (see ligament section and Table 3–1).

Other Stabilizers

- Negative intra-articular pressure may add stability.
- Numerous other structures may aid static and/or dynamic stability, including the coracoacromial (CA) ligament (static) and LHBB tendon (dynamic).

Dynamic Stabilizers

❑ Rotator Cuff

- Joint compression created by coordinated activity of rotator cuff is the primary dynamic stabilizer of the glenohumeral joint.
- Rotator cuff and deltoid paralysis caused by brachial plexopathy results in unstable joint and subluxation/dislocation.
- Acute traumatic rotator cuff tear can lead to rapid dysfunction and arthropathy due to instability during motion.

❑ Other Stabilizers

- LHBB tendon likely helps stabilize the GH joint in the abducted/externally rotated position.
- The scapulothoracic articulation is dynamically stabilized by muscles that indirectly stabilize the glenohumeral joint ("ball on a seal's nose"). Various other structures may act as static or dynamic stabilizers.

Anatomy and Biomechanics Questions

1. What is the principal stabilizing function of the anterior band IGHL?
   A. Limits anterior/inferior translation in 90 degrees of abduction/ER.
   B. Limits anterior/posterior translation in 45 degrees of abduction/ER.
   C. Limits inferior translation and external rotation in adduction.
   D. Limits superior/posterior translation in 90 degrees of abduction/ER.
   E. Limits inferior translation in extreme abduction.

2. Which statement best describes the coracoclavicular (CC) ligaments?
   A. Control primarily anterior/posterior translation.
   B. Are not involved in displaced distal third clavicle fractures.
   C. Conoid is more lateral than trapezoid.
   D. Are injured in all types of AC joint injuries.
   E. Conoid is more medial than trapezoid.

3. Which statement about shoulder osteology is most correct?
   A. Head is retroverted 35 degrees to transepicondylar axis of elbow.
   B. Glenoid is anteverted 5 degrees on average.
   C. The most common os acromiale is the basi-acromion.
   D. Biceps tendon runs medial to the lesser tuberosity.
   E. Coracoid process is origin of pectoralis minor.

4. Which statement about the glenoid is most correct?
   A. Normal glenoid is inverted pear shape.
   B. Glenoid labrum acts as a chock block to deepen the glenoid.
   C. Bony articulation of head and glenoid is highly conforming.
   D. Glenoid version is always opposite humeral head version.
   E. Negative intra-articular pressure is the main stabilizer of the shoulder.

■

Diagnosis

- The shoulder presents a fascinating diagnostic challenge, with relatively subtle points of history, physical examination, and imaging affecting management.
- The diagnosis of each condition is covered in its respective subsection, but general points are discussed here.
- Each surgeon develops his/ her own sequence and style, but the general approach must be quite comprehensive, or diagnoses will be missed.

History

- History may be tailored to the presentation; common presentations include the young and/or competitive athlete, the middle-aged and/or recreational athlete, the active older patient, and the sedentary middle-aged or older patient.
- In younger and/or competitive athletes, sporting history is the key, including throwing or overhead sports, seasonal schedule, pitching frequency, off-season activity, and other provocative activities.
- In middle-aged and/or recreational athletes, sporting history is also important. The possibility of a low-energy injury that has not gone away or is periodically exacerbated is important. Sudden changes in activity level or sport (i.e., the "weekend warrior"), or nonspecific aches and pains due to variable conditioning should be considered.
- The active older patient is similar in this regard. Work-related activities, including heavy labor performed with the arms over the head, and work-related low-energy injuries that have not abated, are important.
- In both sedentary and active older patients, the pattern and nature of pain (e.g., night pain in rotator cuff disease), exacerbating and inciting events (e.g., possible pop in biceps pathology), and medical comorbidity become increasingly important (e.g., diabetes in adhesive capsulitis). A thorough history narrows the differential diagnosis so that nonspecific imaging findings common in this age group are not mistaken for pain generators.

Physical Examination

- Specific muscle testing and provocative maneuvers are the key to examination (Table 3–2).
- The examination may be tailored as the history suggests for common presentations, but a thorough general examination is essential, given the frequency of overlapping pathology and the subtlety of testing.
- Cervical spine disorders may cause referred pain to the shoulder and upper extremity. The spine should be considered an essential part of the examination.
- Inspection and provocative maneuvers for other less common problems are essential, given the complexity of the shoulder.
- Scapular winging may be lateral (spinal accessory nerve palsy affecting trapezius) or medial (long thoracic nerve palsy affecting serratus anterior) and accentuated by a push-up maneuver against a wall.
- Scapulothoracic crepitus (snapping scapula syndrome) may manifest as painful crepitus at the scapulothoracic articulation that is exacerbated by elevation of the shoulder and

Table 3–2 Muscle Testing for Shoulder Injuries

Examination	Technique	Significance
Impingement/Rotator Cuff		
Impingement sign	Passive FF > 90 degrees	Pain = impingement syndrome
Impingement test	Same after subacromial injection	Relief of pain = impingement syndrome
Hawkins test	Passive FF 90 degrees and internal rotation	Pain = impingement syndrome
Jobe test	Resisted pronation/FF 90 degrees	Pain = supraspinatus lesion
Drop-arm test	Maintain FF in plane of scapula	Inability = supraspinatus lesion
Hornblower sign	Resisted maximum ER/abduction 90 degrees	Pain = infraspinatus/(post)supraspinatus lesion
Rubber band sign	Resisted maximum ER/slight abduction	Pain = infraspinatus lesion
Liftoff test	Arm in internal rotation behind back	Inability to elevate from back = subscapularis lesion
Modified liftoff test	Resisted arm held off back	Inability to keep elevated off back = subscapularis lesion
Belly-push test	Elbow held anterior with abduction pressure	Inability to hold elbow forward = subscapularis lesion
Instability		
Apprehension test	Supine abduction 90 degrees and ER	Apprehension = anterior instability
Relocation test	Apprehension with posterior force	Relief of apprehension = anterior instability
Load-and-shift test	Anterior/posterior force on humeral head	Degree of translation = laxity vs. instability (see Table 3–4)
Modified load-and-shift test	Supine load/shift with elbow bending	Degree of translation = laxity vs. instability (see Table 3–4)
Jerk test	Post force with arm adduction and FF	"Clunk" = posterior subluxation
Sulcus sign	Inferior force with arm at side	Increased acromiohumeral interval = inferior laxity vs. instability (see Table 3–4)
Labrum/Biceps		
Active compression test	Adduction 10 degrees, FF 90 degrees, maximum pronation	Pain with resistance = SLAP lesion
Anterior slide test	Hand on hip, joint loading	Pain with resistance = SLAP lesion
Crank test	Full abduction, humeral loading, rotation	Pain = SLAP lesion
Speed test	Resisted FF in scapular plane	Pain = bicipital tendinitis
Yergason test	Resisted supination	Pain = bicipital tendinitis
Miscellaneous		
Spurling maneuver	Lateral flexion, rotation, cervical loading	Cervical spine pathology
Wright test	Extension/abduction/ER of arm with neck rotated away	Loss of pulse and reproduction of symptom(s) = thoracic outlet syndrome

ER, external rotation; FF, forward flexion; SLAP, superior labrum from anterior to posterior.
From Miller M: Review of Orthopaedics: Expert Consult: Online and Print, 5th ed. Philadelphia, Saunders, 2008.

relieved by shoulder stabilization. It may be caused by an osteochondroma (most common bony cause; diagnosed by computed tomography [CT]) or elastofibroma (most common soft tissue cause; diagnosed by magnetic resonance imaging [MRI]).

- Adhesive capsulitis is a diagnosis based on physical examination and history; it is typically self-limited over a 1- to 2-year period. Patients may have a history of diabetes (bilateral), surgery, or trauma. Patients present with painful decreased range of motion in all planes, and passive range is equal to active range, especially in external rotation, because the condition is characterized by painful stiffness, not weakness. Treatment is conservative although arthroscopic release may be required in some cases.

Imaging

- Plain film radiography is an essential tool, and numerous specific views are useful for particular diagnoses (Table 3–3).
- MRI (possibly with gadolinium arthrography) is the standard for soft tissue diagnosis.
- CT is useful for fractures and is the standard for evaluating bony Bankart lesions when operative management is being considered.
- Ultrasonography has emerged as an important tool for rotator cuff disease, because the cuff is sufficiently superficial to be well visualized in many patients. However, the results are highly operator dependent.

Special Studies

❑ Diagnostic Injections

- Diagnostic injections with local anesthetic are useful in the subacromial space,

Table 3–3 Radiographic Views and Signs

View/Sign	Findings	Significance
View of supraspinatus outlet	Acromial morphology (types I-III)	Type III acromion associated with impingement
View of 30-degree caudal tilt	Subacromial spurring	Area below level of clavicle = impingement area
Zanca 10-degree cephalic tilt	AC joint pathology	AC DJD, distal clavicle osteolysis
West Point view	AI glenoid evaluation	Bony Bankart lesion seen with instability
Garth view	AI glenoid evaluation	Bony Bankart lesion seen with instability
Stryker notch	Humeral head evaluation	Hill-Sachs impression fracture
Anteroposterior internal rotation	Humeral head evaluation	Hill-Sachs defect
Hobbs view	SC injury	AP dislocations
Serendipity view	SC injury	AP dislocations
45-degree abduction, true AP	Glenohumeral space	Subtle DJD
Arthrography	Rotator cuff injuries	Dye above cuff = tear
Computed tomography	Fractures	Classification easier
Magnetic resonance imaging ± arthrography	Soft tissue evaluation	Labral, cuff, muscle tears

AC, acromioclavicular; AI, anteroinferior; AP, anteroposterior; DJD, degenerative joint disease; SC, sternoclavicular.
From Miller M: Review of Orthopaedics: Expert Consult: Online and Print, 5th ed. Philadelphia, Saunders, 2008.

glenohumeral joint, acromioclavicular joint, and biceps tendon sheath to help narrow the differential diagnosis.
  - For example, AC joint disease may be mistaken for biceps pathology on physical examination. Injection should provide significant immediate relief if the pathology is intra-articular.
  - In the presence of a full-thickness rotator cuff tear, the subacromial space and glenohumeral joint communicate, mitigating the diagnostic benefit of injections in this setting.
- ❑ Electromyography and Nerve Conduction Velocity Testing
  - Electromyography and nerve conduction velocity (EMG/NCV) is an essential tool for discriminating cervical spine pathology from shoulder pathology. EMG/NCV should always be ordered with paraspinous muscle testing.
  - EMG/NCV is also essential for the diagnosis of other nerve pathology about the shoulder (such as suprascapular nerve: If lesion is in the suprascapular notch, EMG results will be abnormal in the supraspinatus *and* infraspinatus; if lesion is in the spinoglenoid notch, EMG results will be abnormal in the infraspinatus but *not* the supraspinatus).
- ❑ Arthroscopy
  - Arthroscopy remains the "gold standard" for diagnosis of shoulder disorders. A systematic diagnostic arthroscopy should be performed at the beginning of every surgical arthroscopy to confirm or refine the working diagnosis and include/exclude concomitant pathology.
  - Arthroscopic examination with use of anesthesia and in provocative positions improves the diagnosis by arthroscopy (e.g., the peel-back phenomena in superior labrum anterior to posterior [SLAP]) lesions, biceps tendon subluxation in forward flexion and rotation).
  - However, in the modern era, the preoperative working diagnosis must include a high-probability surgical lesion, and routine arthroscopy for diagnosis only is contraindicated.

"Alphabet Soup" Lesions of the Shoulder

- The shoulder has acquired "alphabet soup" lesions that include diagnoses of instability, rotator cuff disease, and superior labrum pathology. Because they are highly testable and easily confused, they are discussed together in this section on diagnosis.
- Mnemonic: The dictionary defines a *gaffe* as a noticeable mistake. If you do not memorize the alphabet soup lesions, there will be GAPHS (*G*LAD, *A*LPSA, *P*ASTA, *H*AGL, *S*LAP) in the clinic and operating room.
- GLAD: Glenoid labrum articular disruption is a Bankart lesion with a delaminated section of glenoid articular cartilage attached. The cartilage may often lie back down during Bankart repair, requiring no additional surgery for the cartilage itself. Unstable lesions may require additional débridement, but rarely cartilage procedures.
- ALPSA: Anterior labrum periosteal sleeve avulsion is a Bankart lesion that is attached by a periosteal sleeve on the glenoid neck. The lesion displaces medially (and inferiorly) and may scar down. This development is a concern because the injury is hard to identify, and the glenoid rim may appear labral deficient from the posterior viewing portal. Maintain a high index of suspicion, review the MRI, and switch portals to make the diagnosis. For management, the lesion must be aggressively mobilized and capsular tissue

must be included to augment the Bankart repair.

- PASTA: Partial articular-sided tendon avulsions are a common type of partial-thickness rotator cuff tear on the articular rather than bursal side. They have a characteristic appearance at arthroscopy, and the severity (thickness) may be difficult to fully characterize by MRI. They are managed in a variety of ways, including conservative, completion and repair, and transtendinous repair (Snyder).
- HAGL: Humeral avulsion of the glenohumeral ligament is an instability-associated lesion in which the anterior band IGHL is avulsed at or near its humeral insertion and retracts medially (inferiorly). It appears irregular and thickened but may be difficult to diagnose by MRI or arthroscopy. It is difficult to repair arthroscopically.
- SLAP: Superior labrum anterior to posterior is a tear of the superior labrum and, possibly, the LHBB tendon (or other intra-articular structures). This well-known lesion and its many variants are discussed in detail in the section on superior labrum/biceps pathology.
- Other alphabet soup lesions have been coined, and other related injuries fall into this category. For example, the Perthes lesion is a Bankart variant with an intact periosteal sleeve that is not retracted and scarred like an ALPSA lesion. If nondisplaced, it may be difficult to detect by MRI, but imaging in abduction/external rotation (ABER) may help. The P-HAGL lesion is a posterior equivalent of the HAGL lesion. Additional lesions may appear with time, but the GAPHS mnemonic helps with the commonly tested lesions.

Diagnosis Questions

1. The alphabet soup lesion that is least amenable to arthroscopic repair is:
   A. GLAD.
   B. ALPSA.
   C. PASTA.
   D. HAGL.
   E. SLAP.
2. Lateral scapular winging is caused by palsy of the:
   A. Suprascapular nerve.
   B. Long thoracic nerve.
   C. Cranial nerve XI.
   D. Nerve to subclavius.
   E. Axillary nerve.
3. O'Brien test is most accurate for:
   A. AC pathology.
   B. Anterior supraspinatus pathology.
   C. SLAP tear.
   D. Bankart lesion.
   E. Biceps pathology.
4. Adhesive capsulitis:
   A. Is best treated by arthroscopic release.
   B. Is always associated with diabetes.
   C. Is nearly always bilateral.
   D. Is exacerbated by aggressive motion during the freezing phase.
   E. Is characterized by passive range of motion (ROM) greater than active ROM.

Shoulder Arthroscopy

Positioning

- Either beach chair or lateral decubitus positioning may be used. The choice is surgeon preference.
- Protect critical structures such as the axilla, head and neck, and bony prominences with any positioning.

❑ Lateral Decubitus

- The lateral decubitus position may be preferred for posterior instability procedures because of the angle of the posterior/inferior portal.
- Take care to position the arm in sterile fashion in an outrigger arm-holder with proper tension (beginning with 10 lb; excessive weight risks injury) and favorable angle (degree of abduction and forward flexion that the outrigger creates) for the desired procedure.
- Carefully position the beanbag so that the patient does not progressively slump during the procedure and so that full motion of instruments at the anterior portal is not blocked by the bean bag.
- Position the monitor across from the bed at the head of the bed, so that it can be seen while the surgeon is working forwards (facing the head of the patient) and backwards (facing the foot).
  - If the monitor is toward the foot of the bed, most of the procedure must be done backwards (facing the foot); doing so may be disorienting unless the surgeon is accustomed to working this way exclusively.

❑ Beach Chair

- The beach chair position may be preferred for possible conversion to open procedures and for rotator cuff disease repair for some surgeons.
- Take care to position the arm with an arm board so that it does not need to be held to remain on the sterile field, but can be manipulated for better arthroscopic examination. Various complex arm positioners have been marketed, but they are not essential.

- Carefully adjust the beach chair position of the bed so that the patient does not progressively slump during the procedure (especially the head and neck) and so that full motion of instruments is not blocked by the patient's head or drapes.
- Position the monitor across from the bed at the midpoint, so that it can be seen while the surgeon is working forward (facing the head of the patient or standing to the side) and backward (facing the foot).

Portals

- Figure 3–3 demonstrates the position of standard and additional arthroscopic portals about the shoulder.

❑ Standard Portals and Diagnostic Sequence

Posterior Viewing Portal

- Established first, approximately 2 cm distal and 2 cm medial to the posterior/inferior angle of the acromion.
- The portal may be created by using a large-gauge spinal needle to inject the glenohumeral joint with saline, distending the capsule and aiding arthroscope placement with a cannula and blunt obturator.
- The neck of the glenoid and the head of the humerus may be used carefully as landmarks for palpation with instruments to identify the joint, and the capsule may be entered slightly superiorly. Distraction of the arm may help with a tight capsule.

Anterior Working Portal

- Established second, just caudal to the AC joint and lateral to the coracoid. The portal may be created outside-in with the aid of a large spinal needle. Alternatively, the portal may be created inside-out with the use of a switching stick (blindly).
- Care is taken to pass just inferior to the biceps tendon so that instruments do not pass through the tendon but may pass below or above it as needed. The portal should be placed relatively superiorly, especially for Bankart repair, to allow space for the anterior/inferior portal (see later section on additional portals).

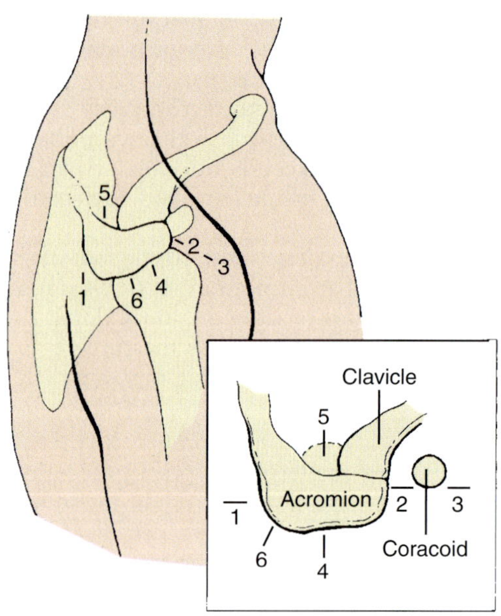

Figure 3–3 Arthroscopic portals of the shoulder. 1, posterior; 2, anterosuperior; 3, anteroinferior; 4, lateral; 5, supraspinus (Nevassier); 6, port of Wilmington. *(From Miller MD, Cooper DE, Warner JJP: Review of Sports Medicine and Arthroscopy. Philadelphia, WB Saunders, 1995, p 135.)*

Lateral Portal

- Established third for working in the subacromial space. May be established 4 cm distal to the lateral border of the acromion and roughly in line with the posterior border of the clavicle.
- Additional anteriorly and posteriorly placed lateral portals may be utilized for a complex rotator cuff repair.
- Portals may be established with the use of a large spinal needle once the arthroscope has been placed into the subacromial space through the posterior view portal or while the scope is in the GH joint in the presence of a large cuff tear, allowing visualization.

Diagnostic Arthroscopy

- The details of the diagnostic scope are surgeon dependent. We outline a few basic features here that follow the order of portal establishment.
- After distention of the capsule with a spinal needle and saline, create the posterior viewing portal. Immediately localize the anterior working portal with a needle, then create it with a blunt instrument and pass a disposable cannula, through which a probe is inserted.
- Inspect the glenohumeral articular cartilage, the anterior labrum, the superior labrum and biceps anchor, the biceps tendon (pass above and pull into the joint with forward flexion), and the articular side of the rotator cuff (including abduction/external rotation).
- The posterior labrum may be inspected in a limited fashion. If better visualization is required, switch the working and viewing portals with a switching stick.
- Reposition the posterior cannula into the subacromial space with the use of a blunt obturator, sweeping the cannula against the undersurface of the acromion to confirm placement. Take care not to place it subcutaneously.
- Either the lateral portal may be established next or the anterior portal cannula may be repositioned for a working portal. The acromion, AC joint, and cuff are inspected after bursectomy for the purposes of exposure.

Additional Portals

- Additional portals are best localized with a spinal needle before creation, because small variations in position greatly affect both the ability to position instruments and the repair.

- The anterior/inferior portal either is placed at the level of the superior border of the subscapularis at the 5 o'clock position. Care is taken so that the position of the drill for anchors is relatively perpendicular to the glenoid rim at 5 o'clock and 4 o'clock.
- The posterior/inferior portal (posterolateral portal) is placed at approximately 7 o'clock for posterior Bankart repair. The portal is localized so that the position of the drill for anchors is relatively perpendicular to the glenoid rim and at 45 degrees lateral to the glenoid face, but also so that a curved or straight retrograde suture passer can achieve the appropriate bite. Erring slightly inferiorly can be helpful.
- The Port of Wilmington portal is placed just anterior to the posterolateral corner of the acromion for SLAP repair. It is critical to accurately position the portal for minimally traumatic and accurate passage through the muscle belly of the rotator cuff into the joint.
- The anterosuperolateral portal is placed just posterior to the anterolateral corner of the acromion for SLAP repair; it is an anterior analogue of the Port of Wilmington portal.
- Numerous other portals are useful, including the Neviaser portal, auxiliary lateral portals for rotator cuff repair, and the subclavian portal for rotator cuff repair.

Suture Passing and Knot Tying

- Numerous highly specialized instruments and repair devices have been introduced for different lesions by a myriad of vendors. We do not seek to survey them all.
- We focus on a few principles of suture passing and arthroscopic knot tying, a core skill in arthroscopic shoulder surgery regardless of pathology, even in the era of knotless repair devices.

❑ Suture Passing

- Most instability and rotator cuff procedures require the use of suture anchors for the attachment of suture to bone. Sutures are then passed to repair soft tissues.
- Anterograde passers place suture by directly piercing through the soft tissue after being loaded with suture. The suture is retrieved after passage, then tied or passed further.
  - The common example is in rotator cuff repair, for which suture is passed with an advanceable and retractable sharpened wire on a grasping device.
  - Multiple manufacturers offer such as device, including the Scorpion (Arthrex, Inc., Naples, FL) and ExpresSew (DePuy Mitek, Inc., Raynham, MA), which feature a disposable nitinol sharpened wire on a reusable handle and grasper.
- Retrograde passers retrieve suture by grasping it after the passer has been placed through the soft tissue. Such passers are used for instability and rotator cuff procedures.
  - The passer must exit the soft tissue relatively close to the suture to be retrieved, or else one risks tearing the tissue. Therefore, the passers come in a variety of sizes and angles, and a grasper may be used to feed the suture for retrieval.
  - Various vendors offer numerous products, including the BirdBeak (Arthrex, Inc.).
- Suture shuttles retrieve suture in a retrograde fashion with the use of a loop of wire or suture.
  - The shuttles come in a variety of shapes and angles, including corkscrews that are left or right turns.
  - The sharpened leading end of the shuttle is passed through soft tissue; then the wire loop and the desired suture limb are retrieved through a cannula, passed through the loop extracorporeally, then retracted to pass the suture limb through the soft tissue.
  - The shuttles are used for instability or rotator cuff repairs.
  - Various vendors offer numerous products, including the Suture Lasso (Arthrex, Inc.).
  - Some surgeons find the handedness of the corkscrew turn of the suture shuttle to be best determined by pathology and side, using an ipsilateral turn for Bankart (anterior) repair and a contralateral turn for SLAP repair and posterior Bankart repair.
- Many innovations in shoulder arthroscopy involve disposable instruments or consumables that can be expensive, including some anterograde passers and suture shuttles. Some surgeons are attempting to return to or adopt techniques for suture passage that minimize the use of consumables, and these techniques can be adapted with alternative instruments.

❑ Knot Tying

- Arthroscopic knot tying can be challenging and underwent extensive research during the development of arthroscopy.
- A knot pusher is an essential device, because knots are tied extracorporeally, then pulled and pushed through a cannula with the aid of a knot pusher.
- Here, no attempt is made to catalog and demonstrate various knots, because the choice is partially arbitrary and surgeon dependent. Almost everyone agrees that one can choose two knots (one sliding and one nonsliding knot technique) and master only them. Although a few knots have been shown to have somewhat less favorable biomechanics, the significance of this finding is unknown.

Basic Knots

- Knots are often categorized into sliding, locking, and sliding/locking types:
  - Sliding knots include the fisherman's knot, Nicky's knot, Roeder knot, and Tennessee slider.
  - Locking knots include the square, easy, and Revo knots.
  - Sliding/locking knots include the Weston, SMC, and modified Roeder knots.
- Numerous other knots have been developed.

Flat Square Knots

- One can tie flat square knots arthroscopically, because these are the gold standard knots tied open.
- One technique for tying flat square knots requires alternating the knot pusher between limbs on every pass, which is effective but cumbersome.
- Another technique uses the knot pusher on the same limb, but flips posts while passing, tensioning the limbs equally when the knot is cinched to tissue. This technique creates reproducible flat square knots arthroscopically.

Backup Knots

- Regardless of the basic knot tied, several studies have shown that *it is necessary to back up any basic knot* with additional knots.
- Of the many possible options, research has shown that *reverse half-hitches on alternating posts* (RHAPs) are the best backup knot.
- Making reverse half-hitches tied by flipping the post without alternating the knot pusher is a practical approach.

Arthroscopy Questions

1. Which statement about arthroscopic instrumentation is most correct?
  A. Antegrade suture passers are best for labral repairs.
  B. Retrograde passers are used only for rotator cuff repairs.
  C. Suture shuttles are of historical interest only.
  D. Most passers are reusable, eliminating the cost of disposables.
  E. Instrumentation is highly surgeon dependent.

2. Which statement about arthroscopic knot tying is most correct?
  A. It is not possible to tie flat square knots arthroscopically.
  B. Sliding/locking knots have replaced other types of knots.
  C. The best backup knot is reverse half-hitches on alternating posts.
  D. It is essential to be versatile and able to tie many types of arthroscopic knots.
  E. Knotless devices for SLAP repair have made knots obsolete for SLAP.

3. Which statement about portals is most correct?
  A. SLAP repair may be performed only through the anterosuperolateral portal.
  B. The posterior/inferior portal is best for Bankart repair.
  C. The anterior portal is used for viewing in posterior Bankart repairs.
  D. The anterior/inferior portal is best for posterior Bankart repairs.
  E. Cuff repair is effective only through the Neviaser portal.

■

Instability

- The shoulder joint is a tradeoff between stability and range of motion, and it is commonly dislocated. Instability is a condition caused by excessive motion of the humeral head about the glenoid fossa during shoulder activity.

Definitions

- TUBS syndrome: Traumatic, unilateral dislocation with a Bankart lesion may require surgery.
- AMBRI syndrome: Atraumatic, multidirectional, bilateral shoulder dislocation/subluxation responds to rehabilitation or, rarely, an inferior capsular shift or plication.
- Anterior (inferior) instability: The most common type of instability associated with a dislocation event, an anterior Bankart or bony Bankart lesion and possibly a Hill-Sachs lesion. The classic mechanism is external rotation in abduction.
- Bankart lesion: Glenoid labrum injury between 3 o'clock and 6 o'clock. A bony Bankart lesion is an anterior/inferior glenoid rim fracture with a Bankart lesion. A variety of surgical options exist (see later).
- Hill-Sachs lesion: Posterior humeral head impaction fracture kissing the anterior glenoid rim after anterior/inferior dislocation. This lesion may engage, causing recurrent locking, catching, or dislocation events. Operative treatment is sometimes indicated, depending on the size, location, and symptoms of the lesion.
- Posterior instability: May be associated with posterior dislocation. Posterior dislocation is less common than anterior (1:10). Management is conservative with posterior Bankart repair (posterior/inferior quadrant or 6 to 9 o'clock) and/or capsular shift reserved for refractory cases.
- 360/270/180-degree lesions: Dislocation and instability are violent events, and injuries may be extensive enough not to fit a single classic

pattern. Classic Bankart injuries (anterior/inferior quadrant) may be combined with posterior Bankart injuries (posterior/inferior quadrant) and/or SLAP tears (superior quadrants). With these larger lesions, it is still advisable to avoid repairing the labrum at 1 to 3 o'clock (variable area; see sections on anatomy and superior labrum/biceps).

- Quadrant locations: The location of labral lesions about the glenoid fossa may be labeled by quadrants: anterior/superior (SLAP and normal MGHL variants), anterior/inferior (Bankart and variants), posterior/inferior (posterior Bankart), and posterior/superior (SLAP extensions and 360/270-degree lesions).
- Clock-face locations: The location of labral lesions about the glenoid fossa may also be labeled by hours on a clock face. The analogy is clearest for the right shoulder. The left shoulder is a mirror-image clock face, a fact that some find confusing. Typical clock positions are SLAP (11 to 1 o'clock), normal MGHL variants (1 to 3 o'clock), Bankart lesions (3 to 6 o'clock, especially 4 to 5 o'clock), posterior Bankart lesions (6 to 9 o'clock), and extensions of SLAP and posterior Bankart lesions and 360/270-degree lesions (9 to 11 o'clock).

Anterior Instability

❑ History
- May reveal a cardinal dislocation event and possibly multiple dislocations/subluxations.
- History is variable regarding the energy of the events and the clarity of whether the joint was classically dislocated/reduced or merely subluxated/unstable during any one event. Subsequent events may occur with less force.
- In a few patients, history may include some element of baseline laxity (TUBS on AMBRI syndrome).
- The true first time dislocation is important to identify, as is the first dislocation event in a chronically unstable shoulder.

❑ Examination
- Complements a full history; reveals signs of anterior instability listed in the history and physical examination section.
- Positive apprehension test and relocation test results are common.
- A load-shift test should be performed to grade the instability (Table 3–4). A sulcus sign may be present.
- The patient should be examined to rule out signs of posterior instability and superior labrum/biceps pathology. The older patient should be assessed for a traumatic rotator cuff tear.
- An examination for generalized laxity (e.g., elbow, knee, thumb to forearm) may be performed.

❑ Imaging
- Because the diagnosis is based on history and examination, imaging aids with operative planning or establishing a baseline for conservative management.
- MRI, possibly with gadolinium arthrography, is essential both for labral characterization and for assessment of concomitant capsular, biceps, and cuff pathology.
- For characterization of bony Bankart lesions, CT is the standard. Plain films, including special views as discussed in the diagnosis section, are essential in the clinic.

❑ Natural History
- Natural history of anterior dislocation varies widely by age.
- Patients with first-time dislocations who are in their teens or 20s have a very high rate of recurrence with conservative management (80%–90%). The recurrence rate decreases with each passing decade, so that patients 50 years or older have a low rate of recurrence.
- Although the management of first-time dislocations is controversial, conservative management is the gold standard for simple dislocations in every age group. Owing to the high recurrence rate in young and athletic patients, there is some evidence to support early operative management for first-time dislocations in such patients.
- Older patients with dislocation are at high risk for traumatic rotator cuff tear, whereas this problem is less common in younger patients (higher index of suspicion for high-energy trauma in the young).

Table 3–4 Grades of Instability

Grade	Anteroposterior Grading Scheme*	Sulcus Grading Scheme†
0	Normal small amount of humeral head translation	Not applicable
1	Humeral head translation to but not over the glenoid rim	Acromiohumeral interval < 1 cm
2	Humeral head translation over the glenoid rim with spontaneous reduction when the applied force is withdrawn	Acromiohumeral interval 1–2 cm
3	Humeral head translation with locking over the glenoid rim	Acromiohumeral interval > 2 cm

*Abnormal (vs. contralateral shoulder): anterior instability = grade 1; posterior instability = grade 3.
†Abnormal (vs. contralateral shoulder) = grade 2.
From Miller M: Review of Orthopaedics: Expert Consult: Online and Print, 5th ed. Philadelphia, Saunders, 2008.

- Conservative Treatment and Rehabilitation
  - Conservative treatment and rehabilitation are a mainstay of management and are equally critical after operative management.
  - May include brief immobilization (in neutral or rotated position), progressive passive range of motion with range limitations to avoid provocation, formal physical therapy, progressive strengthening and cuff exercises, activity modification, and sport-specific rehabilitation (e.g., throwing rehabilitation and mechanics coaching).
  - There is some evidence that for the young patient with a first-time dislocation, bracing in external rotation for 3 to 6 weeks with progressive activity is useful to help decrease the recurrence risk.
- Surgery
  - Numerous procedures have been utilized in patients for whom conservative treatment has failed (Table 3–5).
  - They divide broadly into *soft tissue procedures* and *bony procedures*. The details of procedure selection, standard, and concomitant pathology are complex for any one patient.
  - In summary, much anterior instability can be addressed with arthroscopic Bankart repair, although some injuries, patient populations, and revisions benefit from open soft tissue procedures.
  - Patients with bony glenoid defects may require a bony procedure, especially if the defect is greater than 20% of the maximum anteroposterior (AP) diameter as assessed on CT.
    - Open coracoid bony transfer procedures (Latarjet procedure, in which the coracoid is placed on its side parallel to the glenoid, and Bristow procedure, in which the coracoid is placed on end perpendicular to the glenoid) are the currently preferred methods.
    - Reconstruction with an iliac crest autograft may be needed for large lesions.
  - Large engaging Hill-Sachs lesions may require surgery. Numerous procedures have been described, including rotational osteotomy, open reduction with internal fixation (ORIF) with auto/allograft, bone transfer procedures (e.g., less tuberosity and subscapularis transfer) and remplassage (tenodesis of the infraspinatus to a Hill-Sachs lesion).
  - Progressive and intensive rehabilitation with supervised increasing activity levels for 3 months or more, depending on goals and activity level, is essential.
- Recurrent Instability
  - May occur because of failure of rehabilitation that has been insufficient, poorly advanced, or not complied with.
  - Early recurrence may occur with a repair failure as a result of an underappreciated bony lesion that was addressed only with a soft tissue repair.
  - Patients may experience late recurrence with a new injury or because of poor compliance with lifelong rehabilitation and activity modification. Seizure disorders are notorious for causing recurrence.
- Stiffness
  - Stiffness is the other end of the spectrum from recurrent instability but is equally problematic.
  - Failure of rehabilitation may result in adhesive capsulitis. Unlike in some other joints, the concept of stiff but stable does not apply in the shoulder, and shoulders with stiffness will function very poorly unless managed appropriately (see section on adhesive capsulitis).
  - Overtightening with anterior soft tissue procedures (Putti-Platt) may cause not only poor range of motion in external rotation but also early anterior arthrosis that can be debilitating. Z-lengthening may be required.

Other Types of Instability

- Posterior Instability
  - History may reveal a posterior dislocation caused classically by seizure, electric shock,

Table 3–5 Treatment of Shoulder Instability

Procedure	Essential Features	Comments/Complications
Bankart	Reattachment of labrum (and inferior glenohumeral ligament complex) to glenoid	Gold standard
Staple capsulorrhaphy	Capsular reattachment and tightening	Staple migration/articular injury
Putti-Platt	Subscapularis advancement with capsular coverage	Decreased external rotation, degenerative joint disease
Magnuson-Stack	Subscapularis transfer to greater tuberosity	Decreased external rotation
Boyd-Sisk	Transfer of biceps laterally and posteriorly	Nonanatomic, recurrence
Bristow/Latarjet	Coracoid transfer to inferior glenoid	Non-union, migration, labral tears
Bone block osteotomy	Anterior bone block	Non-union, migration, articular injury
Capsular shift	Inferior capsule shifted superiorly"pants over vest"	Overtightening, gold standard for multidirectional instability

From Miller M: Review of Orthopaedics: Expert Consult: Online and Print, 5th ed. Philadelphia, Saunders, 2008.

excessive ethanol use, or high-energy trauma. Internal rotation, adduction, and posteriorly directed axial load are possible mechanisms, including the overpull of the posterior musculature and subscapularis in seizure and shock.
- Physical examination may show positive results of the jerk test and load-shift test as well as loss of passive external rotation. Examination for anterior instability, generalized ligamentous laxity, and concomitant pathology is performed (see section on physical examination and Table 3–4).
- Conservative management and rehabilitation are focused on progressive motion and rotator cuff strengthening to improve abduction/external rotation and avoid provocative internal rotation/adduction. Immobilization, if any, is classically performed with a "gunslinger" type sling, which holds the arm in abduction/external rotation.
- Surgical management of those in whom conservative management fails includes posterior Bankart repair, posterior capsular shift, and other arthroscopic or open procedures.
- The Kim lesion is an avulsion of the posterior/inferior labrum associated with posterior or multidirectional instability that may be hard to diagnose by MRI and arthroscopy.

❑ Multidirectional Instability
- In multidirectional (Neer) instability of the shoulder, there is instability in the inferior direction as well as in the anterior or posterior direction (or both).
- History may show subluxation with minimal trauma (e.g., while sleeping) even without an initial traumatic dislocation. Complaints may be bilateral. In the appropriate setting, a diagnosis of Marfan syndrome (fibrillin 1 gene, autosomal dominant) or Ehlers-Danlos syndrome (numerous forms, collagen genes, often autosomal dominant) may be considered.
- Physical examination reveals instability in multiple planes with both inferior instability (sulcus sign) and anterior and posterior provocative maneuvers (load-shift, jerk). Generalized ligamentous laxity may be evident in the knees, elbows, and wrists. Pectus excavatum, arachnodactyly, and scoliosis may be assessed in the appropriate clinical setting.
- Management is conservative and focused on rehabilitation and behavior/activity modification.
- Surgery, which is reserved for only very refractory cases, consists of inferior capsular shift. Voluntary dislocation is an especially difficult management problem and should be treated conservatively.

Instability Questions

1. Which of the following is not a classic complication of instability?
  A. Overtightening after open anterior advancement.
  B. Recurrent instability in Bankart repair with undiagnosed bony Bankart lesion.
  C. Adhesive capsulitis after excessive postoperative immobilization.
  D. Traumatic rotator cuff tear in an elderly patient after dislocation.
  E. New posterior dislocation after standard anterior Bankart repair.

2. Which statement is most true of multidirectional instability?
  A. Is not often associated with laxity in other joints.
  B. Is not associated with genetic conditions.
  C. Is best treated conservatively.
  D. Is not treated surgically.
  E. Is often associated with voluntary dislocation and secondary gain.

3. Which statement regarding history and physical findings is most true?
  A. The patient with a first-time dislocation is never a surgical candidate.
  B. Self-reduction events are never real instability without ER reduction.
  C. Dislocation in a 65-year-old patient is not concerning because it will not recur.
  D. A first-time dislocation in a 25-year-old patient is unlikely to recur.
  E. Recurrence after prior surgery may not indicate a new injury.

Rotator Cuff Disease

- Rotator cuff disease represents *a continuum* from subacromial impingement/bursitis through partial-thickness tear, full-thickness tear, and massive tear, to cuff tear arthropathy. This is an age-related degenerative process.
- Many older patients have asymptomatic tears as *incidental* findings.
  - Some of these patients progress to having symptoms, and the *development of symptoms is correlated with the progression of the tear.*
  - However, some patients remain asymptomatic even with tear progression, and this relationship is incompletely understood.
- Rotator cuff surgery may be performed for pain, pain and function, or function alone.
- Twenty-eight percent of patients older than 60 years, and 65% of those older than 70 years, have full-thickness tears.

- In the patient with a symptomatic full-thickness tear, there is a greater than 50% chance of an asymptomatic contralateral tear of some type. Of patients with asymptomatic tears, 50% experience symptoms at 3 years.
- Many partial-thickness tears begin on the articular *not* the bursal side, and they may or may not be associated with a hooked acromion. To explain this fact, a wash-wringer effect has been proposed, in which the tendon is squeezed between two "rollers": the humeral head and the undersurface of the acromion (hooked or not).
- Articular-sided partial tears in the athlete involved in overhead sports are thought to result from tension failure in this subgroup.
- *A traumatic rotator cuff tear* in any age group represents an especially problematic variant, which may be associated with massive tears, severe loss of function, and rapid progression to arthrosis.
- Traumatic tears should be repaired urgently, not electively. A high index of suspicion must be maintained in the traumatized patient with shoulder pain, normal radiographs, and a limited examination. Active range of motion may be severely limited. The older patient with a dislocation or subluxation event is at especially high risk.
- *Calcific tendinitis* is an idiopathic condition typically of the supraspinatus tendon. Slightly more common in women, it is managed conservatively and is self-limited. Arthroscopy is rarely indicated.

Diagnosis

- ❑ History
  - Reveals an insidious onset of pain, which may be intermittent and may partially remit with conservative therapy or activity modification.
  - Pain may be exacerbated by overhead arm activity, and night pain is possible.
  - An inciting event may or may not be present, except in traumatic tears, for which an event precedes pain and loss of function.
  - The chief complaint may be pain or weakness.
- ❑ Physical Examination
  - Complements a full history and reveals the signs of impingement and/or rotator cuff disease listed in the history and physical examination sections of this chapter.
  - The presence of Neer impingement sign (and positive test result after injection) and positive results of both Hawkins test and specific muscle testing are common.
  - The patient should be examined to rule out signs of biceps/superior labrum pathology and AC joint pathology.
- ❑ Imaging
  - The diagnosis is often suspected from the history and physical findings, and imaging serves to confirm it, to assist with operative planning, or to establish a baseline for conservative management.
  - MRI is useful to assess tear thickness, size, retraction, geometry, and fatty atrophy, all important surgical parameters. It is also good for assessing concomitant pathology, especially that of the superior labrum/biceps and AC joint.
  - Ultrasonography is now an important alternative to MRI for assessment of cuff disease (see earlier section on diagnosis).
  - Plain radiographs are essential in the clinic. The AP view is examined for AC arthritis, superior migration, and an alternative diagnosis of primary glenohumeral degenerative joint disease. The axillary lateral view is examined for joint space narrowing and glenoid version/wear. The acromial outlet view is useful for assessing acromial morphology, and a cephalad view for AC pathology.

Natural History

- Is a critical issue, as discussed earlier. The diagnosis of symptomatic cuff disease involves a careful correlation of history, physical examination, and imaging findings as well as exclusion of alternative diagnoses.
- Careful correlation is needed due to the high rate of asymptomatic cuff tears in older patients and the possibility of additional diagnoses in the cervical spine, shoulder, and upper extremity.

Treatment

- Conservative treatment and rehabilitation are a mainstay of management.
- Most patients show response to a combination of injections, formal therapy with cuff-specific strengthening, and activity modification with ADL strategies. This statements is true of cases spanning the spectrum from simple impingement to irreparable massive tears with arthropathy.
- Surgery is reserved for patients in whom conservative management proves ineffective, usually after a trial of 3 to 6 months or longer.

- ❑ Subacromial Decompression
  - Impingement symptoms may respond to subacromial decompression with bursectomy with or without acromioplasty; however, some studies have shown no improvement of surgical results over results with physical therapy alone.
  - Decompression may or may not include resection of the CA ligament. This issue is controversial, because resection could predispose the humeral head to superior migration in the setting of subsequent massive tear.
  - Figure 3–4 shows the spectrum of acromial morphology.

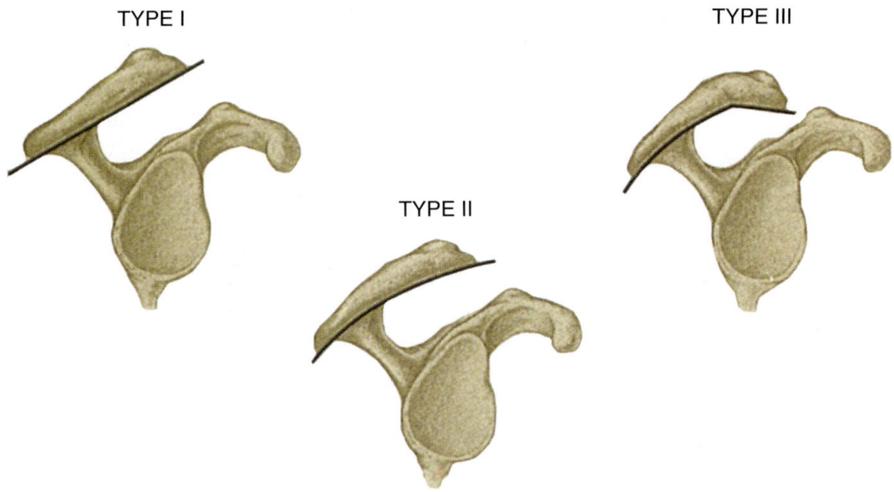

Figure 3–4 Acromion morphology is classified on the basis of the supraspinatus outlet view as originally described by Bigliani. *(From Esch JC: Shoulder arthroscopy in the older age group. Op Tech Orthop 1:200, 1991.)*

- Care is taken to assess for AC pathology preoperatively, because it might be an adjacent pain generator that could be easily addressed at the same setting.

❑ Rotator Cuff Repair

- For any one patient, determining the repair strategy may be complex. Some basic principles are presented here.
- Correctly determining the *tear geometry* is absolutely essential, because it guides the repair sequence and pattern. Many tear patterns, including crescent, U, V, L, reverse L, complex, delaminated, partial, and retracted/massive, have been described.
- Some basic suturing patterns are broadly useful:
  - *Margin convergence* is a side-to-side (tendon-to-tendon) suturing pattern that can covert more complex tear patterns (e.g., L, reverse L) into simpler (crescent-type) patterns.
  - Most repairs involve *suture anchors* into the cuff footprint, then simple or mattress sutures passed through the cuff with suture passers (see arthroscopy section). Transosseous tunnels are also used instead of anchors.
  - *Double row* is a term used for a specific type of arthroscopic repair involving medial and lateral rows of anchors and a criss-crossing mattress suture–type repair. The goal is to restore the footprint and improve healing.
- For *partial-thickness tears,* several methods have been described, including débridement, completion and repair, and transtendinous repair.
- For *massive (>5 cm or >2 tendons) and retracted tears,* mobilization of the remaining cuff is essential to restore the footprint and decrease tension at the repair. Mobilization is accomplished by several techniques, including elevation with sharp elevators, anterior interval slide, and, especially, posterior interval slide.
  - With *posterior interval slide,* care is taken to preserve the suprascapular nerve, which is at risk medially. If full lateralization of the cuff cannot be achieved, medialization of the footprint by 5 to 10 mm is possible. Fatty atrophy and retraction past the glenoid are harbingers of poor reparability.
  - Simple débridement, including treatment of other pain generators such as the biceps tendon and synovitis, is an alternative for massive cuff tears with only mild arthropathy, and research supports its effectiveness. It may be preferable to attempting a tenuous repair that requires a protracted rehabilitation for uncertain results. Some evidence shows that function and pain relief after repair of massive tears are poorly correlated with the integrity of the repair.
- For *subscapularis tears,* management is controversial.
  - Repair may be performed open or arthroscopically (technically challenging) for symptomatic full-thickness tears.
  - Partial-thickness tears may be treated without repair; they may be related to biceps tendon pathology at the superior margin of the subscapularis.
- Revision arthroscopic repair is possible for failed repairs but is technically difficult with diminished outcomes in comparison with primary repair. Tendon transfers are also possible, with or without arthroplasty.
- Arthroscopic rotator cuff repair has broadly equivalent results to, and is less invasive than, open repair. The idea that arthroscopic repair therefore represents a new gold standard for management is controversial.

Postoperative Course

- ❑ Rehabilitation
  - A comprehensive rehabilitation program is mandatory after rotator cuff repair. Many protocols extend over 3 months or more and include limited active range of motion for 6 weeks.
  - The rehabilitation is rigorous, and failure of rehabilitation puts the patient at high risk for poor functional outcome and repair failure.
  - It is essential to counsel the patient regarding the need for protracted rehabilitation when discussing the options for treatment, because decompression and débridement require much less rehabilitation than cuff repair.
  - Expectations must be tailored to patient functional demands but also to the *size and retraction* of the tear.
  - The repair of a massive, retracted tear can be attempted, but the patient should be counseled about the higher failure rate of and lower functional outcome for a successful repair.
  - *Stiffness* may is associated with failure of rehabilitation and adhesive capsulitis, a difficult problem in the context of a cuff repair needing rehabilitation.

Recurrence

- Recurrent tear may occur for a number of reasons. Loss of function and pain are the primary reasons to consider recurrence or additional pathology.
- Some research has shown that functional outcome is only partially correlated with repair integrity at medium-term follow-up, a puzzling finding that is still under investigation.

Rotator Cuff Disease Questions

1. Which of the following is least true of cuff tear geometries?
A. An L tear is repaired in part with margin convergence.
B. A U tear is best repaired by tendon-to-bone technique alone.
C. A reverse L tear is repaired with anchors alone.
D. Crescent tears are common.
E. Small delaminations may be debrided.

2. The statement least true regarding massive and retracted tears is:
A. Arthroscopic repair is technically challenging.
B. Mobilization is achieved by posterior interval slide.
C. Symptoms are determined by repair success.
D. The footprint may be medialized to achieve repair.
E. Double-row technique is essential.

3. The main advantage of simple débridement for massive tears is:
A. Improved pain relief and no difference in functional measures.
B. Decreased rate of arthropathy.
C. Improvement in ability to perform ADLs.
D. Minimal rehabilitation and immobilization.
E. Diminished hardware costs.

4. The size of a cuff tear is:
A. Small if < 1 cm.
B. Medium if 1–3 cm.
C. Large if 3–5 cm.
D. Massive if > 5 cm.
E. All of the above.

■

Superior Labrum/Biceps Pathology

- The superior labrum, biceps anchor, and LHBB are considered as a group because they are anatomically related.
- Pathology of these structures may sometimes be functionally related, and treatment may overlap (e.g., type IV SLAP tear).
- *SLAP tears* are tears of the superior glenoid labrum, which may be of several types and include various other structures (Fig. 3–5).
- The mechanism of SLAP tears classically involves overhead sports, but other mechanisms are common. Associations with instability and rotator cuff disease depend on the mechanism and patient age group.
- Biceps pathology is most often a degenerative tendinosus of the intra-articular portion of the LHBB tendon. It is a continuum from biceps fraying through tendon split tears, severe fraying, bicipital groove stenosis, and biceps dislocation from the groove (requires a subscapularis tendon rupture), to tendon rupture (so-called autotenotomy).
- Biceps pathology may exist with SLAP tears (type IV tear), impingement, and rotator cuff tears (superior subscapularis partial tear and anterior supraspinatus leading-edge tear).

Diagnosis

- ❑ History and Physical Examination
  - History is related to sport and throwing history in the athlete or to exacerbating or inciting events in any age or activity group.
  - A complete biceps tear with a distal stump (distally migrated muscle belly) that exits the groove may result in a sudden pop and "Popeye deformity."
  - Physical examination includes provocative testing (O'Driscoll dynamic labral shear test and O'Brien test for SLAP tears, and Speed and Yergason tests for biceps pathology; see Table 3–2).

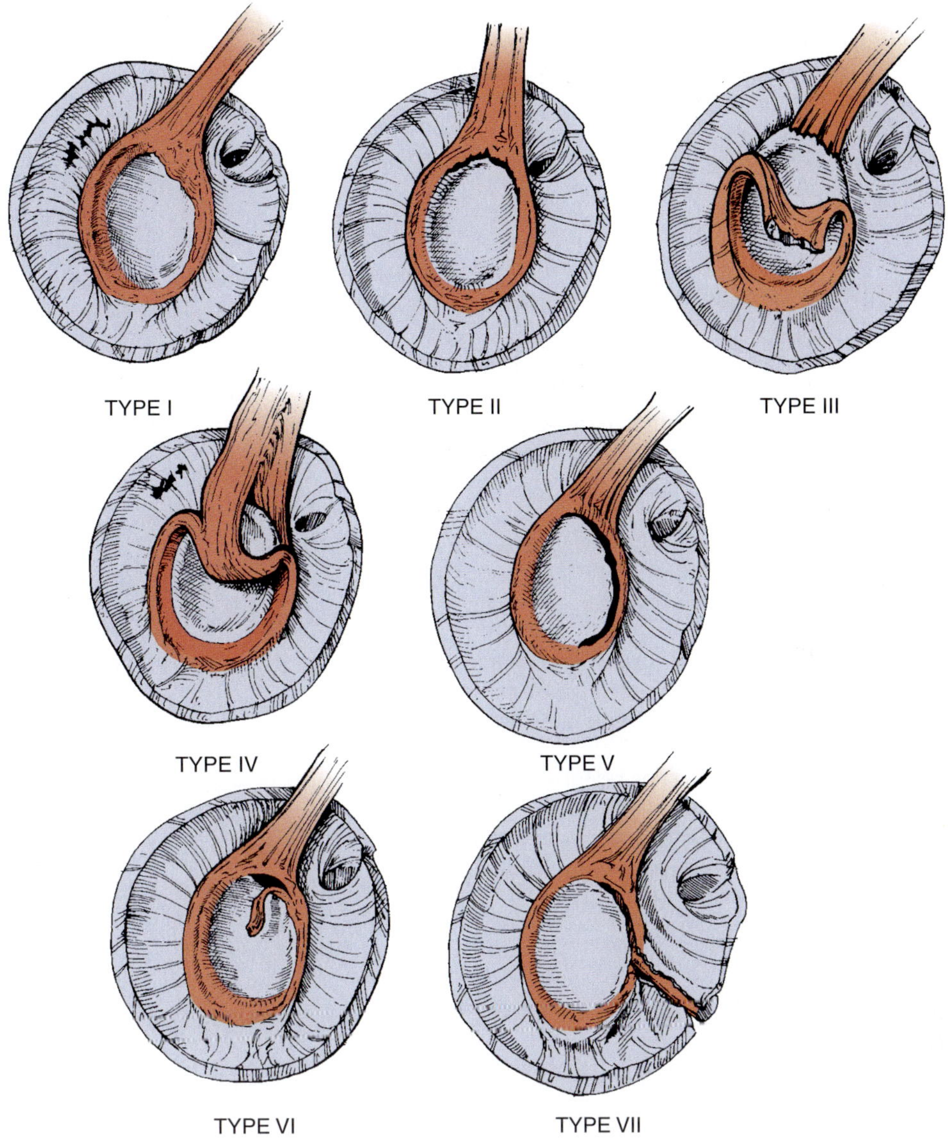

Figure 3–5 Anterior and posterior lesion types I to VII of the superior labrum. *(From, Osborne JR, Warner JJP, Fuy FH, et al: MRI-Arthroscopy Correlative Atlas. Philadelphia, WB Saunders, 1997, p 157.)*

- Examination must be careful and systematic because many physicians believe that SLAP tears/biceps pathology can be easily confused with cuff, AC, and other labral pathology.

❑ Imaging
- Imaging focuses on MRI with gadolinium arthrography. MRI diagnosis can be challenging, and there is a normal recess about the biceps anchor that may be mistaken for a SLAP tear.
- Incomplete tears of the tendon can be difficult to assess, especially at the bicipital groove, where the tendon takes a 90-degree turn, causing MRI artifact (magic angle effect). Because subluxation at the groove can be dynamic, MRI may underestimate pathology in this region, depending on arm position.
- Subscapularis tears and AC arthrosis should be sought on MRI.

❑ Arthroscopic Diagnosis
- Arthroscopy is the gold standard for diagnosis and may change the management relative to the preoperative plan.
- The biceps anchor should be carefully probed for stability, and abduction/external rotation may aid diagnosis.
- The biceps tendon is inspected for the subtle color changes of tendinosus, and it is subluxated with the use of a probe into the joint to inspect its intra-articular course and its stability and gliding in the groove.
- Inspecting the superior subscapularis and anterior edge of the supraspinatus may identify kissing lesions.

Treatment

❑ Conservative Management

- Conservative management is often effective, depending on the functional goals of the patient.
- Athletic injuries may respond to modification of goals. Injuries in older patients may respond to injections and activity modification.
- Although injection of the biceps sheath in the groove may be attempted, injection of the biceps tendon, whether intra-articular or in the groove, should be avoided because of the risk of rupture.
- In selected patients, the risk of biceps rupture may be acceptable if injections provide relief and surgery is to be avoided.

❑ SLAP Repair

- SLAP repair is indicated for an unstable biceps anchor (type II) or an unstable anchor with extension to the biceps (type IV).
- Repair is indicated for a SLAP tear as part of a 360/270/180-degree lesion (type V) and a SLAP tear with capsular trauma (type VII).
- SLAP repair is accomplished with the use of special portals (e.g., Port of Wilmington, anterosuperolateral), suture anchors, suture passers (e.g., corkscrew shuttles), and arthroscopic knot tying.
- The treatment of SLAP tears evolved in the arthroscopic era and is performed arthroscopically (Table 3–6).
- For SLAP repair, a progressive protocol carefully advances the athlete to return to throwing over 4 to 6 months.

❑ Débridement

- Débridement is indicated for superior labral fraying (type I) and labral bucket-handle tears that do not involve the tendon (type III).
- It is also indicated for fraying along the entire course of the tendon that is not severe.

❑ Tenotomy

- *Tenotomy* is a form of complete débridement of the intra-articular biceps tendon. It is indicated for severe biceps pathology for which conservative management has failed and that does not require tenodesis.
- Indications for *tenotomy versus tenodesis* are controversial and surgeon dependent. Patients who have lower functional demands, do not object to possible deformity, or will not tolerate the rehabilitation of a tenodesis may be candidates for tenotomy. Informed consent and discussion of tenodesis are important.
- Intra-articular tenotomy does not always result in migration of the tendon into the upper arm, and some studies have measured the force required for migration (≈100 Newtons).

❑ Tenodesis

- Tenodesis is reserved for patients with end-stage biceps pathology who are not candidates for tenotomy. Indications include biceps pathology and SLAP tears in patients older than 40 years and some types of SLAP tears in younger athletes (type IV).
- Numerous tenodesis procedures are described, from arthroscopic suturing into the rotator interval to bony tenodesis with a screw.
- Options include arthroscopic versus mini-open, proximal (in the groove) versus distal (under pectoralis tendon), keyhole/bone tunnel versus device-based, and suture anchors versus interference screws (see Golish et al, 2008a).
- Considerable biomechanical and some clinical studies compare these methods, but ultimately the choice is surgeon dependent.
- The tenodesis method also depends on how the presence of other pathology affects the rehabilitation protocol, which determines how much tenodesis strength is needed (e.g., rotator cuff repair).

Table 3–6 Superior Labral and Biceps Tendon Injuries

Type	Description of Injury	Treatment
I	Biceps fraying, intact anchor on superior labrum	Arthroscopic débridement
II	Detachment of biceps anchor	Reattachment/stabilization
III	Bucket-handle superior labral tear; biceps intact	Arthroscopic débridement
IV	Bucket-handle tear of superior labrum into biceps	Repair or tenodesis of tendon, on basis of symptoms and condition of remaining tendon
V	Labral tear + SLAP	Stabilization of both
VI	Superior flap tear	Débridement
VII	Capsular injury + SLAP	Repair and stabilization

SLAP, superior labrum from anterior to posterior.
From Miller M: Review of Orthopaedics: Expert Consult: Online and Print, 5th ed. Philadelphia, Saunders, 2008.

Superior Labrum/Biceps Pathology Questions

1. Which statement about SLAP repairs is most true?
   A. Open repairs are the gold standard, but arthroscopic repairs are possible.
   B. Repair is indicated for all types of tears that are symptomatic.
   C. Arthroscopic repair is best done by new bioabsorbable anchors.
   D. Repair is extended from 11 o'clock down to 3 o'clock.
   E. Tenodesis is an alternative for some tear patterns and patients.
2. Tenodesis of the long head of the biceps brachii tendon:
   A. Is possible by insertion of a bioabsorbable interference screw into the humerus.
   B. Is possible by suture alone.
   C. Is not always necessary due to the pullout strength of the tendon from the capsule.
   D. Depends on rehabilitation plans determined by other pathology (e.g., cuff).
   E. All of the above.
3. Which of the following statements about biceps pathology is least true?
   A. May include dislocation of the tendon from the groove seen on MRI.
   B. May be associated with partial-thickness subscapularis tears.
   C. Is always treated with tenotomy alone if a cuff repair is performed.
   D. Device-based tenodesis has load-to-failure superior to tenotomy.
   E. Is diagnosed by arthroscopic examination in addition to physical examination and MRI.
4. Which of he following is the most correct sequence of repair for a SLAP tear?
   A. Anchors, suture passing, rim débridement, Port of Wilmington portal, reexamination.
   B. Rim débridement, Port of Wilmington portal, anchors, suture passing, tying.
   C. Port of Wilmington portal, anchors, suture passing, tying, rim débridement.
   D. Rim débridement, anchors, suture passing, Port of Wilmington portal, tying.
   E. Any of the above.

Clavicle Disorders

Acromioclavicular Joint

❑ Acromioclavicular Separation

- AC separation is among the most common sports-associated injuries, typically involving athletes in their second and third decades.
- Direct injury results from a blow to the shoulder in which the acromion is driven downward and medially disrupts the stabilizing ligaments. Indirect injury may occur with a fall onto the elbow or outstretched hand.
- The capsular ligaments fail first. Rupture of the coracoclavicular ligaments leads to vertical instability and AC joint dislocation.
- Figure 3–6 demonstrates the classification according to this progressive sequence of injury.
- Deforming forces include the sternocleidomastoid muscle, which causes superior displacement of the clavicle, and the weight of the arm, which causes inferior displacement of the acromion and scapula.

Diagnosis

- History of a fall directly onto the shoulder or outstretched arm generally precedes AC joint injury, with subsequent localized pain over the joint, deformity, or pain or heaviness of the arm.
- Physical examination should be performed with the patient standing to accentuate any asymmetry or deformity.
- Tenderness over the AC joint may be present in mild injuries (types I and II). Deformity, prominence of the distal clavicle, or skin tenting may be apparent in more severe injuries.
- Type III injuries are usually manually reducible, whereas types IV through VI are not.
- Neurologic status should be carefully assessed because traction injury to the brachial plexus or axillary nerve may occur with AC separation.
- Associated injuries, including fractures of the acromion, clavicle, coracoid process, or ribs, pulmonary contusion, and pneumothorax, should be considered.

Imaging

- Consists of plain radiographs, which should include standing AP views of both shoulders for comparison.
- Zanca view, in which the x-ray beam is directed 10 to 15 degrees cephalad, aids in visualization of the AC joint.
- Axillary views may reveal anterior or posterior displacement of the distal clavicle.
- An AP radiograph of both shoulders with 10 to 15 pounds strapped to each may demonstrate vertical instability with CC ligament disruption.

Treatment

- Treatment of AC joint injuries depends on severity.

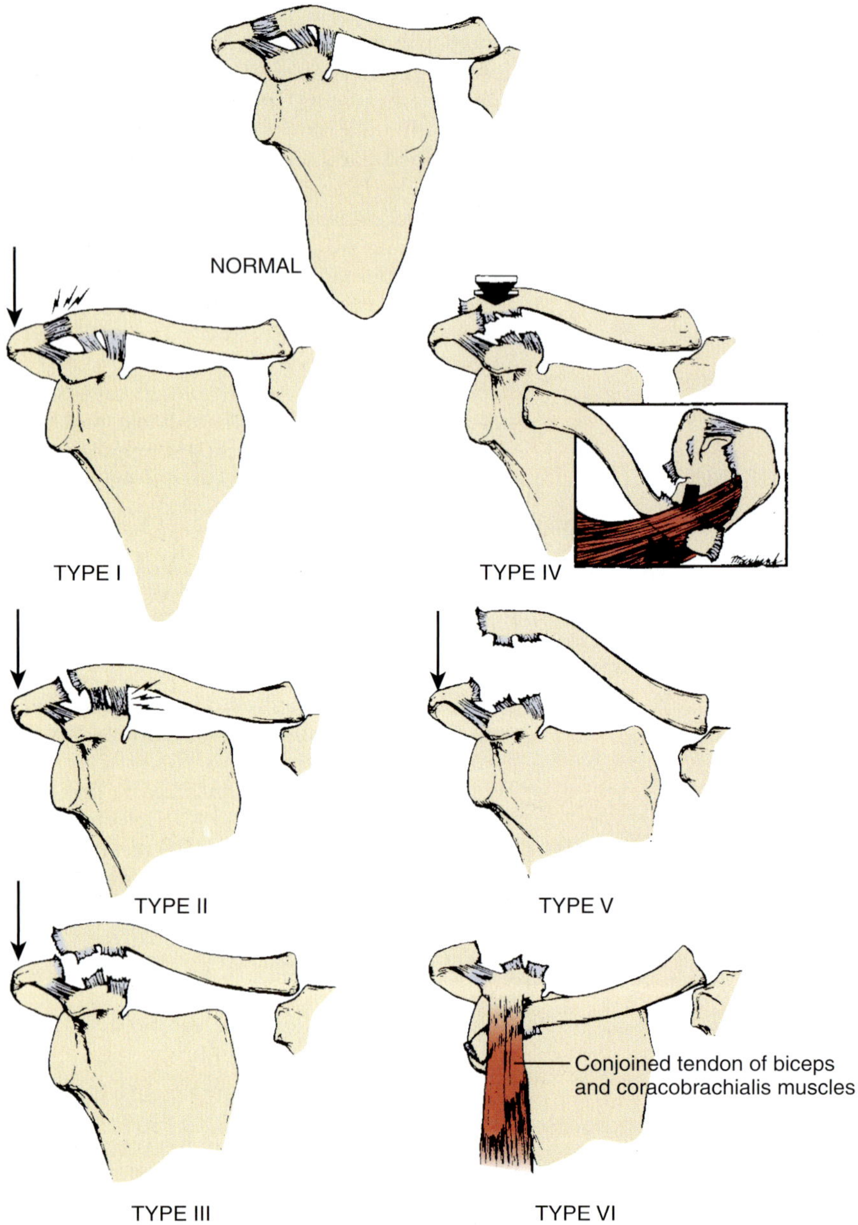

Figure 3–6 Classification of acromioclavicular (AC) separations. Type I injuries involve only an AC sprain. Type II injuries are characterized by a complete AC tear but intact coracoclavicular (CC) ligaments. Type III injuries involve both the AC and CC ligaments, with a CC distance of up to 100% greater than that of the opposite shoulder. Type IV injuries are associated with posterior displacement of the clavicle through the trapezius muscle. Type V injuries involve superior displacement, with a CC distance of more than twice that of the opposite side. This injury is usually associated with rupture of the deltotrapezial fascia, leaving the distal end of the clavicle subcutaneous. Type VI injuries are rare and are defined on the basis of inferior displacement of the clavicle below the coracoids. *(From Rockwood CA Jr, Young DC: Disorders of the acromioclavicular joint. In Rockwood CA Jr, Matsen FA III [eds]: The Shoulder, 2nd ed. Philadelphia, WB Saunders, 1998, p 495.)*

- Type I and II injuries are treated conservatively, with ice, sling, and activity restrictions until symptoms resolve.
- Type III injuries may be managed conservatively or operatively, depending on the treating physician, hand dominance, occupation, sports participation, and risk for re-injury.
- Type IV through VI injuries generally require operative intervention.

SURGICAL MANAGEMENT

- Operative intervention for AC joint separation aims to address the displacement, instability, and pain caused by the injury.
- After open or closed reduction of the AC joint, operative fixation consists of reconstruction of the torn CC ligaments, fixation of the AC joint, or fixation of the clavicle to the coracoid process.
- CC ligament reconstruction addresses the vertical and medial/lateral instability caused by disruption of the conoid and trapezoid ligaments.
- The distal clavicle may be resected to reduce pain, although this procedure may exacerbate instability.
- Numerous specific reconstructions have been proposed:

- The modified Weaver-Dunn procedure involves transfer of the coracoacromial ligament to the distal clavicle.
  - The CA ligament is detached from deep surface of acromion with or without attached bone, in an open procedure or arthroscopically.
  - This construct may be augmented with screw fixation, suture loops or cerclage, or tendon graft.
- Anatomic reconstruction with tendon graft employs semitendinosus autograft or allograft inserted through bone tunnels in the clavicle with or without interference screws.
  - The graft may be wrapped around the coracoid or passed through bone tunnels.
  - This technique has demonstrated solid biomechanical properties and good clinical results.
  - Fracture through bone tunnels is a possible complication.
- With ORIF, coracoclavicular fixation to allow soft tissue healing may be obtained with a screw or suture loops securing the distal clavicle to the coracoid process.
  - This technique may used alone or to augment a ligament reconstruction.
  - Staged removal may be planned.
  - Acromioclavicular fixation using threaded or smooth K-wires has largely been abandoned owing to the risk of pin migration.
  - Internal fixation of the AC joint may be obtained with distal clavicle hook-plates. This technique may also be used to augment ligament reconstruction.

COMPLICATIONS

- Complications depend on extent of injury and method of treatment.
- Nonoperatively treated minor AC joint separations may be complicated by residual deformity with prominence of the distal clavicle, early or late arthrosis, chronic pain, distal clavicle osteolysis, or recurrent instability.
- Complications from operatively treated AC joint separations include hardware failure or cutout, iatrogenic injury to adjacent neurovascular structures, aseptic reaction to implants, and early or late fracture from instrumentation or bone tunnel placement.

❑ Acromioclavicular Joint Arthritis

- Large loads from the upper extremity transmitted to the axial skeleton through the small surface area of the AC joint predispose it to arthritis.
- Primary AC arthritis is common (up to 57% of elderly patients).
- AC joint arthritis may also be post-traumatic.

Diagnosis

- History of intermittent or progressive pain exacerbated by activities such as overhead lifting, washing the opposite axilla, or reaching for a wallet may be present. Pain at night or painful subjective crepitus may also be present.
- Physical examination reveals point tenderness and prominence. Reproduction of pain with the cross-body adduction of the arm is a good provocative test. Patients should be examined for superior labral biceps, cuff, and glenohumeral pathology, which may be easily confused with AC joint arthritis.
- Imaging of the arthritic AC joint demonstrates degenerative changes such as joint space narrowing, osteophytosis, sclerosis, and subchondral cysts. A Zanca view, in which the x-ray beam is aimed 10 to 15 degrees cephalad, provides an unobstructed view of the joint.
- Diagnostic injection is helpful. Injection must take account of the inferomedial to superolateral slope of the joint, the narrow entry point of the arthritic joint, and the small intra-articular space (≈1 mL injection volume).

Treatment

- Conservative treatment is the standard of care, including activity modification, physical therapy, and nonsteroidal anti-inflammatory drugs. Corticosteroid injections into the joint may provide relief.
- Operative treatment consists of arthroscopic distal clavicle resection (or, less commonly, open resection).
  - Arthroscopic resection should resect approximately 1 cm of distal clavicle to avoid residual impingement without detaching the CC ligaments.
  - A bur or aggressive shaver is inserted into the joint through the anterior working portal, which can be repositioned directly into the joint. A localizing needle may be used.
  - The superior and posterior capsule (AC ligaments) should be preserved to prevent anterior/posterior instability.
  - Residual symptoms may result with incomplete or inadequate resection. The anterior/superior margin is at risk because of the angle of the bur during arthroscopic resection.

❑ Distal Clavicle Osteolysis

- A condition of insidious aching pain in the AC joint region most commonly seen in weight-lifters or patients with history of AC joint injury.
- Results from repetitive microtrauma sustained by the subchondral bone of the distal clavicle such as from a bench press.

- History reveals shoulder pain exacerbated by exercises that stress the AC joint, such as a bench press, push-ups, or overhead activities.
- Physical examination usually demonstrates point tenderness over the distal clavicle or AC joint but, generally, no joint instability and full shoulder range of motion.
- Imaging should include the unaffected side for comparison; findings may be normal or may demonstrate lucency of the distal clavicle. Technetium Tc 99m-MDP (methylenediphosphonate) bone scanning shows increased uptake in the distal clavicle. MRI may reveal bone marrow edema in the distal clavicle (increased T2 signal).
- Treatment is focused on activity modification. Otherwise, treatment is similar to that for AC arthritis. Operative management is occasionally necessary.

Sternoclavicular Joint Injuries

- Sternoclavicular injuries are rare, representing less than 3% of injuries to the shoulder girdle.
- The medial clavicular physis remains open well into the third decade, and thus, suspected dislocations in patients younger than 25 years may represent *physeal injuries.*
- Injury to the SC joint may represent a minor ligament sprain with no displacement, subluxation with partial ligament disruption, or complete dislocation with displacement of the medial clavicle.
- *Anterior dislocation,* the more common direction of dislocation, may result indirectly from forces transmitted through the clavicle from impact on the anterolateral shoulder, with the first rib acting as a fulcrum.
- *Posterior dislocation* is less common because of the stabilizing posterior capsule and sternoclavicular ligaments; it may result from direct impact to the anteromedial clavicle or a blow to the posterolateral shoulder with indirect force transmitted through the clavicle.
- The proximity of vital mediastinal structures, including the brachiocephalic vasculature, trachea, and esophagus, make posterior SC dislocation a potentially life-threatening injury. Thus prompt diagnosis and treatment are critical.

❑ Diagnosis

- History reveals a high-energy mechanism such as a motor vehicle collision, sporting impact, or fall from a height. The patient may complain of sternal pain or deformity.
- A choking sensation, shortness of breath, or difficulty swallowing may occur with posterior dislocations because of compression of the trachea and esophagus.
- Physical examination of suspected sternoclavicular dislocation involves inspection of the chest (including auscultation) and bilateral clavicles for tenderness, deformity, and asymmetry.
- A thorough neurovascular examination is important, given the proximity of the brachial plexus and great vessels, and venous congestion of the neck or upper extremity may be apparent with posterior dislocations. Wright test for thoracic outlet syndrome may be performed.
- Imaging of suspected SC injuries includes an AP view and a serendipity view (40 degrees cephalad) of the chest centered on the manubrium.
  - Computed tomography clearly illustrates the direction and degree of displacement and may demonstrate physeal injury or compression of mediastinal structures. Severe posterior dislocations may require CT angiography.

❑ Treatment

- SC joint sprains and reduced subluxations may be treated conservatively with ice packs and immobilization with a sling or figure-of-eight brace until the pain resolves.

Acute Anterior Dislocations

- Closed reduction may be obtained by placing a bump between the shoulders and applying direct pressure on the anterior clavicle.
- After reduction, the upper extremity should be immobilized in a sling, or a figure-of-eight dressing may be used to help hold the reduction. The reduction may be unstable and difficult to hold with closed means.
- Operative intervention is most often not indicated. Operative treatment may be undertaken in certain circumstances, such as very wide displacement, deformity, and loss of function.

Acute Posterior Dislocations

- Potentially serious injuries with possible associated pulmonary or neurovascular compromise.
- A thorough evaluation is critical. *Vascular or thoracic surgery consultants should be closely available prior to reduction,* in the event of unrecognized vascular injury and cardiac tamponade.
- Early closed reduction may be possible in the supine patient. It is performed with a bump between the shoulders with either abduction or adduction of the affected shoulder and longitudinal traction on the arm. Downward-directed force on the both shoulders may facilitate reduction.
- For difficult reductions, a sterile towel clip may be used to grasp the medial clavicle. Reduced posterior dislocations are generally stable.
- After reduction, the upper extremity should be immobilized in a sling, or a figure-of-eight dressing may be used to help hold the reduction.

- Operative treatment may be required for irreducible dislocations or if pain or popping persists after reduction.
  - A variety of methods has been described to secure the SC joint using capsular repair, ligament reconstruction, or internal fixation across the joint.
  - Minimal violation of the anterior capsule is critical to prevent anterior instability. Wire and pin fixation is contraindicated because of risk of migration. Hardware is used with caution.
- *Physeal injuries* of the medial clavicle may be treated conservatively, except in the event of irreducible posterior displacement with symptomatic compression of vital mediastinal structures.

Complications and Chronic Dislocations

- *Chronic dislocations* are treated operatively only in patients who complain of persistent pain or functional limitation.
  - Resection of the medial head of the clavicle with preservation of the sternoclavicular ligaments may alleviate the pain of chronic dislocation.
- Complications of *anterior dislocations* include poor cosmesis and late arthrosis.
- *Posterior dislocations* may result in injury to mediastinal structures, including disruption or compression of the great vessels, brachial plexus, trachea, and esophagus.
- Hardware complications may occur in operatively treated sternoclavicular dislocations, with numerous reports of migration of K-wires or Steinmann pins into the heart, great vessels, and lungs.

Clavicle Fractures

- One of the most commonly fractured bones in the body, the clavicle may be fractured from a direct blow or indirectly from impact to the outstretched arm or shoulder.
- Clavicle fractures occur most commonly in males younger than 30 years, and implicated mechanisms include sporting injuries, motor vehicle crashes, and falls.
- Depending on the location of the fracture, the primary deforming forces include the SC muscle (superior displacement of the proximal fragment), the weight of the arm (inferior displacement of the distal fragment), and the pectoralis major and trapezius muscles (shortening).

❑ Classification

- Classification of clavicle fractures is based on the anatomic location of the injury:
  - Middle third (diaphyseal) fractures are most common, accounting for 80% to 85% of fractures.
  - Medial third fractures are least common, accounting for 5% of fractures.
  - Lateral third fractures account for 10% to 15% of clavicle fractures and are further subdivided on the basis of location, displacement, and integrity of coracoclavicular ligaments (Fig. 3–7):
    - Type I: Nondisplaced fracture with intact coracoclavicular ligaments.
    - Type II: Displaced fracture medial to the coracoclavicular ligaments.
    - Type IIA: Intact coracoclavicular (conoid and trapezoid) ligaments attached to the distal fragment.
    - Type IIB: Interligamentous fracture between the conoid and trapezoid ligament, in which the conoid is torn and the intact trapezoid remains attached to the nondisplaced distal fragment.
    - Type III: Intra-articular fracture involving the AC joint.

❑ Diagnosis

- History of acute pain and deformity occurring after impact or a fall onto the shoulder or arm typically indicates fracture of the clavicle.
- Physical examination by observation and palpation is usually revealing because of the subcutaneous location of the clavicle.

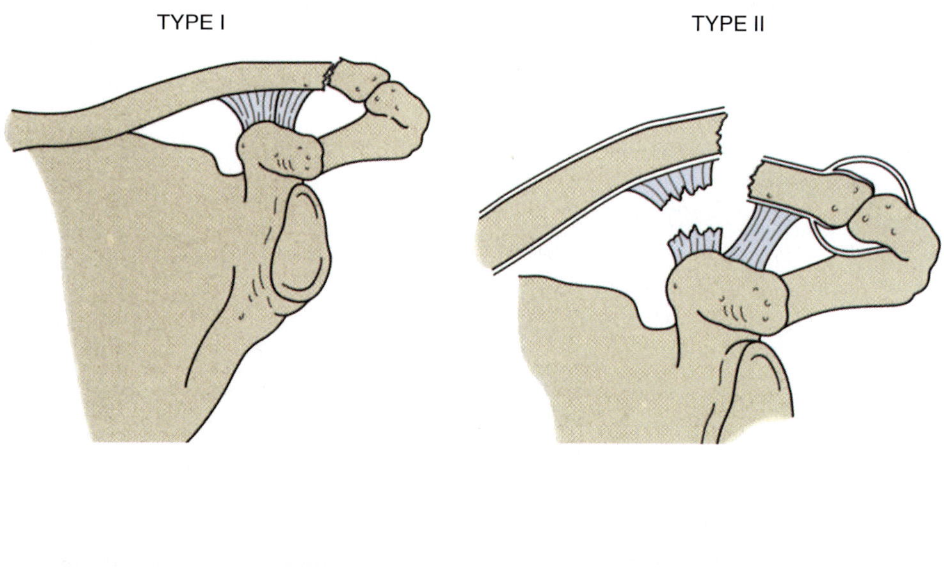

Figure 3–7 When the distal end of the clavicle is fractured, the ligaments may either remain intact and maintain apposition of the fracture fragments (type I) or rupture, allowing wide displacement of the fragments (type II). *(Redrawn from Rockwood CA, Freen DP, eds: Fractures, vol 1, 4th ed. Philadelphia, JB Lippincott, 1996.)*

    - Shoulder asymmetry, pain and ecchymoses over the clavicle, and splinting of the injured arm are present.
    - Skin tenting may occur with displacement, and penetration of the sharp proximal fragment through the platysma may endanger the overlying skin.
  - The neurovascular status of the upper extremity should be carefully assessed and documented.
  - Imaging consists of plain radiography. An AP view of the clavicle and/or chest is useful but may not reveal the extent of comminution and displacement, which may be obscured by the underlying ribs and scapula. A 20- to 30-degree cephalad view provides a clearer image of the clavicle.

- ❑ Treatment
  - Treatment of clavicle fractures continues to evolve and is based on location of the fracture and the degree of displacement.
  - Historically, most clavicle fractures were treated *conservatively*. Owing in part to randomized clinical trials, there has been a trend toward ORIF of displaced midshaft fractures.
  - Nonoperative treatment is typically used for nondisplaced or minimally displaced fractures regardless of location. A variety of different braces includes simple sling, sling and swath, figure-of-eight braces, and Velpeau wraps.
  - A simple sling provides good clinical results with higher patient satisfaction and fewer skin complications.

Operative Treatment

MIDSHAFT FRACTURES

  - Considerable controversy persists as to the surgical treatment of midshaft clavicle fracture. Indications include open fractures, skin tenting, neurovasculature damage, polytrauma, associated scapulothoracic dissociation, and *shortening greater than 2 cm, displacement of 100%, and significant comminution*.
  - For closed midshaft fractures with displacement greater than 100% of bone diameter, a randomized clinical trial showed improved Constant-Murley Shoulder Outcome score; disabilities of the arm, shoulder, and hand (DASH) score; union rate; and patient satisfaction at 1 year (McKee, 2007) with ORIF vs. nonsurgical treatment.
  - Open reduction and internal fixation with a superiorly placed plate is the most widely used technique.
    - Because of the prominence of the superiorly based plates, subsequent hardware removal is often required.
    - Anterior plating is also possible and may be less prominent.
    - Intramedullary fixation is challenging because of the sigmoid shape of the clavicle but provides less soft tissue disruption and hardware prominence.
    - Some biomechanical evidence indicates that superior plating is more rigid than anterior plating or intramedullary fixation (Golish et al, 2008b).

OTHER CLAVICLE FRACTURES

  - Few indications exist for operative treatment of medial clavicle fractures, such as irreducible posterior fracture displacement causing neurovascular compromise.
  - Open reduction and subsequent stabilization with a Balser plate or suture have been described.
  - Displaced distal clavicle fractures (type II) that are treated nonoperatively frequently progress to delayed union, non-union, or deformity, which may be acceptable in older or sedentary patients. Resultant arthrosis may cause pain, requiring late distal clavicle resection.
  - Younger patients with type II distal clavicle fractures are generally treated operatively.
  - Open reduction and internal fixation with a plate-and-screw construct may be used for fracture configurations possessing a distal fragment large enough to hold at least two screws.
  - For smaller distal fragments or vertically unstable fractures, a plate that crosses the AC joint and fixes to the acromion or a hook-plate that engages the undersurface of the acromion may be used.
  - Fractures with significant displacement of the medial fragment should always be treated with coracoclavicular ligament repair, reconstruction, or fixation with a screw, graft, suture, or a combination of techniques to reduce the fracture and secure the displaced medial fragment to the coracoid process.
  - Distal clavicle resection may be indicated for comminuted intra-articular fractures or for persistent AC joint pain after distal clavicle fracture.

- ❑ Complications
  - Complications of clavicle fracture include early or late neurovascular compromise, non-union, malunion with resultant deformity or loss of function, and early or late AC or SC joint arthrosis.
  - Non-union is more frequently seen in fractures with initial shortening or displacement greater than 2 cm, in older patients, and with refractures, inadequate immobilization, and distal third fractures.

- Operative treatment of clavicle fractures frequently results in prominent or painful hardware, requiring reoperation for hardware removal. Refracture may also occur regardless of treatment.

Clavicle Disorders Questions

1. Which of the following radiographic views in which the x-ray beam is directed 15 degrees cephalad is helpful in diagnosing acromioclavicular joint pathology?
   A. Zanca view.
   B. Serendipity view.
   C. Axillary view.
   D. Anteroposterior stress view.
   E. Lateral chest view.

2. All of the following are associated with clavicle fracture non-union *except*:
   A. Fracture of the distal third.
   B. Initial shortening of greater than 2 cm.
   C. Immobilization with a sling.
   D. Refracture.
   E. Elderly patient.

3. An 18-year-old high school lacrosse player complains of left shoulder pain after diving for a shot. She reports landing directly on her left shoulder. Examination reveals prominence of the distal clavicle and localized tenderness. The patient has full active and passive range of motion at the shoulder. Stress radiographs demonstrate AC joint separation with 100% displacement. What type of AC joint separation has this patient sustained, and which structures are likely disrupted?
   A. Type II; acromioclavicular ligaments, coracoclavicular ligaments.
   B. Type III; acromioclavicular ligaments, coracoclavicular ligaments.
   C. Type II; acromioclavicular ligaments only.
   D. Type V; acromioclavicular ligaments, coracoclavicular ligaments.
   E. Type III; coracoclavicular ligaments only.

4. A 20-year-old college football player complains of sternal pain after being tackled during a football game. He also describes a choking sensation and inability to catch his breath. On physical examination, there is asymmetry, with the left clavicle appearing more prominent. He is tender to palpation over the right clavicular head and has diminished pulses in the right upper extremity. After appropriate plain radiographs are obtained, a CT scan would likely show:
   A. Posterior subluxation of the right SC joint.
   B. Midshaft right clavicle fracture.
   C. Right clavicular medial physeal fracture with posterior displacement of the clavicle.
   D. Anterior dislocation of left SC joint.
   E. Sternal fracture.

■

Glenohumeral Arthrosis

Primary Glenohumeral Arthritis

❑ Diagnosis
- Progressive osteoarthritis (OA) of the shoulder parallels that of other joints.
- Patients complain of diffuse pain that is slowly progressive and is exacerbated by range of motion.
- Physical examination reveals reduced range of motion and crepitus.
- Disease progression includes fibrillation of cartilage, asymmetrical joint space narrowing, osteophyte formation, subchondral sclerosis, complete loss of joint space, and bony erosion (posterior glenoid).
- Joint space narrowing is well-appreciated on the axillary lateral views but its appearance may be deceptive on the AP view. The AP view should be examined for superior migration (cuff arthropathy), inferior osteophytes, and AC pathology.
- MRI is useful to rule out an incompetent rotator cuff, because pain and stiffness may limit examination of muscle function.

❑ Treatment
- For patients with primary glenohumeral arthrosis, conservative management with injections and activity modification is a mainstay of treatment.
- Patients for whom conservative management fails may be surgical candidates.
- The role of simple débridement is controversial, but it may be useful if combined with capsular releases (to improve ROM), synovectomy (to reduce inflammatory burden), or treatment of other pain-generating structures (biceps tenodesis/tenotomy).
- Concomitant pathology such as AC disease and subacromial impingement may respond to surgery.

Arthroplasty
- Arthroplasty is considered for patients for whom conservative management has failed and who have intractable symptoms.
- Candidates for arthroplasty must have a functional rotator cuff and deltoid, with reasonable functional demands.
- Hemiarthroplasty is well accepted, especially for the younger patient with higher functional demand, limited glenoid arthrosis, or, possibly, even severe glenoid arthrosis with loss of glenoid bone stock.
- Hemiarthroplasty with nonprosthetic glenoid arthroplasty is performed by débridement alone ("ream and run") or by interposition with fascia, although later evidence shows rapid degradation of interposed soft tissue.
- Total shoulder arthroplasty was introduced by Neer. Some studies have shown better outcomes with total arthroplasty than with

hemiarthroplasty in some populations. This achievement comes at the expense of additional complexity, especially in the revision setting.
- Fixation of the glenoid component is a key issue. Aseptic loosening of glenoid components is unfortunately common.
- Both peg and keel designs have been used, and the choice is controversial. Keels are known to be associated with prevalence of radiolucent lines, which may be of unknown significance as an isolated finding.
- Most designs are cemented, but some ingrowth prostheses exist. In either case, the management of glenoid bone stock is critical in the revision setting.

Cuff Tear Arthropathy

❑ Diagnosis and Classification
- Classification of the severity of cuff tear arthropathy includes elements of physical examination, imaging, and a knowledge of the pathophysiology. All patients may be weak on provocative maneuvers, with variable degrees of stiffness and limited active range of motion, pain, and crepitus.
- Type I (centered) consists of arthrosis in the context of an incompetent cuff but with minimal superior migration. The anterior restraints are intact, and there may be acetabularization of the CA arch and femoralization of the humerus. Some medial erosion of the glenoid may be present.
- In type II (decentered), the hallmark is severe superior migration of the humeral head. There may be compromised anterior restraints and minimal stabilization by the CA arch.
- Type III (unstable) is characterized by incompetent anterior structures, anterior/superior escape, and no stabilization by the CA arch. Significant bony erosions may be present.

❑ Treatment
- For patients with cuff tear arthropathy, conservative management with injections and activity modification is a mainstay of treatment.
- Patients in whom conservative management fails may be surgical candidates. The role of simple débridement is controversial, but many believe that débridement for severe arthropathy is of limited value (except for the elimination of other pain-generating structures, such as the biceps tendon). The possible exception is the débridement of massive tears with only mild arthrosis (see rotator cuff discussion).
- Arthroplasty is considered for patients in whom conservative management has failed and who have intractable symptoms and a functional deltoid. Candidates for hemiarthroplasty must have an intact CA arch.

Hemiarthroplasty
- Recommended for patients younger than 70 years who retain active forward flexion to 90 degrees, with an intact CA arch.
- Anatomic heads are preferred of sufficient size to limit excessive anterior/posterior translation. Large head prostheses have been designed, but the current practice is to avoid overstuffing.
- Cuff tear hemiarthroplasties are designed for cuff arthropathy with a large head arc (>180 degrees) to accommodate articulation with the acromion as well as glenoid.
- Anterior/superior escape is a severe problem following hemiarthroplasty involving compromise of the CA arch; it may be associated with previous subacromial decompression and resection of the CA ligament.

Reverse Total Shoulder Arthroplasty
- Recommended for patients older than 70 years who may have limited active forward flexion (pseudoparalysis) or an incompetent CA arch.
- Current designs (originating with the design due to Grammont) involve a 2/3-sphere attached to the glenoid (glenosphere) atop a glenoid baseplate (metaglene), which is fixed to the glenoid by screws. The humeral component includes a stem (cemented), a neck, and a polyethylene socket.
- The reverse design recruits the deltoid for better abduction due to a longer lever arm by medializing the center of rotation. The glenoid baseplate is tilted slightly inferiorly relative to the glenoid face to avoid scapular notching. Newer designs have lateralized the center or rotation to decrease scapular notching and improve the function of the remaining rotator cuff (subscapularis, teres minor).
- Glenoid bone loss due to severe arthrosis, ill-advised reaming, or revision is a potentially serious problem. Severe glenoid bone loss may require salvage with resection arthroplasty.
- Standard unconstrained total shoulder arthroplasty is contraindicated because of superior migration of humeral head, which leads to edge loading and rocking of the glenoid component.
- Superior migration in total shoulder arthroplasty results in rapid glenoid loosening, requiring revision. Constrained total shoulder designs attempted to compensate for this complication, but are of historical interest only because they have a high revision rate.

Glenohumeral Arthrosis Questions

1. Which of the following is least true about hemiarthroplasty for cuff arthropathy?
   A. Incompetent CA ligament is a contraindication.
   B. Large head prosthesis is a key design feature.
   C. Some prosthetic heads have a large arc to articulate superiorly.
   D. Is functionally superior to reverse total arthroplasty.
   E. Is superior to conventional total shoulder arthroplasty.
2. Which of the following is true about reverse arthroplasty for cuff arthropathy?
   A. The Grammont design medializes the center of rotation.
   B. Baseplate rocking leads to early loosening with superior migration.
   C. Has uniformly superior outcomes to hemiarthroplasty for all patients.
   D. Is recommended for younger patients because of improved function.
   E. Is technically as difficult as hemiarthroplasty.
3. Which of the following is true of arthroplasty for primary GH arthritis?
   A. The results of total arthroplasty are worse than those of hemiarthroplasty.
   B. Interposition hemiarthroplasties are clearly better than hemiarthroplasty alone.
   C. Keel-based glenoids are superior to peg-based designs.
   D. PMMA cement may be used on the glenoid side.
   E. Press-fit stems on the humeral side are the standard of care.
4. In the diagnosis of primary GH arthritis, which of the following is least important?
   A. Joint space narrowing assessed on the axillary lateral view.
   B. Assessment of cuff integrity and deltoid function.
   C. Assessment of AC joint and subacromial impingement as pain generators.
   D. Hand dominance in the setting of intractable pain.
   E. Limited range of motion with painful crepitus.

■

The Thrower's Shoulder

- Overhead sports and competitive throwing in particular are severe tests of shoulder anatomy and biomechanics.
- Competitive throwers are subject to shoulder injury. Some pathology, such as glenohumeral internal rotation deficit (GIRD), is nearly unique to throwers and overhead athletes. Lesions such as SLAP tears are classic in throwers and athletes competing in overhead sports.
- Figure 3–8 shows the phases of throwing. Maximum forces are encountered in deceleration and late-cocking phases (see Fig. 4–12).
- Coaching focused on throwing biomechanics improves performance and mitigates injury risk.

Internal Impingement

- *Internal impingement* is repetitive contact of the greater tuberosity with the posterior/superior glenoid in abduction/external rotation. Such contact causes impingement on the rotator cuff and posterior/superior labrum/capsule.
- It is seen in competitive throwers and is a pathologic variant of normal shoulder biomechanics, in which impingement exists but is nonpathologic.
- Patients complain of posterior shoulder pain exacerbated by throwing.
- Repetitive microtrauma to the posterior band of the IGHL and posterior capsule may result in contracture. Competitive throwing results in increased external rotation and decreased internal rotation (humeral retrotorsion), which is a normal adaptation to long term throwing.
- GIRD is diagnosed as a loss of 30 degrees of the total arc of rotation (external rotation + internal rotation) relative to the contralateral side.
- GIRD, which is due to posterior capsular contracture, alters the biomechanics of throwing, shifting the center of rotation of the humeral head posteriorly and superiorly.
- GIRD is treated with the sleeper stretch, in which the patient lies in lateral decubitus with

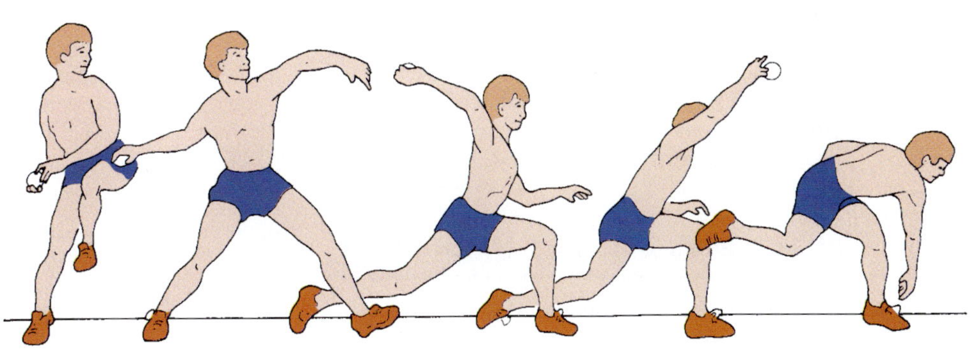

Figure 3–8 Glenohumeral arthrosis, the thrower's shoulder. *(From Miller MD, Cooper DE, Warner JJP: Review of Sports Medicine and Arthroscopy. Philadelphia, WB Saunders, 1995, p 123.)*

Table 3–7 Pitch Count Recommendations for Youth Baseball

Age (yrs)	Pitch Count			
	Per Game	Per Week	Per Season	Per Year
9–10	50	75	1000	2000
11–12	75	100	1000	3000
13–14	75	125	1000	3000

From Miller M: Review of Orthopaedics: Expert Consult: Online and Print, 5th ed. Philadelphia, Saunders, 2008.

the injured arm down, using the well arm to progressively internally rotate the injured arm, stretching the posterior capsule.

- Posterior SLAP tears or posterior labral lesions may result from an increase in the "peel-back" mechanism of the biceps on the superior glenoid.
- Articular-sided partial rotator cuff tears of the posterior supraspinatus or infraspinatus may result from increased external rotation and force before the otherwise normal impingement mechanism occurs, leading to injury from repetitive trauma.
- Management is conservative. In some throwers for whom conservative management has truly failed, posterior capsular release with SLAP repair followed by extensive rehabilitation may be an option.
- Many patients also have scapular dyskinesis and prominence of the inferior medial border of the scapula, or scapular malposition, inferior medial winging, coracoid tenderness, scapular dyskinesis (SICK) syndrome. This is clearly demonstrated by asymmetry on physical examination.

Little Leaguer's Shoulder

- Little Leaguer's shoulder is a Salter-Harris I fracture of the proximal humeral physis occurring in young pitchers.
- Failure to limit pitch counts and inadequate rest both between games and throughout the year (off-season pitching) contribute. Early adoption of breaking pitches may be a factor.
- Radiographs may demonstrate widening of the proximal humeral physis in comparison with the contralateral side. MRI can confirm the diagnosis.
- Treatment is conservative, including rest, activity modification, and pitching mechanics. Return to play is contemplated only when symptoms have resolved completely.
- Table 3–7 demonstrates pitch count recommendations for various age groups.

The Thrower's Shoulder Questions

1. GIRD and SICK syndrome in the young thrower may be treated by:
A. Pitch count moderation.
B. Off-season rest.
C. Sleeper stretch.
D. Throwing coach and scapular mechanics.
E. All of the above.

2. Highest stresses in throwing are in:
A. Late cocking and deceleration.
B. Wind-up and follow-through.
C. Cocking only.
D. Acceleration only.
E. None of the above.

References and Resources

Burkhart, S.S., Lo, I.K., 2006. Arthroscopic rotator cuff repair. J. Am. Acad. Orthop. Surg. 14, 333–346.

Burkhart, S.S., Lo, I.K., Brady, P.C., 2006. Burkhart's View of the shoulder: A Cowboy's Guide to Advanced Shoulder Arthroscopy, second ed. Lippincott, Williams & Wilkins, Philadelphia.

Canadian Orthopaedic Trauma Society, 2007. Nonoperative treatment compared with plate fixation of displaced midshaft clavicular fractures: A multicenter, randomized clinical trial. J. Bone Joint Surg. Am. 89, 1–10.

DeLee, J.C., Drez Jr., D., Miller, M.D. (Eds.), 2009. DeLee & Drez's Orthopaedic Sports Medicine, third ed. Saunders Elsevier, Philadelphia.

Ecklund, K.J., Lee, T.Q., Tibone, J., Gupta, R., 2007. Rotator cuff arthropathy. J. Am. Acad. Orthop. Surg. 15, 340–349.

Elhassan, B., Endres, N.K., Higgins, L.D., Warner, J.J., 2008. Massive irreparable tendon tears of the rotator cuff: Salvage options. Instr. Course Lect. 57, 153–166.

Elkousy, H., Hammerman, S.M., Edwards, T.B., et al., 2006. The arthroscopic square knot: A biomechanical comparison with open and arthroscopic knots. Arthroscopy 22, 736–741.

Gartsman, G.M., 2008. Shoulder arthroscopy, second ed. Saunders Elsevier, Philadelphia.

Gartsman, G.M., Edwards, T.B., 2008. Shoulder Arthroplasty. Saunders Elsevier, Philadelphia.

Golish, S.R., Caldwell 3rd, P.E., Miller, M.D., et al., 2008. Interference screw versus suture anchor fixation for subpectoral tenodesis of the proximal biceps tendon: A cadaveric study. Arthroscopy 24, 1103–1108.

Golish, S.R., Oliviero, J.A., Francke, E.I., Miller, M.D., 2008. A biomechanical study of plate versus intramedullary devices for midshaft clavicle fixation. J. Orthop. Surg. 3, 28.

Heyworth, B.E., Williams 3rd, R.J., 2009. Internal impingement of the shoulder. Am. J. Sports Med. 37, 1024–1037.

Lo, I.K., Burkhart, S.S., 2004. Arthroscopic revision of failed rotator cuff repairs: Technique and results. Arthroscopy 20, 250–267.

Lo, I.K., Burkhart, S.S., Chan, K.C., Athanasiou, K., 2004. Arthroscopic knots: Determining the optimal balance of loop security and knot security. Arthroscopy 20, 489–502.

Mckee, Canadian orthopaedic trauma society, 2007.

Miller, M.D., 2008. Review of Orthopaedics, fifth ed. Saunders Elsevier, Philadelphia.

Miller, M.D., Cole, B.D., 2004. Textbook of Arthroscopy. Saunders Elsevier, Philadelphia.

Miller, M.D., Chabra, A.B., Hurwitz, S.R., et al., 2008. Orthopaedic Surgical Approaches. Saunders Elsevier, Philadelphia.

Tonino, P.M., Gerber, C., Itoi, E., et al., 2009. Complex shoulder disorders: Evaluation and treatment. J. Am. Acad. Orthop. Surg. 17, 125–136.

CHAPTER 4

Elbow

LUKE S. OH

Anatomy and Functional Biomechanics

Joint Articulations

- The elbow joint is composed of three articulations:
  - Ulnohumeral:
    - Ginglymus (hinge) joint.
    - Transmits 40% of an axial load.
    - Primary passive stabilizer of elbow near terminal extension (< 20° of flexion) and terminal flexion (> 120° of flexion)
  - Radiocapitellar:
    - Trochoid (pivot) joint.
    - Transmits 60% of an axial load.
  - Proximal radioulnar.

Bones

❑ Distal Humerus

- Arch composed of two condyles that contain the articular surfaces of:
  - Trochlea, which articulates with the ulna.
  - Capitellum, which articulates with the radial head.
- Medial epicondyle is the proximal attachment site for:
  - Medial collateral ligament (MCL) complex.
  - Flexor-pronator muscles of forearm:
    - Pronator teres.
    - Flexor carpi radialis.
    - Palmaris longus.
    - Flexor carpi ulnaris.
- Lateral epicondyle is the proximal attachment site for:
  - Lateral collateral ligament (LCL) complex.
  - Extensor-supinator muscles of forearm:
    - Extensor carpi radialis longus.
    - Extensor carpi radialis brevis.
    - Extensor carpi ulnaris.
    - Extensor digiti minimi.
    - Anconeus.
    - Supinator.

❑ Proximal Ulna (Fig. 4–1)

- Olecranon.
- Coronoid process.
  - Anteromedial coronoid essential for prevention of posterior subluxation.
- Sublime tubercle:
  - Distal attachment site of the anterior bundle of the medial collateral ligament.

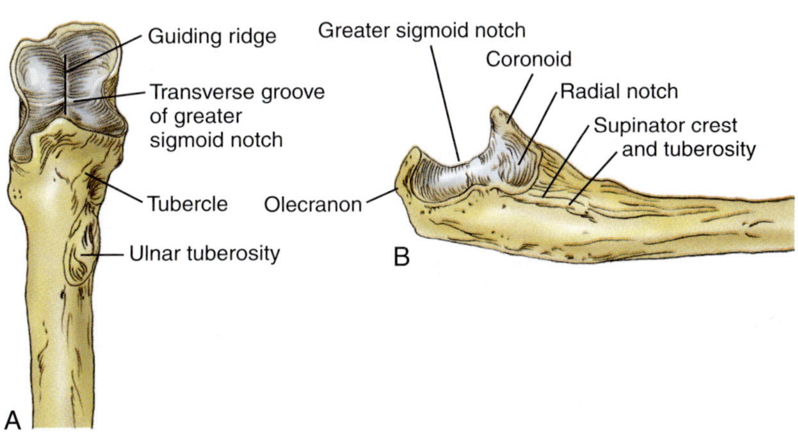

Figure 4–1 Proximal ulna. **A**, Anterior aspect of the proximal ulna demonstrating the greater sigmoid fossa with the central groove. **B**, Lateral view with landmarks. *(From Morrey BF: Anatomy of the elbow joint. In Morrey BF, Sanchez-Sotelo J [eds]: The Elbow and Its Disorders, 4th ed. Philadelphia, Saunders Elsevier, 2009, p 16.)*

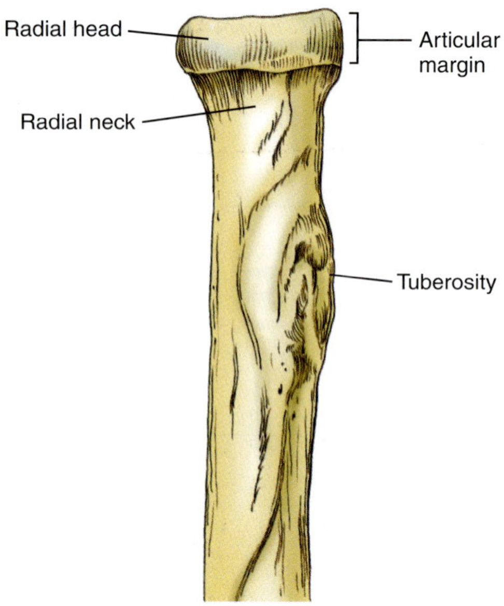

Figure 4–2 Proximal aspect of the radius demonstrating the articular margin for articulation with the olecranon, the radial neck, and tuberosity. *(From Morrey BF: Anatomy of the elbow joint. In Morrey BF, Sanchez-Sotelo J [eds]: The Elbow and Its Disorders, 4th ed. Philadelphia, Saunders Elsevier, 2009, p 15.)*

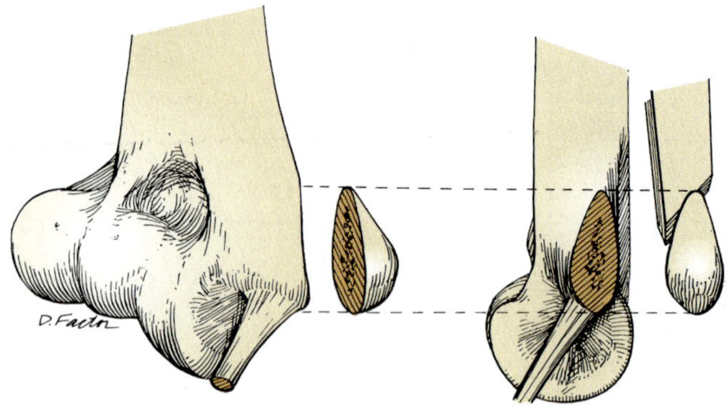

Figure 4–4 Depiction of the medial aspect of the distal humerus with the medial epicondyle removed. The humeral attachment of the ulnar collateral ligament is located in the anteroinferior surface of the medial epicondyle. *(From Morrey BF: Anatomy of the elbow joint. In Morrey BF, Sanchez-Sotelo J [eds]: The Elbow and Its Disorders, 4th ed. Philadelphia, Saunders Elsevier, 2009, p 33.)*

- ❑ Proximal Radius (Fig. 4–2)
  - Radial head is the secondary stabilizer to valgus stress, especially important in the MCL-deficient elbow.

Ligaments

- ❑ Medial Collateral Ligament Complex (Fig. 4–3)
  - Composed of three bundles:
    - Anterior bundle:
      - Humeral attachment: Medial epicondyle, which accounts for the middle two thirds of the anteroinferior surface (Fig. 4–4).
      - Ulnar attachment: Sublime tubercle. Anterior bundle of the MCL Complex is often referred to as the Ulnar Collateral Ligament (UCL).
      - At 90° of elbow flexion, the anterior bundle crosses the elbow at a 45° angle from the anteroinferior surface of the medial epicondyle to the sublime tubercle.
      - Primary restraint to valgus force during the arc of throwing motion from 30° to 120° of flexion.
      - Subjected to near-failure tensile stress during acceleration phase of throwing.
      - Is composed of anterior and posterior bands, which tighten in reciprocal fashion during flexion and extension.
    - Posterior bundle:
      - Fan-shaped structure.
      - Is not vulnerable to valgus overload unless the anterior bundle is completely disrupted.
    - Transverse bundle, also called the "ligament of Cooper," contributes little to elbow stability.
- ❑ Lateral Collateral Ligament Complex (Fig. 4–5)
  - Composed of:
    - Lateral ulnar collateral ligament:
      - Humeral attachment: lateral epicondyle.
      - Ulnar attachment: crista supinatoris.
      - Demonstrates isometry; tight in both flexion and extension.
      - Primary lateral stabilizer of elbow to varus stress.
      - Deficiency results in posterolateral rotatory instability.
    - Radial collateral ligament.
    - Annular ligament, which keeps the radial head in contact with the ulna.
    - Accessory lateral collateral ligament, which stabilizes the annular ligament during varus stress.
  - Not discrete structures but thickenings of the lateral capsule, similar to glenohumeral ligaments in the shoulder (Fig. 4–6).

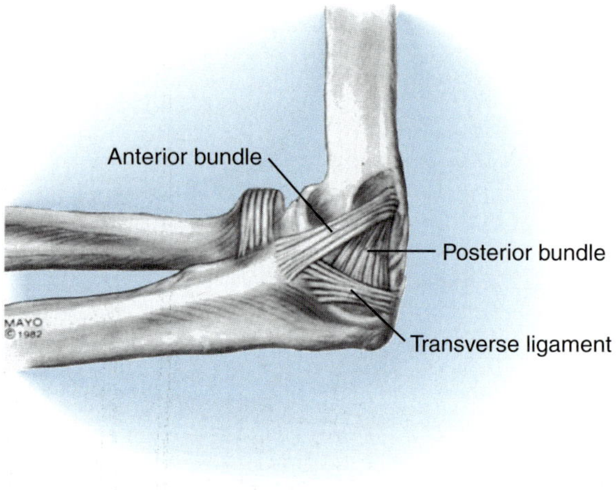

Figure 4–3 Medial collateral ligament (MCL) complex. The classic orientation of the medial collateral ligament, including the anterior and posterior bundles, and the transverse ligament is shown. This last structure contributes relatively little to elbow stability. *(From Morrey BF: Anatomy of the elbow joint. In Morrey BF, Sanchez-Sotelo J [eds]: The Elbow and Its Disorders, 4th ed. Philadelphia, Saunders Elsevier, 2009, p 21. Used by permission of the Mayo Foundation for Medical Education and Research. All rights reserved.)*

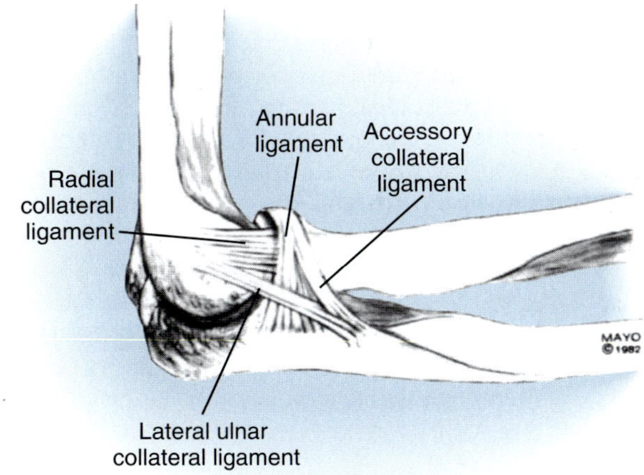

Figure 4–5 Lateral collateral ligament complex. Schematic representation of the lateral collateral ligament complex showing several portions, one of which, termed the radial collateral ligament, extends from the humerus to the annular ligament. This is the portion that is implicated is clinical instability. *(From Morrey BF: Anatomy of the elbow joint. In Morrey BF, Sanchez-Sotelo J [eds]: The Elbow and Its Disorders, 4th ed. Philadelphia, Saunders Elsevier, 2009, p 22. Used by permission of the Mayo Foundation for Medical Education and Research. All rights reserved.)*

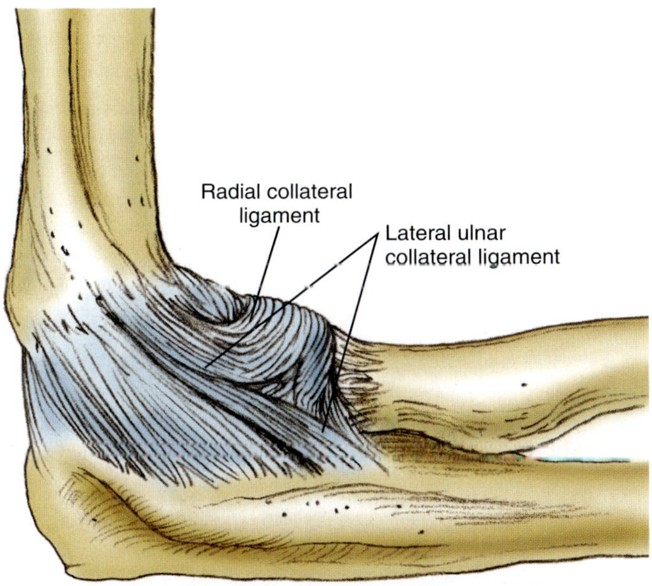

Figure 4–6 Artist's rendition of lateral collateral complex showing the thickening of the lateral ulnar collateral ligament with a more discrete insertion at the tubercle of the supinator. In life, the supinator origin obscures the ligament, making it unnoticeable unless the supinator muscle has been removed. *(From Morrey BF: Anatomy of the elbow joint. In Morrey BF, Sanchez-Sotelo J [eds]: The Elbow and Its Disorders, 4th ed. Philadelphia, Saunders Elsevier, 2009, p 23.)*

Muscles

- Although the bones and ligaments are passive stabilizers of the elbow, the muscles around the elbow are the active stabilizers.

❑ Anterior
- Biceps:
  - Primary supinator of forearm in addition to contributing to elbow flexion.
  - Despite a large cross-sectional area, the mechanical advantage of the biceps as an elbow flexor is less than expected for its size because it crosses the elbow relatively close to the axis of rotation.
- Brachialis:
  - Elbow flexor with largest cross-sectional area.
  - Poor mechanical advantage because it crosses the elbow close to the axis of rotation.
  - Lateral portion of brachialis covers the radial nerve, an important issue during arthroscopic anterior capsulectomy.

❑ Posterior
- Triceps:
  - Powerful elbow extensor.
  - Long and lateral heads of the triceps are innervated by proximal branches of the radial nerve prior to the nerve entering the radial groove. Therefore, radial nerve injuries isolated to the midportion of the humerus usually do not affect the function of the lateral and long heads of the triceps.

Medial

- Flexor-pronator muscles:
  - In combination with shoulder internal rotators, flexor-pronator muscles provide dynamic stabilization during the throwing motion that protects the UCL.

❑ Lateral
- Extensor-supinator muscles.
- Brachioradialis, the elbow flexor with the greatest mechanical advantage.

Nerves

❑ Ulnar Nerve (Fig. 4–7)
- Derived from the medial cord of the brachial plexus (C8 and T1 nerve roots).
- For test-taking purposes, there are no motor branches of the radial nerve above the elbow joint. However, experienced elbow surgeons have on occasion encountered a motor branch to the triceps.
- Traverses through the cubital tunnel and rests against the posterior portion of the MCL.
- Cubital tunnel retinaculum:
  - Forms the "roof" of the cubital tunnel.
  - Flattens with elbow flexion, decreasing the volume of the cubital tunnel (Fig. 4–8).
  - Congenital ulnar nerve subluxation results from absence of the cubital tunnel retinaculum.

❑ Radial Nerve
- Derived from the posterior cord of the brachial plexus (C6-C8 nerve roots, variable contribution of C5 and T1 nerve roots).
- "Kamineni's Rule":
  - The radial nerve crosses the lateral aspect of the humerus approximately 1.7× (range 1.4×–2.0×), the transcondylar distance from the lateral epicondyle (Kamineni et al, 2009).

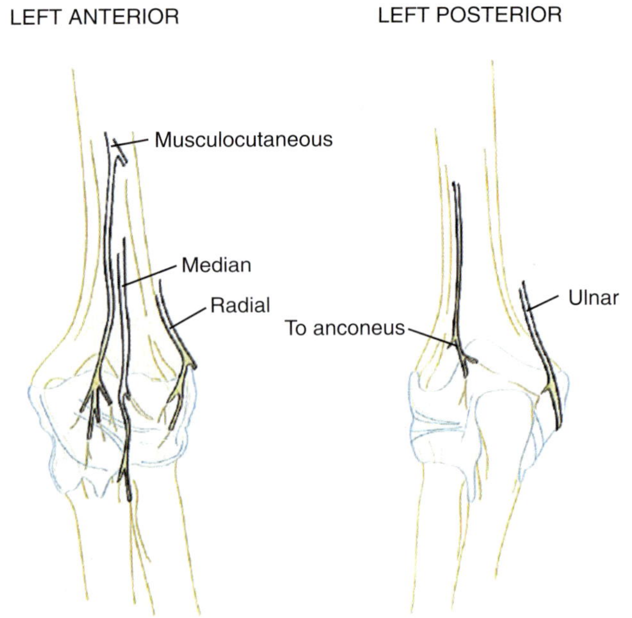

Figure 4–7 Nerves. A typical distribution of the contributions of the musculocutaneous radial median and ulnar nerves to the joint capsule. *(From Gardner E: The innervation of the elbow joint. Anat Rec 1948;102:161.)*

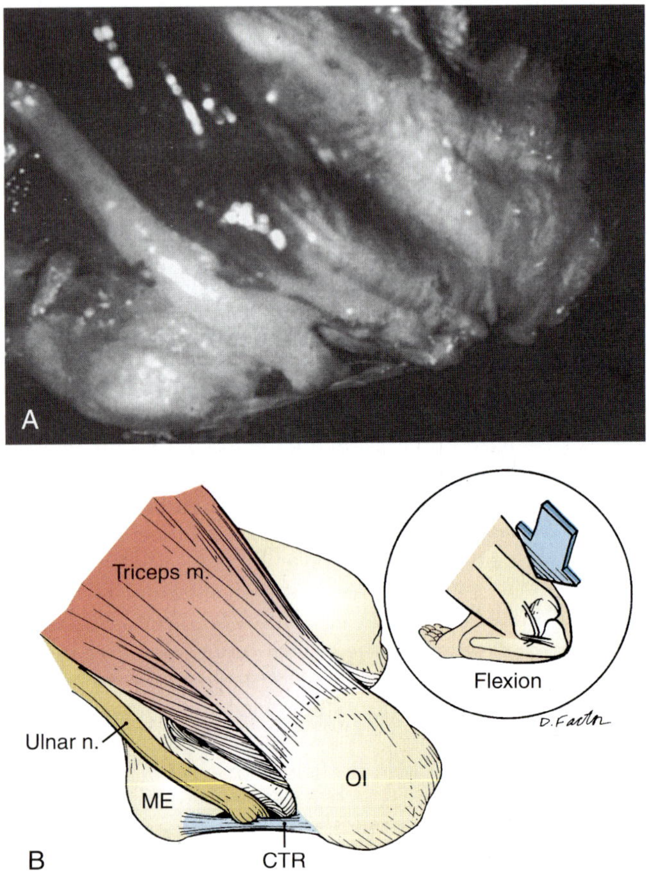

Figure 4–8 A and B, With elbow flexion, the cubital tunnel flattens and may compress the ulnar nerve. CTR, cubital tunnel retinaculum; ME, medial epicondyle; OI, olecranon. *(From O'Driscoll SW, Horri E, Carmichael SW, Morrey BE: The cubital tunnel and ulnar neuropathy. J Bone Joint Surg 1991;73B:613.)*

- "Gerwin' rule":
  - As the radial nerve courses from proximal to distal in the posterior compartment, the nerve is located approximately 21 cm from the medial epicondyle, along the medial border of the triceps and 14 cm from the lateral epicondyle along the lateral border of the triceps.

❑ Median Nerve
- Derived from C5-C8 and T1 nerve roots.
- In the antecubital fossa, it courses medial to the biceps tendon and brachial artery, and then courses distally deep to the bicipital aponeurosis.

Blood Vessels

- Arteries (Figs. 4–9 and 4–10):
  - Brachial artery, which lies medial to the biceps tendon, between the bicipital aponeurosis and brachialis muscle.
  - Ulnar artery.
  - Radial artery.
- Veins form "M"-shaped tributaries at the anterior aspect of the elbow (Fig. 4–11).

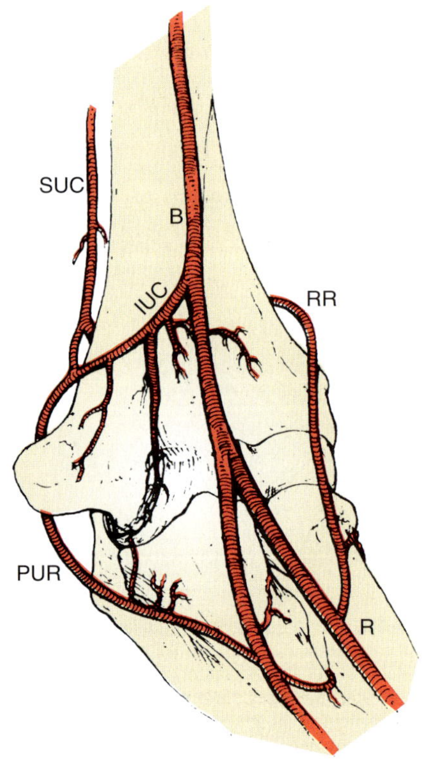

Figure 4–9 Arteries. Illustration of the anterior extraosseous vascular anatomy demonstrating the medial arcade and the relationship of the radial recurrent (RR) artery to the proximal aspect of the radius. The inferior ulnar collateral (IUC) artery provides perforators to the supracondylar region, medial aspect of the trochlea, and medial epicondyle before it courses posteriorly to anastomose with the superior ulnar collateral (SUC) and posterior ulnar recurrent (PUR) arteries. The RR artery provides an osseous perforator to the radius as it travels proximally and posterior. B, brachial artery; R, radial artery. *(Redrawn from Yamaguchi K, Sweet FA, Bindra R, et al: The extraosseous and intraosseous arterial anatomy of the adult elbow. J Bone Joint Surg 1997;79A:1654.)*

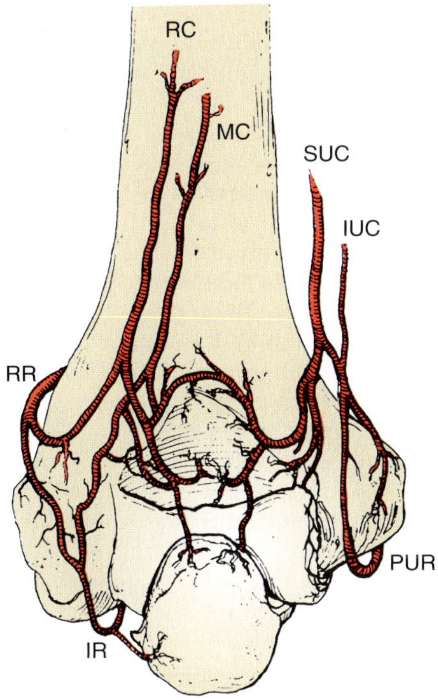

Figure 4–10 Illustration of the posterior collateral circulation of the elbow. There are perforating vessels on the posterior aspect of the lateral epicondyle, in the olecranon fossa, and on the medial aspect of the trochlea. The tip of the olecranon is supplied by perforators from the posterior arcade in the olecranon fossa. The superior ulnar collateral (SUC) artery is seen terminating in the posterior arcade. IR, interosseous recurrent (artery); IUC, inferior ulnar collateral (artery); MC, middle collateral (artery); PUR, posterior ulnar recurrent (artery); RC, radial collateral (artery); RR, radial recurrent (artery). *(Redrawn from Yamaguchi K, Sweet FA, Bindra R, et al: The extraosseous and intraosseous arterial anatomy of the adult elbow. J Bone Joint Surgery 1997;79A:1655.)*

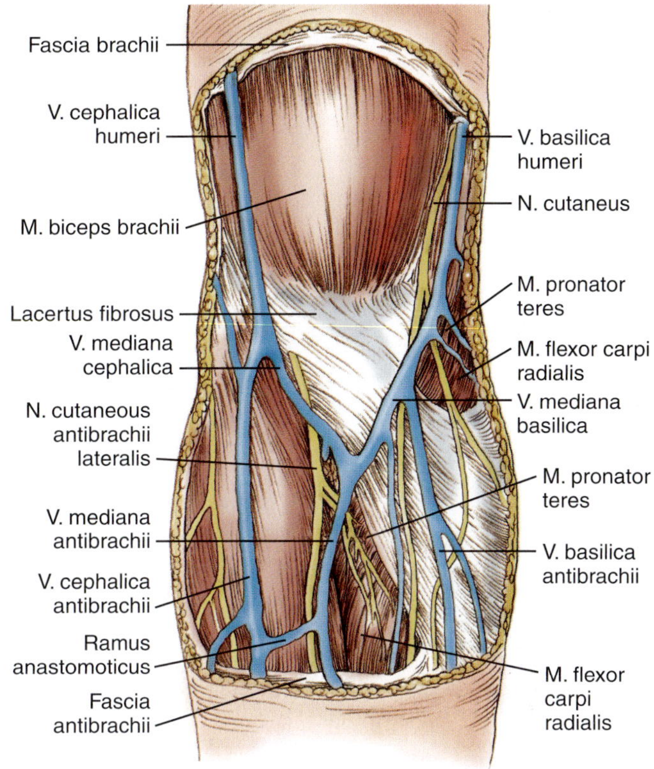

Figure 4–11 Veins form "M"-shaped tributaries at the anterior aspect of the elbow. The superficial venous pattern of the anterior aspect of the elbow demonstrates a rather characteristic inverted M pattern formed by the median cephalic and median basilic veins. M, musculus/musculi; N, nervus/nervi; V, vena/venae. *(Redrawn from Anson BJ, McVay CB: Surgical Anatomy, vol 2, 5th ed. Philadelphia, WB Saunders, 1971.)*

Elbow Biomechanics in Pitching

- Examination of biomechanics of the throwing motion offers insight into spectrum of elbow injury.

❑ The Six Phases of Throwing (Fig. 4–12)
- Wind-up.
- Early cocking.
- Late cocking.
- Acceleration.
- Deceleration.
- Follow-through.

❑ Valgus Extension Overload Syndrome (Fig. 4–13)
- Result of a combination of a large valgus load and rapid elbow extension.

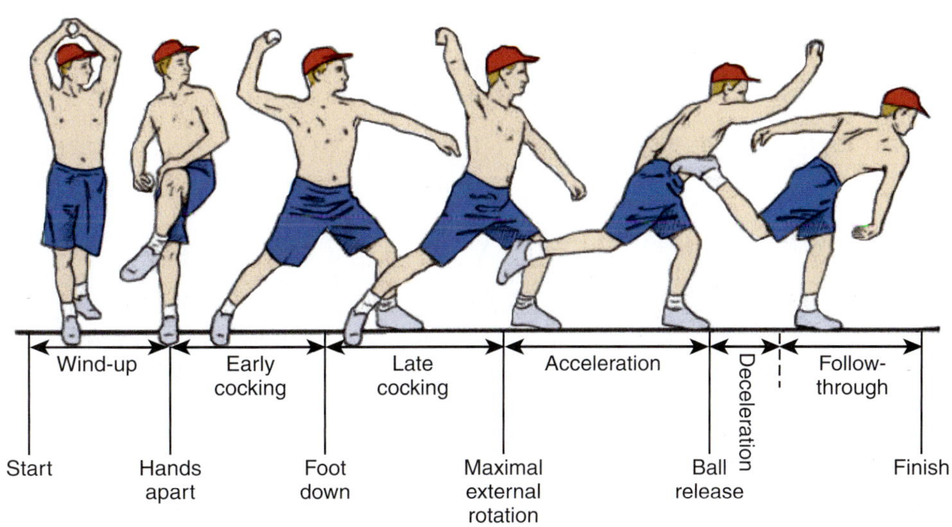

Figure 4–12 The six phases of throwing (indicated by *arrows*). *(From DiGiovine NM, Jobe FW, Pink M, Perry J: An electromyographic analysis of the upper extremity in pitching. J Shoulder Elbow Surg 1992;1:15-25.)*

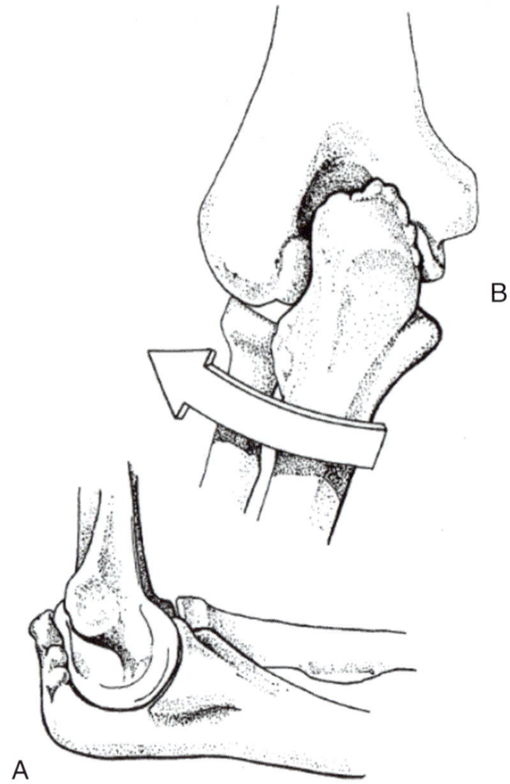

Figure 4–13 Valgus extension overload syndrome. Lateral (A) and posterior (B) views demonstrating valgus force (*arrow*) on the elbow with posteromedial olecranon osteophyte formation. *(From Cain EL Jr, Dugas JR, et al: Elbow injuries in throwing athletes: a current concepts review. Am J Sports Med 2003;31:621-635.)*

- Basic pathophysiologic model for many common elbow injuries in the throwing athlete:
  - Medial tension injuries.
  - Lateral compression injuries.
  - Posterior shear injuries.

❑ Effect on Medial Elbow
- The medial elbow experiences tensile forces with valgus force during throwing.
- The highest valgus force is applied to elbow during late cocking/early acceleration phase (64 newton-meters [N-m]).
- Ultimate strength of the UCL is 33 N-m.
- Valgus force on medial side with a single pitch exceeds the ultimate strength of the UCL.
- However, the UCL does not rupture from a single pitch, because shoulder internal rotation and forearm pronation provide dynamic stabilization.
- Therefore, rehabilitation/strengthening of flexor-pronator muscles for dynamic stabilization is important after UCL injury/surgery.
- Over time, repetitive near-failure loads cause microtrauma to the UCL that may result in UCL insufficiency.
- In the Mayo Clinic experience, only approximately 11% of UCL reconstructions performed were for isolated UCL insufficiency without associated medial elbow disorders (Fig. 4–14) (Smith, 2005).
  - Concomitant medial-sided elbow injuries may include:
    - Ulnar neuritis/neuropathy.
    - Flexor-pronator tendonitis.
    - Medial epicondylitis (medial epicondyle apophysitis in skeletally immature athlete).

❑ Effect on Lateral Elbow
- The lateral elbow experiences compressive forces with valgus force during throwing.

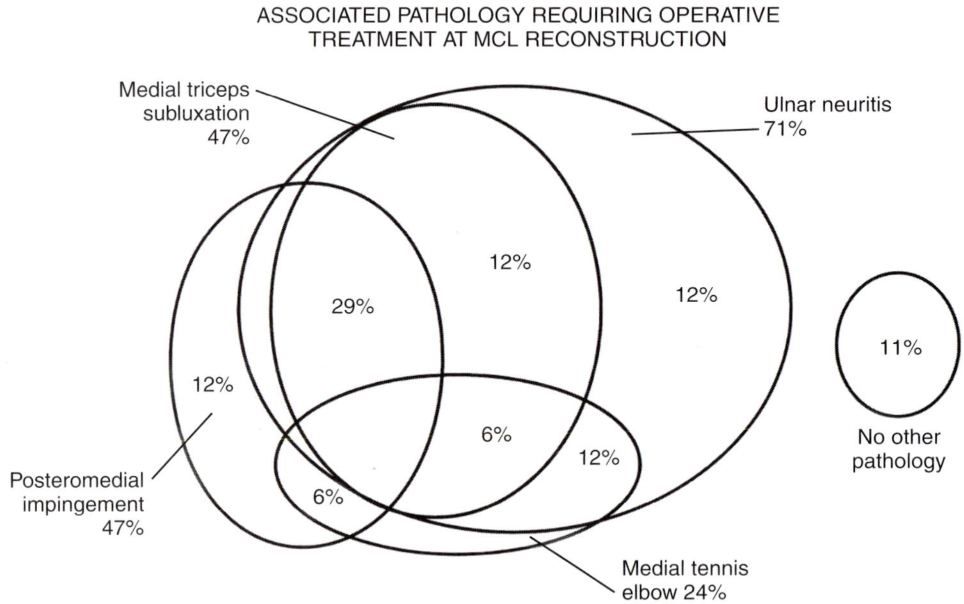

Figure 4–14 In the Mayo Clinic experience, only approximately 11% of MCL reconstructions performed were for isolated MCL insufficiency without associated medial elbow disorders. *(With permission from Mayo Foundation for Medical Education and Research. All rights reserved.)*

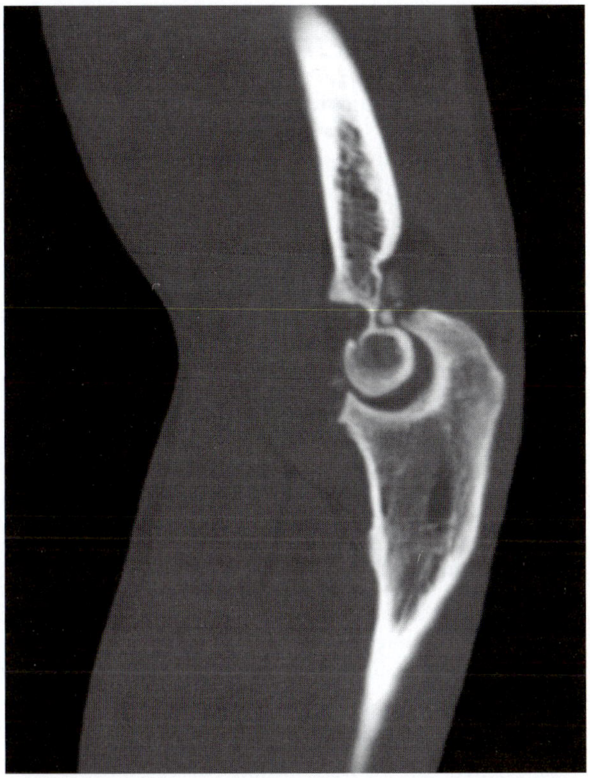

Figure 4–15 Posteromedial olecranon osteophytes may subsequently result in loose bodies. *(© Luke S. Oh, MD.)*

- During the acceleration phase, the elbow extends at a velocity as high as 3000 degrees per second.
- The radiocapitellar articulation experiences up to 500 N of compressive force.
- Degenerative changes in the radiocapitellar joint may develop over time.
- In adolescents, osteochondritis dissecans (OCD) of the capitellum may develop.

❑ Effect on Posterior Elbow
- The posterior elbow experiences shear forces.
- Posteromedial olecranon osteophytes may subsequently result in loose bodies (Fig. 4–15).
  - The most common reason for elbow surgery in baseball players.
- Posteromedial trochlea chondral lesion is a "kissing lesion" caused by posteromedial olecranon osteophytes.

Anatomy and Functional Biomechanics Questions

1. The proximal attachment of the anterior bundle of the medial collateral ligament in the elbow:
A. Is located at the prominence of the medial epicondyle.
B. Has a broad, fan-shaped footprint.
C. Is located in the middle two thirds of the anteroinferior surface of the medial epicondyle.
D. May tether the ulnar nerve and should be released during ulnar nerve transposition.
E. Is often avulsed in patients with posterolateral rotatory instability.

2. Insufficiency of which of the following structures has been identified to be most responsible for posterolateral rotatory instability of the elbow?
A. Radial collateral ligament.
B. Lateral ulnar collateral ligament.
C. Annular ligament.
D. Anterior bundle of the medial collateral ligament.
E. Posterior bundle of the medial collateral ligament.

3. Which of the following statements is FALSE?
A. Only approximately 11% of UCL reconstructions performed are for isolated UCL insufficiency without associated medial elbow pathology.
B. The highest valgus torque experienced by the medial aspect of the elbow during a single baseball pitch exceeds the ultimate strength of the ulnar collateral ligament.
C. Shoulder internal rotation and forearm pronation provide important dynamic stabilization that protects the ulnar collateral ligament during a baseball pitch.
D. The majority of ulnar collateral ligament injuries are not acute, complete tears but rather chronic or acute-on-chronic injuries that may or may not be associated with a "pop" along the medial elbow.
E. Athletes with ulnar collateral ligament injuries should be urged to have early surgical reconstruction of the ligament.

History, Physical Examination, and Imaging

History

❑ Location of Symptoms
- Generating a list of differential diagnoses of common conditions based on location of elbow symptoms is a useful strategy in the evaluation of elbow pathology. Many of these conditions are reviewed separately under their own headings later in the chapter.
- Medial symptoms:
  - UCL insufficiency.
  - Medial epicondylitis.
  - Ulnar neuritis/neuropathy.
  - Subluxating medial triceps.
- Lateral symptoms:
  - Osteochondritis dissecans.
  - Posterolateral rotatory instability (PLRI).
  - Radial head/neck fracture.
  - Lateral epicondylitis.
  - Synovial plicae.
- Anterior symptoms:
  - Distal biceps injury.
  - Distal humerus physeal injury.
  - Synovitis.
  - Capsular strain.

- Posterior symptoms:
  - Posteromedial impingement.
  - Fractured olecranon osteophytes.
  - Loose bodies.
  - Olecranon bursitis.
  - Triceps injury.

❑ Mechanism of Injury
- Once a list of differential diagnoses is generated, understanding the mechanism of injury helps narrow the list.
- Recognize that different sports may predispose athletes to certain types of injuries:
  - Baseball pitchers and javelin throwers apply a large valgus stress to the medial elbow, compressive stress to the lateral elbow, and shear forces to the posteromedial olecranon.
    - In baseball pitchers, it is particularly important to note the phase of throwing in which symptoms are elicited. For example, the UCL is not the source of pathology if pain in the medial elbow is experienced outside of the late cocking and early acceleration phases.
    - Other aspects of the patient's history worthy of documentation, especially in pitchers with a chronic injury, include changes in the thrower's accuracy, velocity, stamina, and strength as well as recent changes in the training regimen.
  - Gymnasts often lock their elbows in order to support their body weight and have a higher incidence of osteochondritis dissecans than other athletes.
  - Wrestlers and snowboarders may sustain elbow dislocations when attempting to break a fall with the upper extremity.

❑ Mechanical Symptoms
- History of catching or locking suggests presence of possible loose bodies, an articular cartilage flap, or synovial chondromatosis.
- Osteochondral loose bodies may not always be easily detected on plain radiographs, especially if the bony component is a thin crescentic piece attached to a larger cartilaginous loose body.

❑ Neurovascular Complaints
- Important to review the history for pathology affecting nerve function and vasculature, including numbness, tingling, radiation of pain, cold intolerance, weakness, and tendency to drop objects.

❑ Neck/Shoulder/Wrist Problems
- It is important to take a thorough history regarding the joints above and below the injured elbow. At times, primary pathology in the shoulder or wrist may contribute to compensation by the elbow, which may result in an overuse condition in the elbow.
- Cervical spine pathology may cause radiation of pain or may affect the upper extremity in a more global fashion, including at the elbow.

❑ Prior Elbow Injuries and Treatment
- Supracondylar or lateral condyle fracture in childhood may result in delayed complications if there was malunion, for example.
- History of prior and/or current treatment, including effective and ineffective conservative treatment modalities to date as well as any type of surgical procedures performed in the past, should be obtained.

Physical Examination

❑ Inspection

Swelling/Effusion
- Joint effusion is characterized by loss of the dimple in the lateral triangular soft spot created by radial head, capitellum, and coronoid.

Deformity
- If cubitus varus or cubitus valgus is present, measure the amount of varus or valgus with a goniometer.

Contracture
- Not uncommon for asymptomatic flexion contracture to develop in baseball pitchers over the course of their careers.
- Contracture is associated with progressive osteoarthritis of the elbow.

Carrying Angle
- By convention, carrying angle is measured at full extension with the forearm fully supinated. Because the carrying angle becomes angulated toward varus with flexion, the carrying angle cannot be accurately measured in a patient with a flexion contracture.
- Normal carrying angle: 11° valgus in men and 13° valgus in women.
- Asymptomatic baseball pitchers often have increased carrying angle in the throwing elbow.

❑ Range of Motion

Extension-Flexion
- Normal: 0 to 140°.
- Functional arc for activities of daily living (ADLs): 30 to 130°.
- Measure with a goniometer. Have the patient stand and forward-flex the shoulder so that the humerus is parallel to the ground; then measure elbow flexion and extension (with the forearm in full supination) by placing the goniometer on the lateral aspect of the extremity.

Forearm Rotation
- Normal: pronation 75°, supination 85°.
- Functional arc for ADLs: pronation 50°, supination 50°.
- Measure the axis connecting the radial styloid and ulnar styloid at the wrist while the patient keeps both elbows flexed to 90° and fully adducted against the torso.

Assessment of End Points in Terminal Extension/Flexion

- Firm end points may suggest a bony block from possible heterotopic ossification or osteophytes.
- Soft end points are more likely with arthrofibrosis and capsular contracture.

Crepitus

- Helpful if the source of crepitus can be determined: ulnohumeral vs. radiocapitellar vs. radioulnar joint.

❑ Palpation

- Bony landmarks: Palpate those bony structures involved in pathologic conditions associated with valgus extension overload syndrome (see Fig. 4–13):
  - Medial epicondyle: Assess for possible medial epicondylitis.
  - Lateral epicondyle: Assess for possible lateral epicondylitis.
  - Radial head: Assess for possible fracture, osteophytes.
  - Olecranon: Assess for posteromedial osteophytes, painful triceps insertion.
- Ligaments:
  - UCL: Palpate the UCL with the elbow flexed to approx 60 to 70° in order to allow the muscle mass to move anteriorly and away from the anterior bundle of the MCL complex, enabling easier palpation.
  - LUCL: Palpate for local tenderness with elbow at 90° of flexion.
- Ulnar nerve: Assess for local tenderness, radiation of pain ('Tinel sign at elbow), and mobility/subluxation.

❑ Muscle Strength Testing

- Document strength of relevant muscles using the standard grading system.

❑ Special Diagnostic Tests

- There are provocative tests that are highly sensitive and specific for a given condition in the injured elbow. They are reviewed in subsequent sections during discussions of specific elbow conditions.

Imaging

❑ Plain Radiographs

Standard Anteroposterior/Lateral Views

- Evaluate the fat pad for evidence of subtle or occult intra-articular fracture and presence of arthritic changes, deformity (e.g., cubitus varus/valgus, evidence of healed prior fracture), subtle subluxation, loose bodies, and heterotopic ossification.

Oblique View

- Difficult for assessment of the joint but helpful for detection of subtle fractures (Fig. 4–16).

Axial View

- Radiograph taken perpendicular to the cassette centered over the elbow joint with the elbow flexed to 120°.
- Helpful to assess for the presence of posteromedial osteophytes (Fig. 4–17).

❑ Computed Tomography

- To evaluate bony fractures, tunnel osteolysis after ligament reconstruction, and location of osteophytes.
- Beware that "loose" bodies seen on computed tomography (CT) may not truly be loose and floating in the joint but instead may be tethered or adhered to surrounding soft tissues.
- Also, an osteochondral fragment or loose body may be larger when encountered intraoperatively because the cartilaginous portion is not visualized on the CT scan.

❑ Magnetic Resonance Imaging

- Helpful for a variety of conditions, particularly those involving the soft tissues, but not as reliable in detection of bony pathology such as small osteophytes.

❑ Ultrasonography

- Advantage is the dynamic nature of a sonogram.
- Disadvantage is that the quality of interpretation and the results are heavily operator dependent.

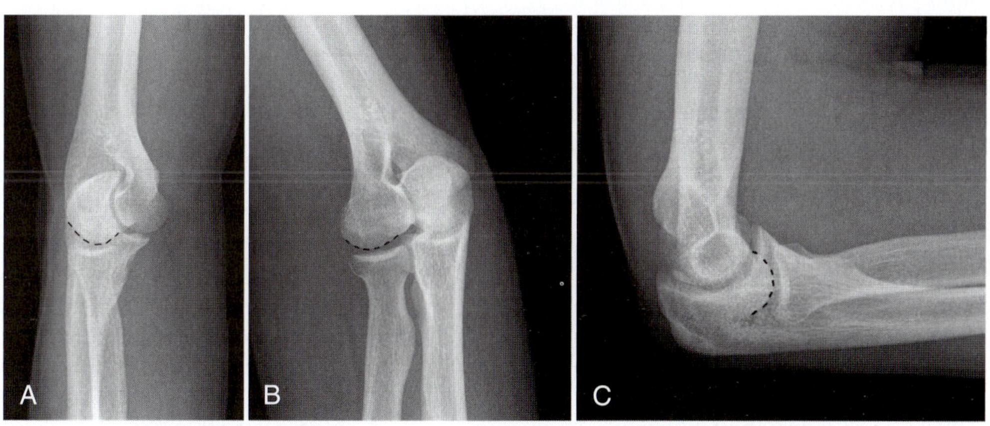

Figure 4–16 In a normal elbow, the radiocapitellar relationship is maintained regardless of the radiographic view. A and B are oblique views and C is a lateral view demonstrating the consistent relationship of the radial head and the capitellum (*dotted line*).

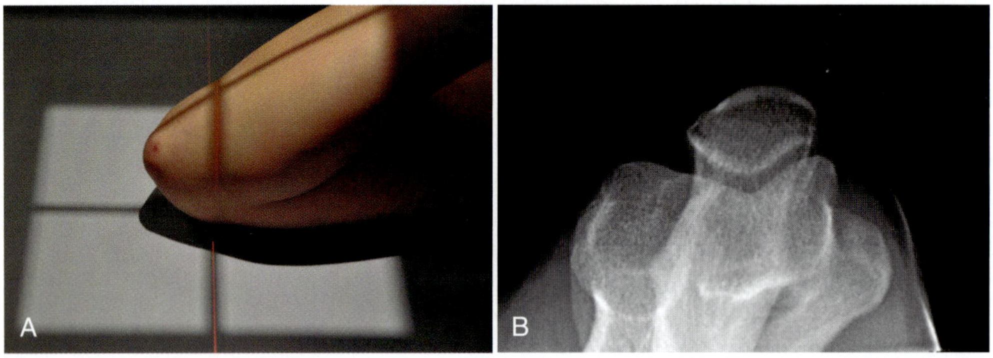

Figure 4–17 Flexion-axial radiograph of the elbow. **A**, The patient's arm is placed on the cassette, with the elbow completely flexed. The x-ray beam is perpendicular to the cassette. **B**, This sunrise view of the elbow is particularly useful for evaluation of posteromedial olecranon osteophytes. *(© Luke S. Oh, MD.)*

History, Physical Examination, and Imaging Questions

1. During which phase of throwing does a baseball pitcher with an ulnar collateral ligament injury classically demonstrate symptoms?
- A. Windup.
- B. Early cocking.
- C. Late cocking/Early acceleration.
- D. Deceleration.
- E. Follow-through.

2. Which of the following statements is FALSE?
- A. The carrying angle of an elbow cannot be accurately measured in a patient with a flexion contracture because the carrying angle becomes angulated toward valgus with flexion.
- B. Asymptomatic pitchers may have an increased carrying angle and a flexion contracture in the throwing elbow that do not affect their performance.
- C. If pain in the medial elbow during throwing is experienced outside the late cocking and early acceleration phases, the ulnar collateral ligament is not the source of pathology.
- D. Palpation of the ulnar collateral ligament is easier when the elbow is flexed to 60 to 70°, because this position allows the medial-sided muscle mass to move anteriorly and away from anterior bundle of the MCL complex.
- E. "Loose" bodies seen on imaging studies may not truly be loose and floating in the joint but may be tethered or adhered to surrounding soft tissues.

■

Medial-Sided Elbow Pain

Ulnar Collateral Ligament Insufficiency

- The anterior band of the MCL complex is the primary passive stabilizer to valgus stress during the throwing motion. (The flexor-pronator muscles and shoulder internal rotators are the primary dynamic stabilizers.) High tensile stresses across the medial aspect of the elbow during the acceleration phase of throwing may result in partial or complete tear of the UCL.
- Occasionally, acute ruptures of the UCL may be associated with a "pop" felt at the medial elbow. These "acute" injuries are more accurately described as acute-on-chronic conditions, in which the UCL tear occurs on an already attenuated ligament.
- More commonly, UCL injuries are associated not with a "pop" but with an insidious onset of pain accompanied by declining performance. Pain arising from the UCL occurs at the point of maximal valgus torque in the elbow during the late cocking and early acceleration phases of throwing. Pain that occurs during other phases of throwing is not attributable to UCL pathology.
- Thorough and careful history and physical examination are important in making an accurate diagnosis as well as to identify any associated injuries that may affect treatment and prognosis.
- In addition to the comprehensive elbow examination outlined previously, special provocative tests aid in the diagnosis of UCL insufficiency.

❑ Special Diagnostic Tests

Static Valgus Stress Test
- Performed with the elbow at 30° of flexion and the forearm fully pronated (Fig. 4–18).
- Because of guarding, it is difficult to assess subtle instability with this maneuver in the office setting. Use of fluoroscopy in the office allows detection of any subtle instability in the awake patient. Fluoroscopic examination with the use of anesthesia provides the most reliable information about elbow stability.
- Most UCL injuries, however, are not associated with frank instability with static valgus stress testing.

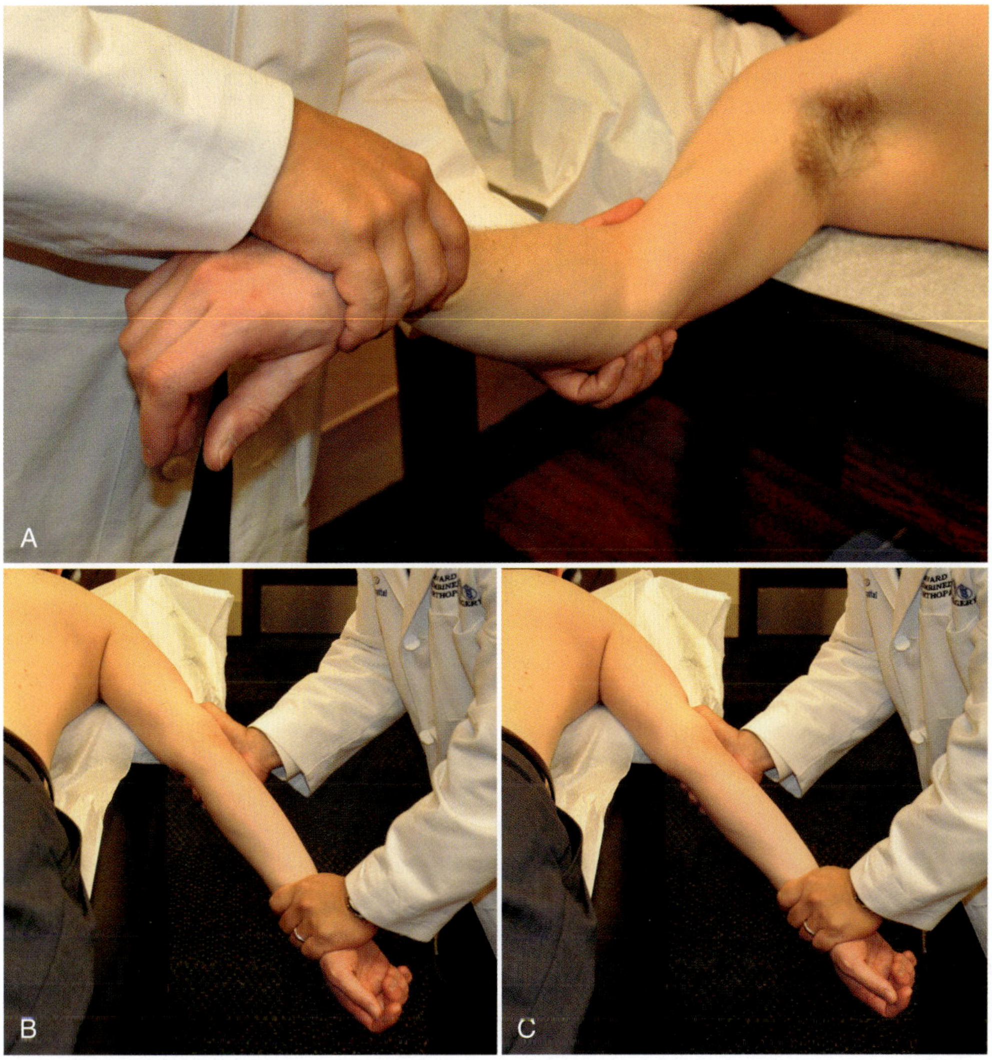

Figure 4–18 A, Supine static valgus stress test performed with the elbow at 30° of flexion and the forearm fully pronation. B and C, To counteract the rotation of the shoulder and humerus created by the forearm pronation, the static valgus stress test performed in the prone positions is advantageous. *(© Luke S. Oh, MD.)*

- Even in the absence of clinical instability with static valgus stress testing, this maneuver may reproduce the medial-sided elbow pain experienced during throwing.
- In an athlete with UCL injury who has been resting the elbow and undergoing conservative treatment, this maneuver may not elicit pain.

Milking Maneuver of O'Brien

- Although the diagram in Figure 4–19 demonstrates an examiner performing the milking maneuver, the original description of this diagnostic maneuver had the patient, not the examiner, apply a static valgus stress by reaching under a flexed elbow and pulling the thumb laterally; a positive result is pain elicited by the maneuver.
- The milking maneuver has been proposed to elicit medial-sided elbow pain from an injured UCL more reliably than the static

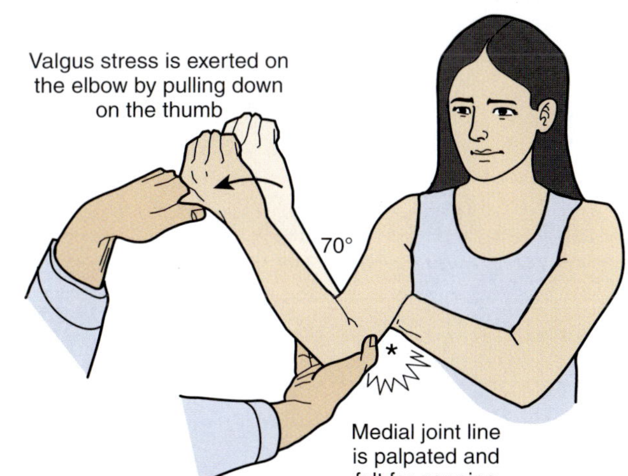

Figure 4–19 Milking maneuver of O'Brien. A positive result is pain (*) at the UCL elicited by the maneuver. *(From Safran M, Ahmad CS, ElAttrache NS: Ulnar collateral ligament of the elbow. Arthroscopy 2005;21:1381.)*

valgus stress test. However, this maneuver may not detect pain generated by UCL injury in patients who have pain only with the addition of shear forces involved in the throwing motion to the valgus torque.

Moving Valgus Stress Test

- Originally described by O'Driscoll and considered to be more reliable in reproducing medial elbow pain arising from UCL pathology, because it recreates not only the valgus stress but also the internal shear stress experienced by the UCL during the throwing motion.
- The moving valgus stress test (MVST) begins with the patient's shoulder abducted to 90° and the elbow at full flexion. While stabilizing the humerus and applying a constant valgus torque to the elbow, the examiner extends the elbow. The patient with UCL pathology experiences maximum pain and/or apprehension as the elbow moves from a flexion angle of 120° to 70°, referred to as the "shear angle." The moving valgus stress test is highly sensitive (100%) and specific (75%) (Fig. 4–20).

❑ Clinical Decision-Making Algorithm for Ulnar Collateral Ligament Injury

- The MVST plays an important role in determining whether or not the UCL is symptomatic (Fig. 4–21).
- UCL injuries occur in a spectrum that may be characterized by three stages:
  - Stage 1: Debonding:
    - Presence of pain without laxity with valgus stress as seen via the arthroscope, except if patient has had asymptomatic laxity as a baseline condition (Fig. 4–22).
  - Stage 2: Partial tear:
    - Pain with mild laxity resulting from chronic attenuation of the UCL.
  - Stage 3: Complete tear:
    - Usually results from an acute-on-chronic rupture of an already attenuated UCL.

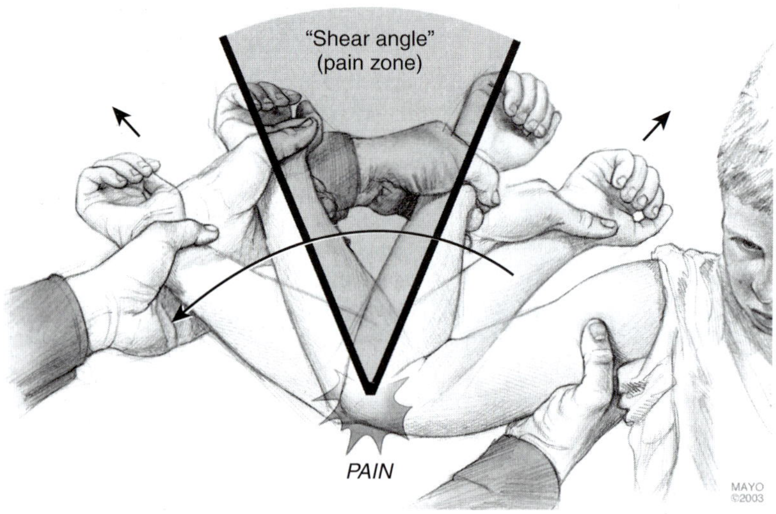

Figure 4–20 Moving valgus stress test. *(With permission from Mayo Foundation for Medical Education and Research. All rights reserved.)*

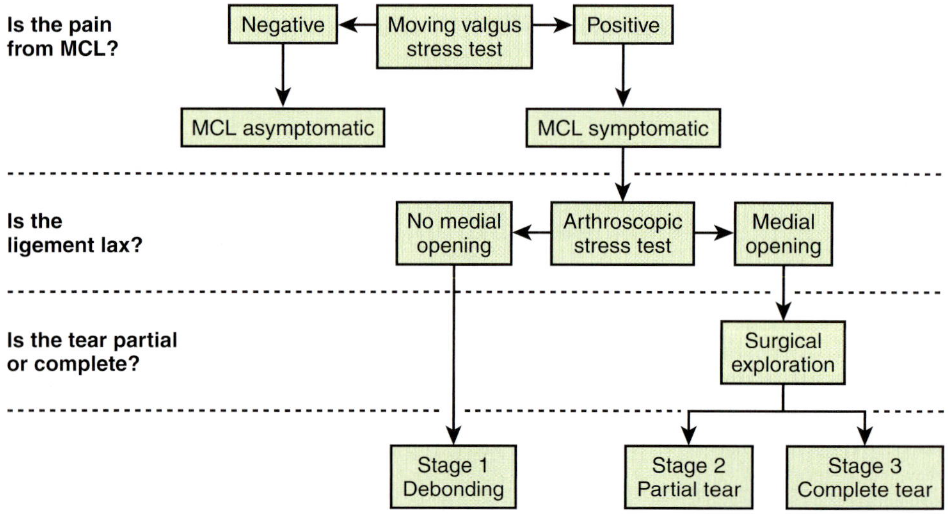

Figure 4–21 The moving valgus stress test plays an important role in determining whether or not the medial collateral ligament (MCL) is symptomatic. *(From Smith AM, O'Driscoll SW: Diagnosing medial elbow pain in throwers. J Musculoskeletal Med 2005;22:305-316.)*

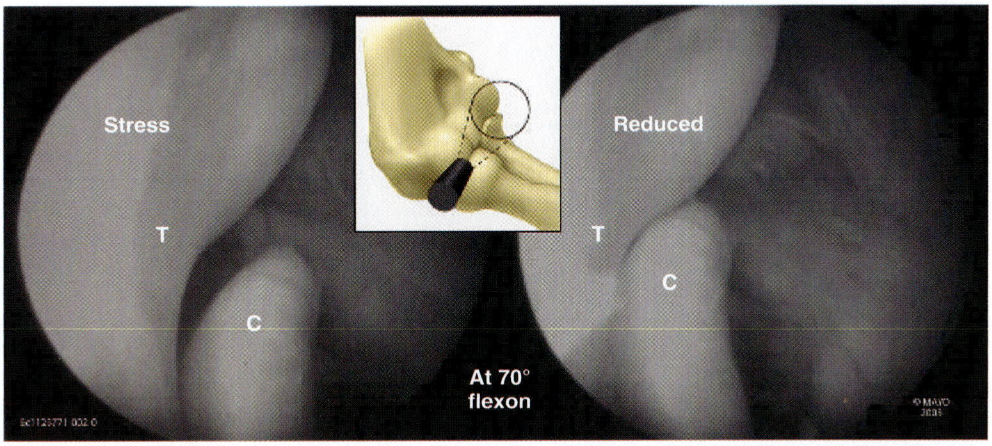

Figure 4–22 Positive arthroscopic stress test result. *Inset,* An arthroscope is placed in the proximal anterolateral portal of the elbow and directed to the medial ulnohumeral joint with the elbow flexed to 70°. *Left,* If the medial collateral ligament is incompetent, valgus stress results in medial ulnar humeral joint opening and is indicated by the gap between the coronoid (C) and the medial trochlea (T). *Right,* With relaxation of the valgus stress, the elbow reduces and the gap disappears (*right*). *(With permission from Mayo Foundation for Medical Education and Research. All rights reserved.)*

❑ Imaging

Plain Radiographs

- Findings frequently normal.
- Possible osteophytes, loose bodies, or changes consistent with early arthritis.
- Possible calcifications in the MCL.

Stress Radiographs

- Not standardized.
- Difficult to interpret because many asymptomatic baseball pitchers have laxity with valgus stress (Fig. 4–23).

Magnetic Resonance Imaging

- Given the greater strength of magnets in the newer magnetic resonance imaging (MRI) machines as well as the increasing number of highly skilled musculoskeletal radiologists, the use of intraarticular contrast is becoming less common. However, in high-level throwing athletes, my preference is to use intraarticular contrast (Fig. 4–24).

❑ Treatment

Conservative

- Rehabilitation and activity modification are recommended as the initial course of treatment.
- It is important to include strengthening of the flexor-pronator muscle group and shoulder musculature in the coordinated rehabilitation program.

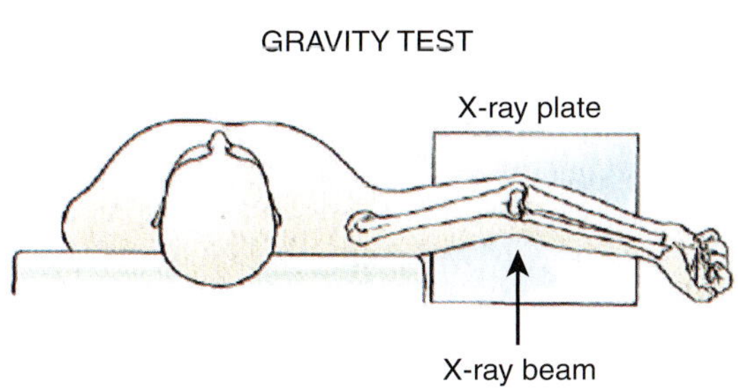

Figure 4–23 Obtaining the gravity stress radiograph. *(Redrawn from Woods GW, Tullos HS, King JW: Elbow instability and medial epicondyle fractures. Am J Sports Med 1977;5:23.)*

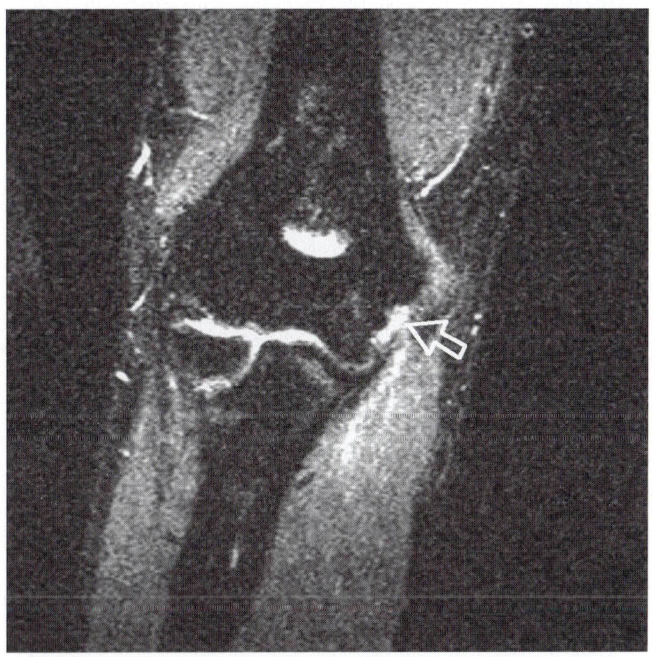

Figure 4–24 Magnetic resonance image with *arrow* indicating ulnar collateral ligament tear. *(© Luke S. Oh, MD.)*

Surgical Repair

- Primary repair of the UCL should not be considered in the throwing athlete.
- Primary repair is appropriate only for the patient with an acute traumatic avulsion of the UCL (due, for example, to weight lifting, wrestling, or mixed martial arts). Beware that in some cases the entire flexor-pronator group may be avulsed in addition to a complete tear of the UCL.

Surgical Reconstruction

- Nonthrowing athletes and some throwing athletes can successfully return to athletic competition without surgical reconstruction.

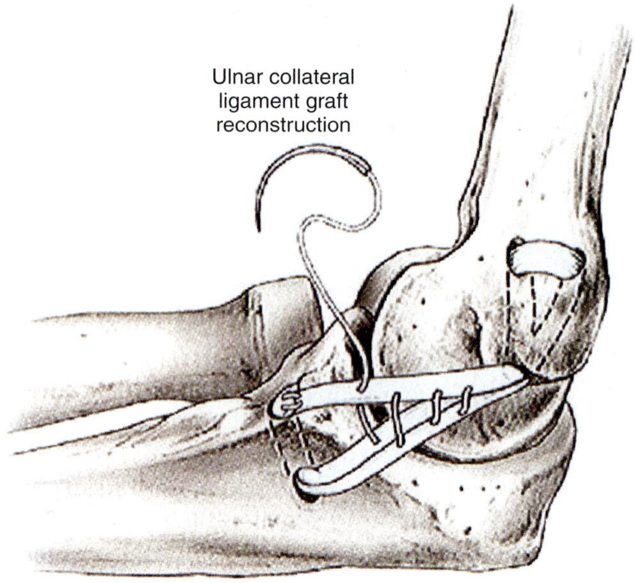

Figure 4–25 Classic Jobe ulnar collateral ligament reconstruction. *(Redrawn from Safran M, Ahmad CS, ElAttrache NS: Ulnar collateral ligament of the elbow. Arthroscopy 2005;21:1381.)*

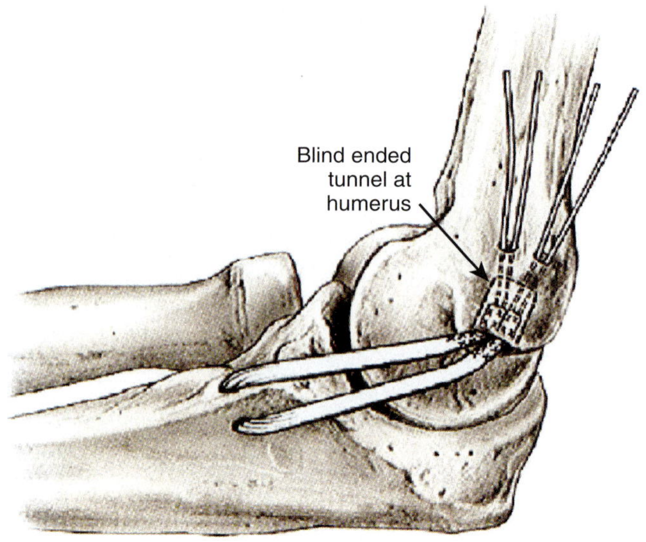

Figure 4–26 Altchek described the "docking" procedure, in which a humeral tunnel is created that would be able to accept the two free ends of the graft after it has been passed through the ulnar tunnel. Sutures on the ends of the graft are passed through drill holes and tied over the bone bridge. The docking technique creates a humeral tunnel that accepts both limbs of the graft, with tensioning performed through superior exit holes. *(From Safran M, Ahmad CS, ElAttrache NS: Ulnar collateral ligament of the elbow. Arthroscopy 2005;21:1381-1395.)*

However, elite throwers are rarely able to perform at the same competitive level. In patients for whom conservative treatment failed, surgical reconstruction may be considered.

- Various techniques have been reported in the literature. All employ a free tendon graft, whether it be palmaris longus autograft, gracilis autograft, or plantaris allograft.
- The original technique described by Jobe wove the tendon graft in a figure-of-8 fashion and sutured it onto itself (Fig. 4–25) (Jobe, 1986).
- Rohrbough et al (2002) described the "docking" procedure, in which a humeral tunnel was created that would be able to accept the two free ends of the graft after it had been passed through the ulnar tunnel. Sutures on the ends of the graft were passed through drill holes and tied over the bone bridge (Fig. 4–26).
- A new technique called the David Altchek Neal ElAttrache Tommy John (DANE TJ) uses interference screw fixation on the ulnar side and the docking technique on the humeral side. This technique is particularly useful in cases of fracture of the sublime tubercle or in the revision setting (Fig. 4–27) (Dines et al, 2007).
- In addition to the method of graft configuration and fixation, there are also different surgical approaches:
  - Early techniques accessed the surgical site via transection of the flexor-pronator origin and performance of a routine transposition of the ulnar nerve.

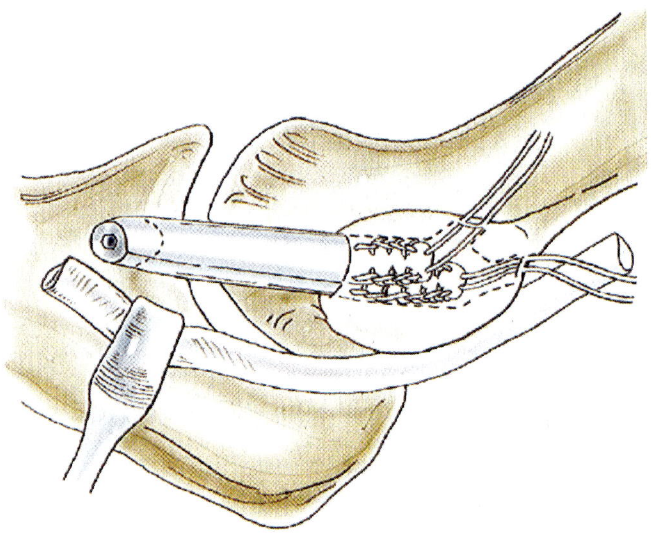

Figure 4–27 Interference screw fixation technique. *(Redrawn from Conway JE: The DANE TJ procedure for elbow medial ulnar collateral ligament insufficiency. Tech Shoulder Elbow Surg 2006;7:36-46.)*

  - Smith et al (1996) demonstrated the safe zone in a muscle-splitting approach that does not require routine transposition of the ulnar nerve. Moreover, not detaching the flexor-pronator origin from the medial epicondyle allows for more aggressive early range of motion (ROM) of the wrist and forearm.

Postoperative Rehabilitation

- Rehabilitation following UCL reconstruction requires a protected and progressive return of ROM during the first 6 weeks after surgery.
- Subsequently, a comprehensive exercise program for the entire upper extremity kinetic chain is initiated in order to optimize dynamic stability of the scapulothoracic, glenohumeral, and ulnohumeral joints.
- At approximately 4 months after surgery, an interval program is started beginning with a distance of 45 ft and then progressing up to 180 ft. Baseball pitchers may begin throwing off the mound at the completion of the interval program.
- After gradual progression to throwing from the mound, most athletes return to competitive pitching 9 to 12 months after surgery.

Medial Epicondylitis

- Medical epicondylitis is less common than lateral epicondylitis but has similar clinical and histologic characteristics.
- It is an overuse condition of the common flexor-pronator origin precipitated by microtears primarily in the pronator teres and flexor carpi radialis.
- Often referred to as "'golfer's elbow" because an overuse condition of the common flexor-pronator origin of the trailing elbow may develop during the golf swing as it pronates the face of the golf club at the time of impact with the golf ball.
- Overuse of the common flexor-pronator group is frequently seen in throwing athletes as well because forearm pronation protects the UCL during each throwing motion in combination with shoulder internal rotation.
- Anatomically, a significant portion of the deep surface of the common flexor tenon is adhered and structurally bonded to the underlying MCL.
  - Therefore, the common flexor tendon experiences valgus stresses similar to those on the UCL during throwing.

❑ Physical Examination

- In medial epicondylitis, physical examination demonstrates tenderness at the common flexor origin, the classic location being anterior and slightly distal to the medial epicondyle with the elbow flexed to 90°. Also, pain can be elicited with resisted pronation or flexion of the wrist.
- Differentiation of pain due to tendinitis of the common flexor-pronator group from pain due to UCL pathology is based on the use of selective provocative physical examination maneuvers. Provocative testing of the common flexor-pronator group does not involve valgus stress, whereas provocative testing of the UCL via the MVST involves applying a constant valgus stress.

Medial Tennis Elbow Shear Test

- O'Driscoll previously described the medial tennis elbow shear test (medial TEST) as having much higher sensitivity and specificity than isolated resistance testing of either wrist pronation or wrist flexion (Fig. 4–28).
- The test is performed by first asking the patient to fully flex the elbow, pronate the forearm, and flex the wrist. The examiner then uses both hands to apply resistance to wrist flexion and forearm pronation, and asks the patient to quickly extend the elbow as if throwing a punch.
- The result is considered to be positive if this provocative maneuver reproduces the patient's medial elbow pain at the common flexor-pronator origin.

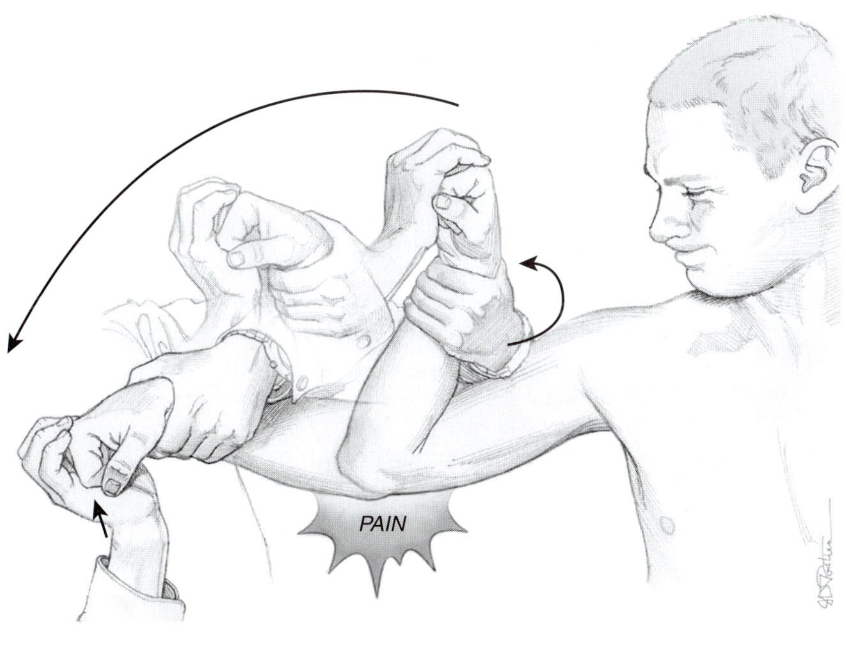

Figure 4–28 The medial tennis elbow shear test (medial TEST) has much higher sensitivity and specificity than isolated resistance testing of either wrist pronation or wrist flexion. *(With permission from Mayo Foundation for Medical Education and Research. All rights reserved.)*

- The high sensitivity and specificity of this maneuver are thought to be due to reproduction of internal shear forces within the common flexor-pronator tendon that cause pain, similar to the manner in which the MVST generates internal shear stress within the UCL that elicits pain.

❑ Treatment
- Nonoperative management is the mainstay of treatment for medial epicondylitis.
- Activity modification and rest are important components of nonoperative management, in addition to oral nonsteroidal anti-inflammatory drugs (NSAIDs), counterforce bracing, and corticosteroid injections.
- Beware of applying ice to the medial elbow. There have been reports of patients who sustained ulnar nerve injury from prolonged application of ice over a large region of the medial elbow.
- Surgery may be considered in patients with recalcitrant medial epicondylitis in whom an extensive period of nonoperative treatment, including avoidance of activities that exacerbate symptoms, has failed.

❑ Ulnar Neuritis
- Ulnar nerve symptoms may manifest as localized pain with paresthesias in the ring and pinky fingers during throwing. More severe involvement may result in pain at rest, diminished sensation along the ulnar nerve distribution, reduced grip strength, atrophy of the interossei, and progressive functional loss.
- Etiology of ulnar nerve injury in the throwing athlete can be attributed to three general types of pathology:
  - Compression, at five classic anatomic areas in the elbow:
    - Arcade of Struthers.
    - Medial intermuscular septum.
    - Cubital tunnel.
    - Fascial origin of the flexor digitorum superficialis.
    - Confluence of the two heads of the flexor carpi ulnaris.
  - Space-occupying lesions:
    - Osteophytes in the cubital tunnel.
    - Thickening of the arcuate ligament.
    - Calcifications of the MCL.
    - Hypertrophy of the medial head of the triceps.
  - Friction:
    - Subluxating ulnar nerve with or without concomitant subluxating medial triceps.
  - Traction:
    - UCL insufficiency and laxity with medial opening of the ulnohumeral joint during throwing may cause a traction injury to the ulnar nerve.
- Irritation of the ulnar nerve may occur in isolation or in combination with other pathology in the medial elbow. Other associated pathology should be treated appropriately and separately from the ulnar neuritis.
- For the patient with isolated ulnar neuritis in whom conservative treatment fails, surgical treatment is indicated. There have been comparable results among the various surgical techniques used in the treatment of ulnar neuropathy.

Subluxating Medial Triceps

- Presenting symptom is medial elbow pain with a snapping sensation when the elbow is flexed more than 90°. Typically observed in the individual with above-average muscle mass, such as a weight-lifter or throwing athlete.
- The pathomechanics of this condition is due to triceps hypertrophy from weight lifting that causes the medial triceps to flare "outward" (i.e., more medially) and necessarily causes subluxation or dislocation of the ulnar nerve. Therefore, in patients with a subluxating medial triceps, careful examination will actually demonstrate two snapping sensations.
- Examination maneuver:
  - The maneuver is best performed with the examiner facing the patient's lateral elbow and palpating the ulnar nerve with the hand closer to the patient's shoulder (Fig. 4–29).
  - With the other hand, the examiner holds the forearm and applies resistance while the patient is asked to actively contract the triceps but to allow the examiner to overcome the patient's active elbow extension, similar to the performance of a "negative" triceps extension exercise.
  - When the elbow reaches approximately 90° of flexion during this eccentric loading of the triceps, the ulnar nerve subluxates and creates a palpable snap that may or may not be painful.
  - In patients with a symptomatic subluxating medial triceps, continued eccentric loading and flexion of the elbow to approximately 120° result in a second palpable snap that is caused by the subluxating medial triceps and is painful.
- Proper diagnosis of this condition had been frequently missed in the past because the snapping sensation in the medial elbow had been attributed to an isolated subluxation of the ulnar nerve.
  - Misdiagnosed patients who undergo an ulnar nerve transposition experience no improvement in symptoms.
  - The appropriate treatment is to perform an excision of the subluxating portion of the distal medial triceps in addition to addressing the ulnar nerve, if symptomatic (Fig. 4–30).
- Because subluxation of the medial triceps is always associated with subluxation or

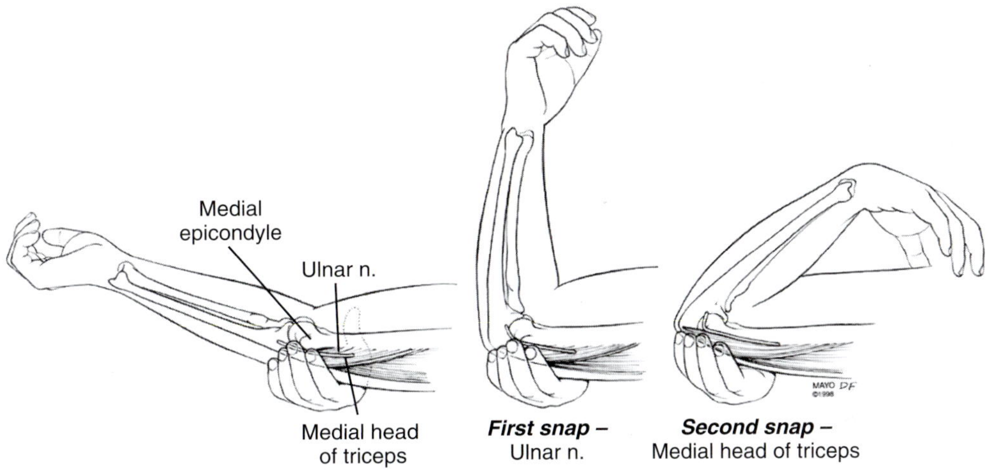

Figure 4–29 Diagnosis of Subluxating Medial Triceps. While palpating the ulnar nerve, the patient is asked to provide resistance while the examiner flexed the elbow. Two separate "snaps" (either audible or palpable sensation) will be present in patients with a subluxating medial triceps. At approximately 90° of flexion, the ulnar nerve will subluxate over the medial epicondyle. At approximately 120° of flexion, the distal medial triceps will subluxate over the medial epicondyle. *(With permission from Mayo Foundation for Medical Education and Research. All rights reserved.)*

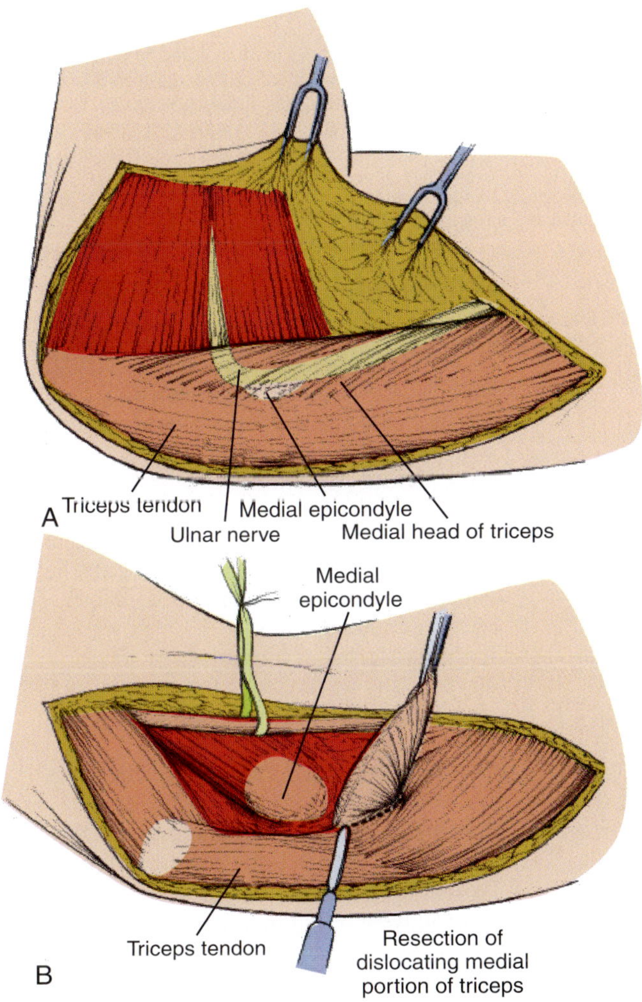

Figure 4–30 Treatment of Subluxating Medial Triceps. **A**, An artist's rendition of an overhanging medial triceps. Misdiagnosed patients who undergo an isolated ulnar nerve transposition will not have relief of symptoms from the subluxating medial triceps. **B**, The appropriate treatment is to perform an excision of the subluxating portion of the distal medial triceps. If the ulnar nerve is symptomatic, then an ulnar nerve transposition may be performed at the same time. *(From Spinner RJ, Goldner RD: Snapping of the medial head of the triceps and recurrent dislocation of the ulnar nerve: Anatomical and dynamic factors. J Bone Joint Surg Am 1998;80:239–247.)*

dislocation of the ulnar nerve, examination for both conditions should be performed when either one is suspected. Depending on severity and/or chronicity of the problem, a patient may have both a painful subluxating medial triceps and ulnar neuritis.

- In addition, symptomatic medial triceps subluxation may occur in combination with a UCL injury, and may be a reason for continued medial elbow pain after an otherwise successful ligament reconstruction.

Medial-Sided Elbow Pain Questions

1. Which of the following statements is/are TRUE?
   A. Both the moving valgus stress test and the medial tennis elbow shear test incorporate application of a valgus stress to the elbow.
   B. Both the moving valgus stress test and the medial tennis elbow shear test incorporate application of shear stress to the elbow.
   C. Both the moving valgus stress test and the medial tennis elbow shear test have a low sensitivity but a high specificity.
   D. The milking maneuver has been proposed to elicit medial-sided elbow pain from an injured UCL more reliably than the static valgus stress test, because the maneuver generates internal shear stress within the ligament.
   E. Subluxation of the medial triceps may not necessarily cause subluxation of the ulnar nerve.

2. An amateur bodybuilder requests a second opinion after having undergone a subcutaneous ulnar nerve transposition performed by another surgeon for a documented dislocating ulnar nerve without ulnar neuropathy. The procedure did not improve the patient's preoperative symptom of painful snapping in the medial elbow at approximately 120° of flexion. Findings of preoperative electromyography (EMG) and

MRI were normal. Which of the following statements about this case is TRUE?

A. If the ulnar nerve transposition had been performed with stabilization of the nerve with fascial slings, the likelihood of this outcome may have been significantly reduced.
B. The patient would benefit most from a revision submuscular ulnar nerve transposition at this time.
C. A second EMG should be ordered because there may now be findings that were not detectable at the time of the preoperative EMG.
D. A diagnostic arthroscopy of the elbow will most likely identify the pathology causing the painful snapping.
E. An open resection of the subluxating medial triceps is indicated.

Lateral-Sided Elbow Pain

Lateral Epicondylitis

- Most common affliction of the elbow, and at least five times more common than medial epicondylitis.
- Overuse injury characterized by pain with resisted wrist extension (e.g., tennis backhand, removing laptop from its bag).
- Frequently affects patients in the fourth and fifth decades of life.
- For tennis players, risk factors include poor backhand technique, a heavy racket, inappropriate grip size, and a racket that is too tightly strung.
- Tenderness located approximately 5 mm distal and anterior to the lateral tip of the epicondyle.
- Classically involves the extensor carpi radialis brevis (ECRB), but may involve the EDC in 50% of cases. Involvement of the extensor carpi radialis longus (ECRL) and extensor carpi ulnaris (ECU) is less common (Fig. 4–31).
- In chronic conditions, *epicondylosis* may be more appropriate term than *epicondylitis*. Pathologic specimens removed during open surgery in chronic cases reveal few inflammatory cells. Rather, there is presence of tendon degeneration characterized by fibroblasts and vascular granulation–like tissue called "angiofibroblastic hyperplasia."
- Radiographic findings are typically normal, but may demonstrate some calcific deposits at the extensor tendon origin.
- MRI is rarely needed to make a diagnosis of lateral epicondylitis/epicondylosis but may be helpful to evaluate for possible concomitant pathology in the lateral elbow.

❑ Initial Treatment

- Activity modification and avoidance of activities that exacerbate the condition, particularly repetitive wrist extension and vibration.
- NSAIDs.

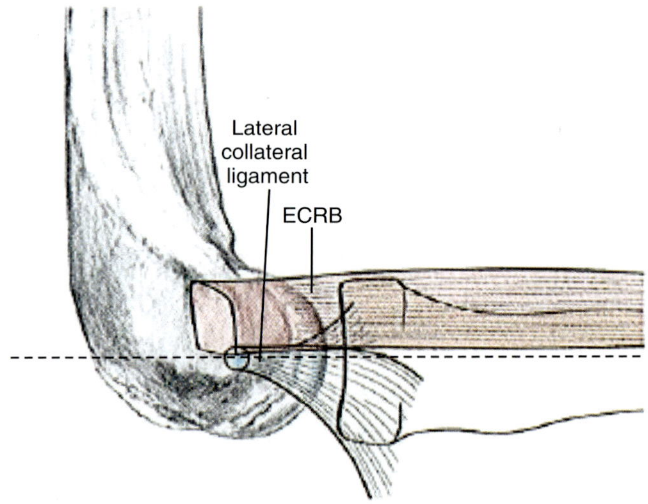

Figure 4–31 Schematic diagram depicting the relationship between the extensor carpi radialis brevis (ECRB) origin at the humerus and the bony landmarks. Note that the ECRB footprint origin is diamond shaped and located between the midline of the joint and the top of the humeral capitellum, beneath the most distal extent of the supracondylar ridge. The tendon does not originate on the epicondyle specifically. Note the relationship between the ECRB origin and the underlying lateral collateral ligament. *(From Cohen MS, Romeo AA: Advanced Techniques: Arthroscopic management of lateral epicondylitis. In Morrey BF, Sanchez-Sotelo J [eds]: The Elbow and Its Disorders, 4th ed. Philadelphia, Saunders Elsevier, 2009, p 611.)*

- Ice.
- Physical therapy:
  - Fatigue of the wrist extensors is implicated as a contributing factor; therefore, a physical therapy program includes gradual strengthening of the wrist extensors along with management of symptoms.
- Corticosteroid injections:
  - Useful in cases in which symptoms are difficult to manage with preceding modalities.
  - Care must be taken not to inject into the substance of extensor tendon, to avoid tendon attenuation.
  - If corticosteroid is administered too superficially in the subcutaneous tissues, skin discoloration and/or atrophy of subcutaneous tissues may result.
  - Transient posterior interosseous nerve (PIN) palsy may be observed if local anesthetic used in combination with the corticosteroid injection seeps through the tissues to reach the nerve.
  - Although there is no real scientific basis for either the safety or the efficacy of repeated corticosteroid injections, use of no more than three corticosteroid injections is recommended as a general rule.
- Counterforce bracing is controversial:
  - Proponents state that bracing reduces extensor muscle fatigue by limiting extensor muscle belly expansion and thereby distributing the force created by wrist extension throughout the muscle belly rather than concentrating the force at the extensor origin.

- Opponents of bracing have encountered patients in whom radial tunnel syndrome developed as a result of using a brace, in whom symptoms were more severe and prolonged than those experienced with lateral epicondylitis.

❑ Surgery

- Surgical intervention may be warranted in patients in whom a coordinated rehabilitation program with various modalities as well as activity modification has failed.
- Some surgeons offer surgery as an option only if the patient has had recalcitrant lateral epicondylitis/epicondylosis for at least a year, because of the understanding that the vast majority of patients with lateral epicondylitis obtain resolution of symptoms from conservative treatment after about a year. Other surgeons offer surgical intervention if there has been no improvement in symptoms after 3 months of conservative treatment.
- The goal of surgery is to remove pathologic tissue.
- Superiority of open or arthroscopic approach is controversial. No clear evidence in the literature demonstrates superiority of one approach over another. Existing reports suggest similar outcome with either approach, with a faster recovery time for the arthroscopic technique.
- Arthroscopic technique may be preferred if there is concern for possible concomitant intra-articular pathology that may need to be evaluated further, such as synovial plicae or early degenerative changes in the radiocapitellar joint.
- Postoperative rehabilitation should include appropriate time for rest and healing; premature return to work or sports should be avoided.

Surgical Complications

- Iatrogenic injury to the LUCL:
  - The LUCL is located posterior to the equator of the radial head, or "below" the equator, when the elbow is flexed to 90 degrees.
  - Iatrogenic release of the LUCL results in posterolateral rotatory instability.
- Incomplete resection of pathology.
  - Inadequate excision of the pathologic tissue at the time of surgery for lateral epicondylitis is associated with poorer outcomes.

Radial Tunnel Syndrome

- Radial nerve entrapment should always be included in the differential diagnosis of lateral epicondylitis.
- Is a more difficult diagnosis to establish than that of lateral epicondylitis. Beware that failed treatment for lateral epicondylitis may be due to misdiagnosis of radial tunnel syndrome or failure to recognize presence of concomitant lateral epicondylitis and radial tunnel syndrome.
- Classic presentation is lateral elbow pain that radiates distally during active forearm rotation. There may be weakness in extension of the elbow and/or wrist; however, there is no sensory deficit.
- Examination reveals tenderness to be more distal than the classic location in lateral epicondylitis.
- Nerve dysfunction may be evaluated with an EMG or nerve conduction study.
- Sites of entrapment:
  - Arcade of Frohse: Midportion of the supinator as the posterior interosseus nerve exits the supinator.
  - Leash of Henry: Radial recurrent vessels.
  - Although the arcade of Frohse and leash of Henry are the classic anatomic sites of entrapment, ganglion cysts or synovitis at the radiocapitellar joint may also cause symptoms of radial tunnel syndrome.
  - Other causes of injury to the radial nerve/PIN are misguided placement of screws during radial head fixation and excessively tight tennis elbow braces.
- Treatment for radial nerve entrapment initially involves activity modification, rest, and time. With failure of nonoperative treatment, surgical decompression may be considered.

Osteochondritis Dissecans

- OCD is an osteochondral lesion originally thought to involve a subchondral inflammatory process that "dissects" a fragment of cartilage with subsequent formation of a loose body. Although no true association with an inflammatory process has been identified, the name remains unchanged.
- Commonly seen in gymnasts and throwing athletes older than 10 years, most commonly in those 10 to 16 years old.
- Etiology thought to be ischemia, trauma, genetic predisposition, or a combination thereof.
- Vascularity of the distal humerus is limited in adolescents. No metaphyseal vessels cross the physis to supply the epiphysis. Instead, a limited number of vessels enter the epiphysis directly. Repetitive valgus loading of the elbow in adolescent throwing athletes may compress the epiphysis of the capitellum and injure the vessels. Histopathologic characteristics of subchondral bone have been shown to be consistent with avascular necrosis.

- Treatment is dictated by clinical findings and the radiographic appearance of the lesion.
- If the lesion is stable without evidence of displacement or fracture of the articular cartilage, nonoperative treatment with activity modification and anti-inflammatory drugs is recommended. Depending on the patient's age, the potential for noncompliance with treatment recommendations, and the severity of symptoms, a brace, splint, or a cast may be indicated.
- If the lesion is unstable, surgical treatment may be required:
  - Mechanical symptoms or locking may suggest presence of loose bodies that require arthroscopic removal. Osteochondral fragments that are either partially detached or at risk for displacement may require excision or surgical fixation with K-wires, Herbert screws, or bioabsorbable implants.
  - A defect in the capitellum may require curettage, microfracture, or anterograde/retrograde drilling with or without bone grafting (Fig. 4–32).

Panner Disease (Fig. 4–33)

- Panner disease is osteochondrosis of capitellum in children younger than 10 years and most commonly between 4 and 8 years.
- Clinical and radiographic manifestations may be similar to those of OCD, but Panner disease is a self-limited condition that resolves with nonoperative treatment and watchful waiting.
- Natural history is favorable, with no residual deformity or long-term sequelae expected.

Snapping Synovial Plicae

- Painful snapping in the posterolateral or anterolateral elbow may be caused by hypertrophic synovial folds (thought to be remnants of the embryonic septae) of the radiocapitellar joint and associated localized synovitis (Fig. 4–34). Symptoms may mimic those of lateral epicondylitis.
- Flexion-pronation test:
  - Painful snapping is elicited with passive flexion between 90 and 110° of flexion with the forearm in pronation.

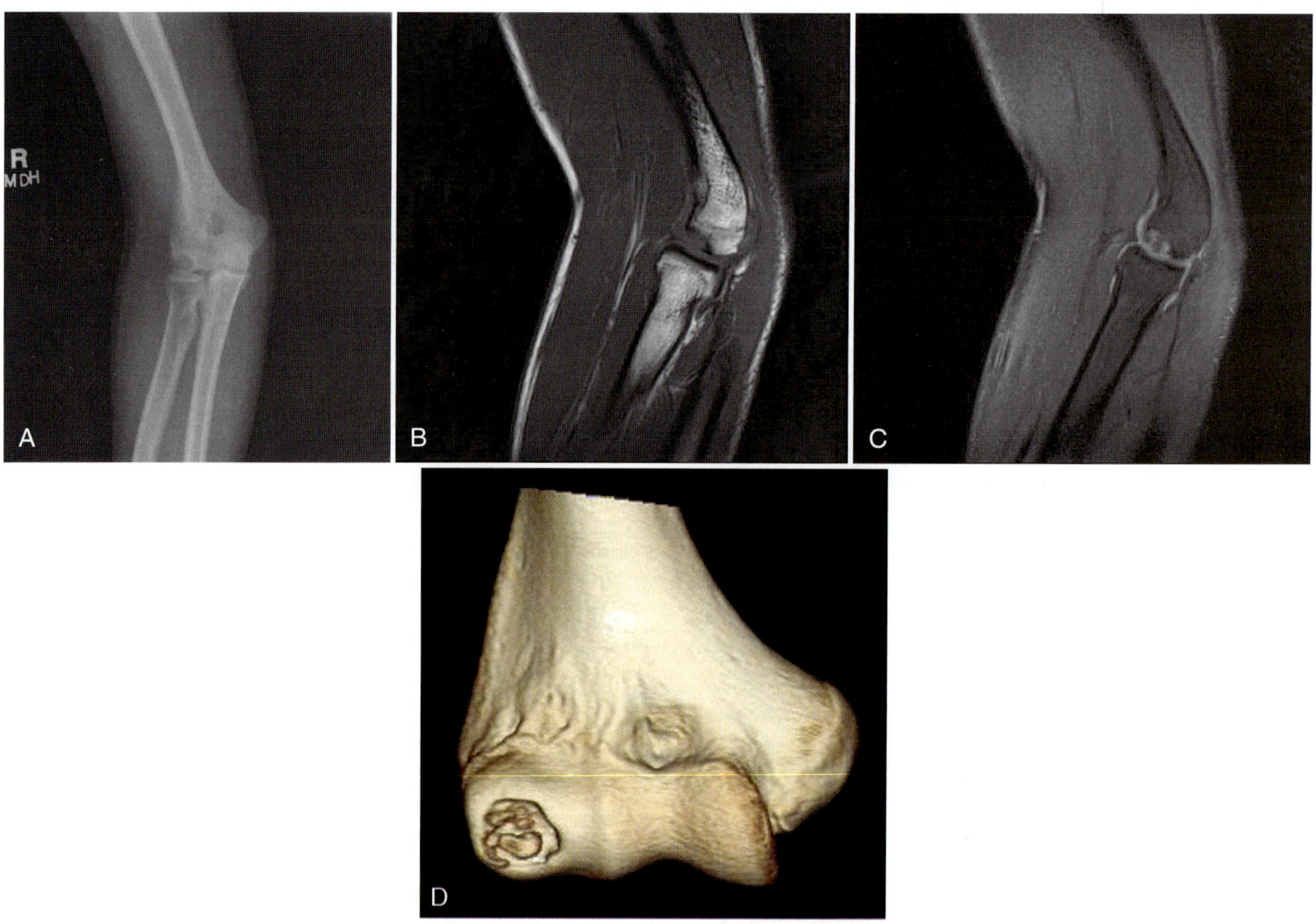

Figure 4–32 Imaging Studies for Osteochondritis Dissecans. **A,** Plan radiograph demonstrates lucency in the capitellum. **B** and **C,** Magnetic resonance imaging of the same lesion as seen on T1 and T2 sequences, respectively. **D,** Computed tomography with 3-D reconstruction demonstrates the fragmentation of the OCD lesion better than other imaging modalities. *(© Luke S. Oh, MD.)*

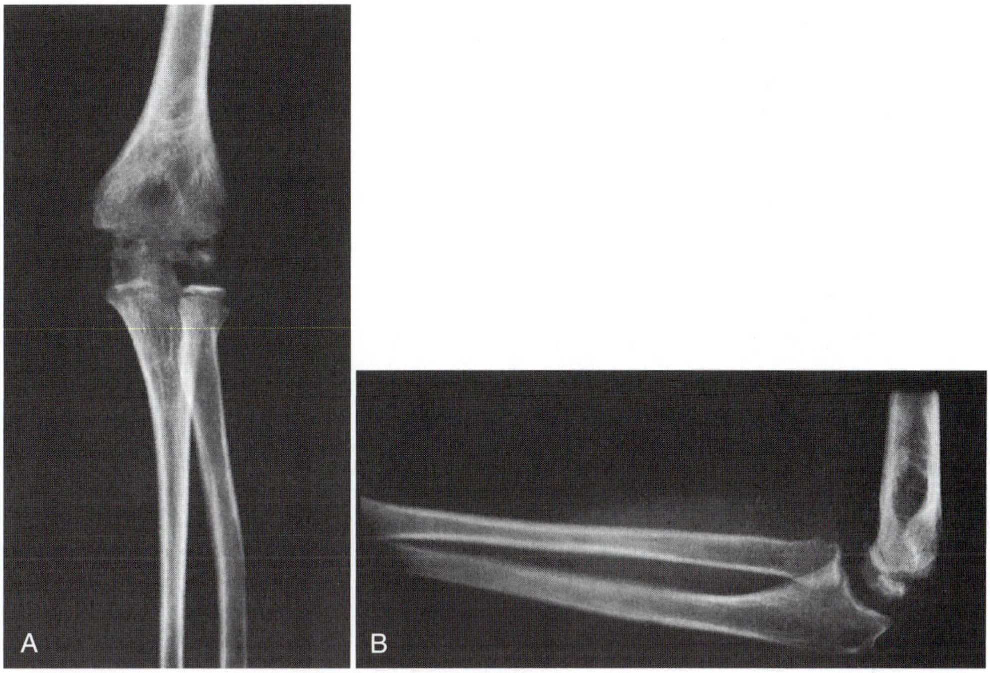

Figure 4–33 Panner disease is an osteochondrosis of the capitellum in children younger than 10 years that resolves with nonoperative treatment. The radiographic findings may be similar to those of osteochondritis dissecans. *(From Shaughnessy W: Osteochondritis Dissecans. In Morrey BF, Sanchez-Sotelo J [eds]: The Elbow and Its Disorders. Philadelphia, Saunders Elsevier, 2009, p 289.)*

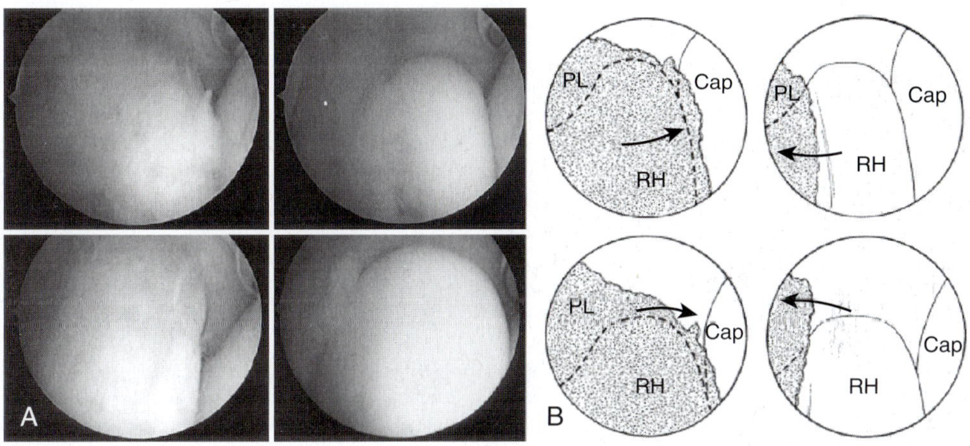

Figure 4–34 Arthroscopic (**A**) and schematic (**B**) views of the plica (PL) falling into the radiohumeral articulation (RH) with extension and retracting back with flexion. Cap, capitellum. *(From O'Driscoll SW, Morrey BF, Korinek S, An KN: Elbow subluxation and dislocation. A spectrum of instability. Clin Orthop Relat Res 1992;280:186-197.)*

- Arthroscopic findings:
  - Lateral plicae have the appearance of an inflamed and thickened extension of the annular ligament that snaps over the radial head during elbow motion (Fig. 4–35).
- Treatment: Arthroscopic excision resolves symptoms.

Posterolateral Rotatory Instability

- PLRI results from lateral collateral ligament complex insufficiency.
- It is the most common pattern of recurrent elbow instability.

❑ Spectrum of Injury
- Stage 1: PLRI:
  - Subluxation of the elbow in a posterolateral direction (Fig. 4–36).
- Stage 2: Perched subluxation:
  - Incomplete dislocation with the coronoid perched underneath the trochlea.
- Stage 3: Dislocation:
  - Complete dislocation of the elbow with the coronoid resting behind the humerus.

❑ Mechanism of Injury
- Traumatic:
  - Subluxation or dislocation.
- Chronic attrition:
  - Cubitus varus deformity.
  - Lateral epicondylitis.
  - Long-term crutch use.
- Iatrogenic:
  - Inadvertent injury to the LUCL during lateral epicondylitis surgery.
  - Repeated corticosteroid injections.

❑ Clinical Presentation
- Lateral-sided elbow pain.
  - Particularly during activities of daily living in the gravity-varus position of the elbow.

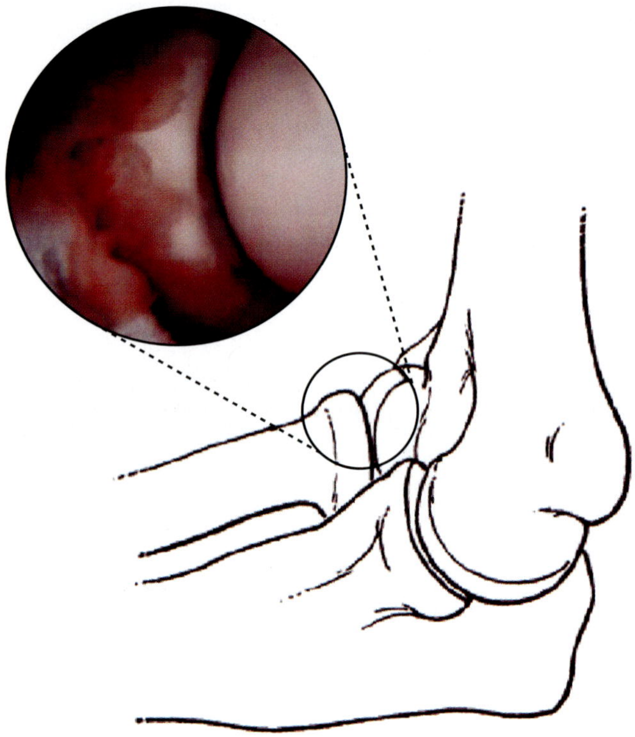

Figure 4–35 Arthroscopic (*inset*) and schematic views of the localized synovitis around the radial head which is commonly seen in cases of snapping synovial plicae. *(From Antuna SA, O'Driscoll SW: Snapping plicae associated with radiocapitellar chondromalacia. Arthroscopy 2001;17:491-495.)*

- Subjective sense of instability.
  - Giving way when push off from a chair to stand.
- Mechanical symptoms.

❑ Physical Examination

- Deformity:
  - Cubitus varus, whether post-traumatic or congenital, is a risk factor for tardy PLRI.
- Surgical incisions:
  - Prior tennis elbow surgery scars that are centered posterior to the midcoronal plane may be associated with iatrogenic sectioning of the LUCL.
- Tenderness over the LCL.
- Apprehension with varus stress:
  - Pure varus stress may cause apprehension but usually does not elicit instability, especially in an awake patient with an element of guarding in the office setting.
- Posterolateral drawer test:
  - Rotatory version of the Lachman test commonly used in the knee.
  - Depending on the patient's level of guarding, a positive result may be elicited in the office setting.
  - Best performed with the patient supine and the upper extremity raised above the patient's head:
    - Bring the shoulder to external rotation and flex the elbow.
    - Stabilize the humerus and rotate the forearm as if to pivot around the MCL while applying gentle axial compression (Fig. 4–37).
- Posterolateral pivot-shift test:
  - The most sensitive physical examination maneuver in the diagnosis of PLRI, but a positive result in the office setting in the awake patient is rare because of guarding. A positive result is most frequently elicited during examination of the patient under anesthesia.
  - Patient is positioned supine with the arm overhead. Steps in this maneuver are similar to those in the pivot shift in the knee:
    - Start with the elbow extended.
    - Supinate the forearm and apply a valgus stress to the elbow.

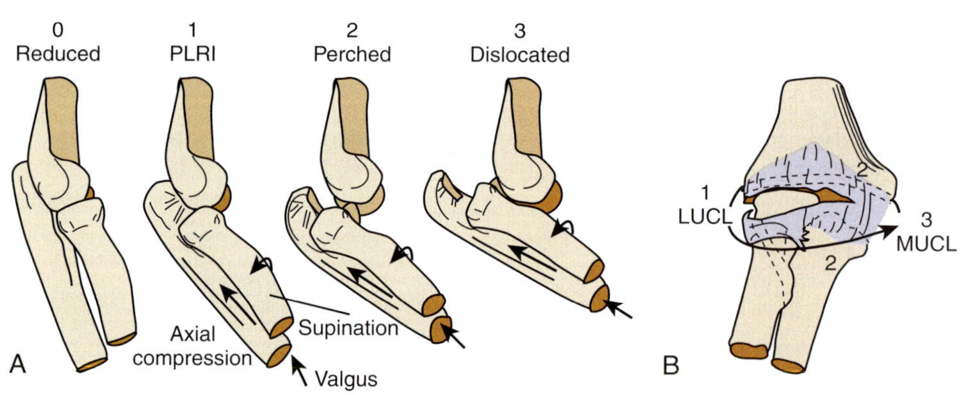

Figure 4–36 A, Elbow instability is a spectrum from subluxation to dislocation. The three stages shown correspond with the pathoanatomic stages of capsuloligamentous disruption shown in B. Forces and moments responsible for displacements are shown. B, Soft tissue injury progresses in a circle from lateral to medial in three stages correlating with those shown in A. In stage 1, the ulnar part of the lateral collateral ligament, the lateral ulnar collateral ligament (LUCL), is disrupted. In stage 2 the other lateral ligamentous structures and the anterior and posterior capsule are disrupted. In stage 3, disruption of the medial ulnar collateral ligament (MUCL) can be partial, with disruption of the posterior medial ulnar collateral ligament only (stage 3A), or complete (stage 3B). The common extensor and flexor origins also are often disrupted. PLRI, posterolateral rotatory instability. *(From O'Driscoll SW, Morrey BF, Korinek S, An KN: Elbow subluxation and dislocation. A spectrum of instability. Clin Orthop Relat Res 1992;280:186-197.)*

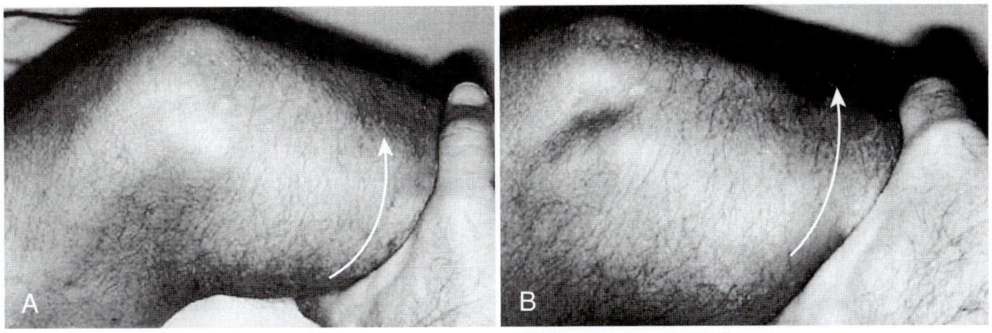

Figure 4–37 The posterolateral rotatory drawer test is similar to the drawer and Lachman tests of the knee. **A,** From the reduced position, the arm is held in the overhead position such that it resembles a leg and the elbow resembles a knee, and the shoulder is in full external rotation in preparation of displacement in the direction of the *arrow*. **B,** The lateral side of the forearm is rotated away from the humerus, pivoting around the medial collateral ligament so that the radius and ulna subluxate away from the humerus, leaving a dimple in the skin behind the radial head. *(From O'Driscoll SW, Morrey BF, Korinek S, An KN: Elbow subluxation and dislocation. A spectrum of instability. Clin Orthop Relat Res 1992;280:186-197. Used by permission of the Mayo Foundation for Medical Education and Research. All rights reserved.)*

    - Begin to flex the elbow by applying axial compression.
    - A positive result consists of a sudden clunk and rotatory shift elicited as the elbow becomes reduced during flexion (Fig. 4–38).
- Chair test:
    - Patient, who is sitting in a chair, is asked to push off on the arm rest to stand up with both forearms in supination and the arms abducted to greater than shoulder width (to apply valgus stress).
    - Apprehension, subluxation, or frank dislocation may occur as the elbow is extended, depending on the severity of the instability.
- Push-up test:
    - Patient is asked to perform an active wall or floor push-up with the arms positioned as for the chair test (forearms supinated and arms abducted to greater than shoulder width).
    - A positive result is apprehension, subluxation, or dislocation with attempted elbow extension.

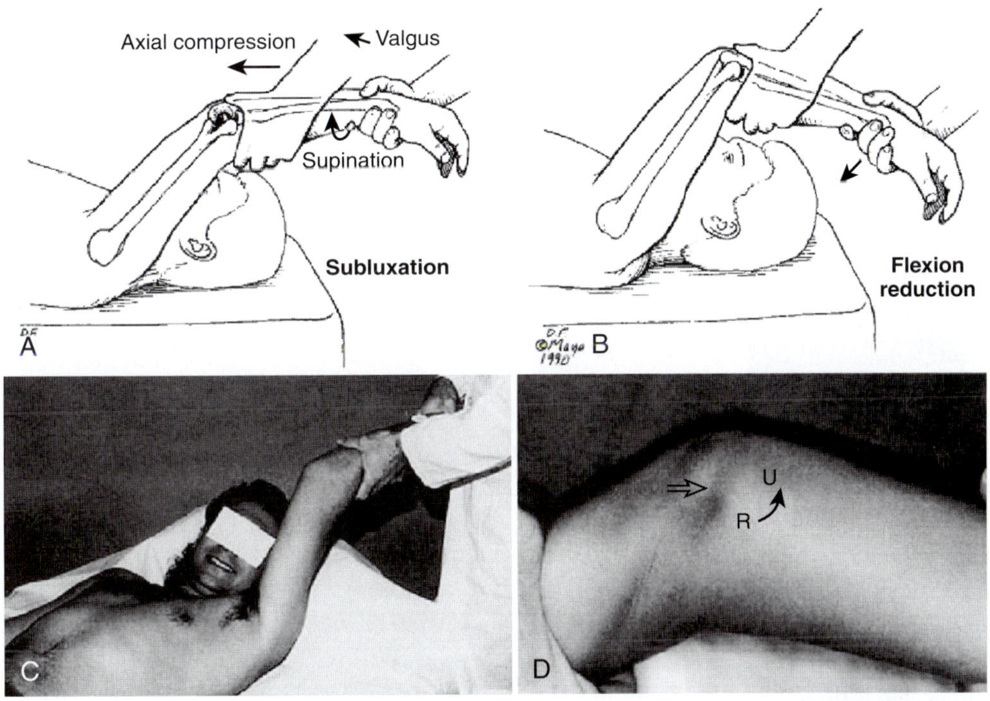

Figure 4–38 **A,** The lateral pivot-shift test of the elbow for posterolateral rotatory instability is performed with the patient supine and the arm overhead. Supination and valgus moments with axial compression are applied during flexion, causing the elbow to subluxate maximally at approximately 40 to 70° of flexion. **B,** Additional flexion produces a palpable visible clunk as the elbow reduces, if the patient is able to relax enough to permit that part of the examination. Unfortunately, the subluxation-and-reduction maneuver is usually not possible in the awake patient. **C,** This creates apprehension in the patient, who feels the sensation that the elbow is about to dislocate. The posterolateral rotatory apprehension test is highly sensitive, with false-negative results having been observed only in patients with profound instability or severe soft tissue laxity. **D,** If the patient is able to relax adequately, or is under general anesthesia, the elbow can be observed to subluxate so that the radius (R) and ulna (U) rotate off the humerus. The skin is sucked in behind the radial head as shown (*arrow*). *(**A** from O'Driscoll SW, Bell DFR, Morrey BF: Posterolateral rotatory instability of the elbow. J Bone Joint Surg 1991;73A:440-446; **B** and **D** from O'Driscoll SW, Morrey BF, Korinek S, An KN: Elbow subluxation and dislocation. A spectrum of instability. Clin Orthop Relat Res 1992;280:186-197; **C** from O'Driscoll SW: Elbow instability. Hand Clin 1994;10:405-415. Used by permission of the Mayo Foundation for Medical Education and Research. All rights reserved.)*

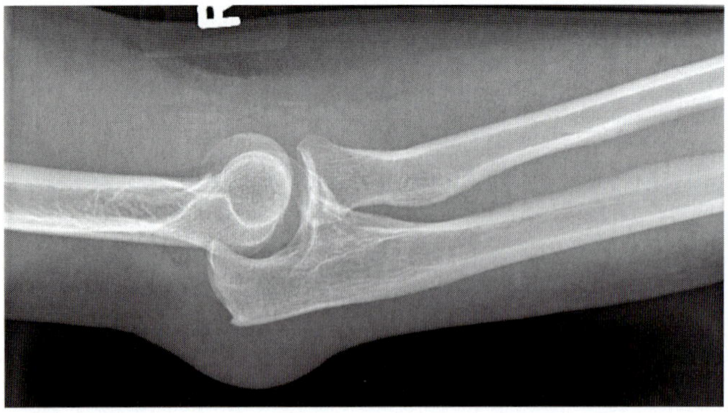

Figure 4–39 Lateral radiograph of a patient with posterolateral rotatory instability demonstrates posterolateral subluxation of the elbow; the radial head and neck are no longer aligned with the center of the capitellum, and the ulnohumeral joint line is widened. *(© Luke S. Oh, MD.)*

❑ Imaging Studies

Plain Radiographs (Fig. 4–39)

- In most cases of PLRI, plain radiographs have normal findings but are useful to assess associated pathology, including cubitus varus and radial head or coronoid fracture.
- In patients with severe insufficiency, there may be evidence of subluxation.

Stress Radiographs or Fluoroscopy

- Best tolerated by the patient under anesthesia.
- Important to assess both medial and lateral stability on the AP view.
- On the lateral view, forced supination and valgus should be applied in order to demonstrate PLRI.

Magnetic Resonance Imaging

- May be useful in assessing soft tissue disruption concomitant with insufficiency of the LCL complex.

Fluoroscopic Examination with Anesthesia

- All of the physical examination maneuvers described previously, as well as stress testing under fluoroscopy, should be performed in the operating room in any patient with elbow instability.

❑ Arthroscopy

- May be used if examination with anesthesia does not reveal a clear diagnosis.
- Various degrees of capsuloligamentous deficiency may be visualized from inside the joint.

❑ Treatment

- Acute traumatic injuries are amenable to primary repair.
- Results of primary repair or imbrication for chronic cases of PLRI are inferior; therefore, reconstruction using a tendon graft is recommended.
  - Important considerations:
    - Preserve capsular flaps to keep the tendon graft extra-articular.
    - Graft placement should be isometric.
    - Pronate the forearm and flex the elbow to 45° when tensioning the graft.
- Any underlying pathology should be addressed:
  - Coronoid or radial head fracture non-union may require either fixation, excision, or prosthetic replacement.
  - Cubitus varus deformity may lead to chronic attenuation of the tendon graft. If cubitus varus is severe, consider a valgus-producing distal humerus osteotomy (Figs. 4–40 and 4–41).

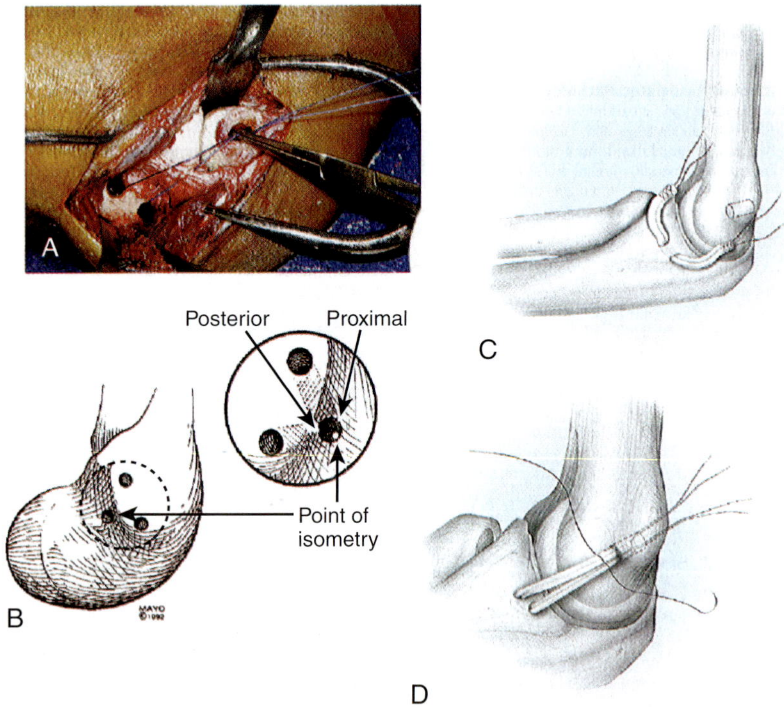

Figure 4–40 Reconstruction of the lateral collateral complex using a tendon graft. **A,** The ulnar tunnel is started at the tubercle of the supinator crest and directed proximally and posteriorly. A suture placed through the ulnar tunnel may be used to confirm the isometricity of the point selected for humeral attachment of the tendon graft. **B,** Two humeral tunnels connect the point of isometry with the anterior and posterior aspects of the lateral humeral column. **C,** The graft is doubled on itself and passed through the ulnar tunnel. **D,** The tendon graft end may be docked into the isometric humeral tunnels and the sutures tied over the humeral epicondyle. *(From Sanchez-Sotelo J: Lateral Collateral Ligament Insufficiency. In Morrey BF, Sanchez-Sotelo J [eds]: The Elbow and Its Disorders, 4th ed. Philadelphia, Saunders Elsevier, 2009, p 675. Used by permission of the Mayo Foundation for Medical Education and Research. All rights reserved.)*

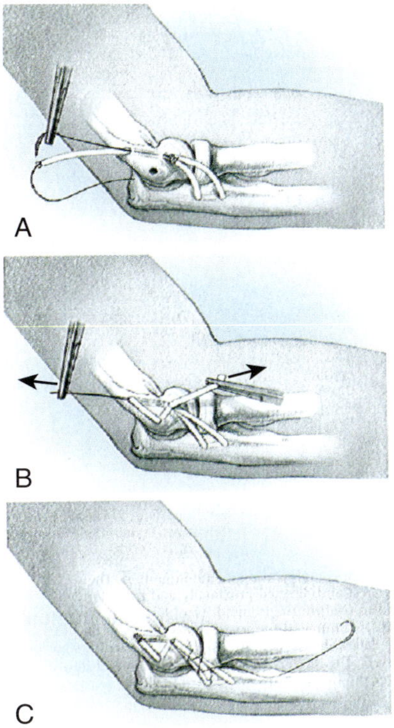

Figure 4–41 A to C, Alternatively (see Fig. 4–40), the two limbs of the graft may be sutured together. One end of the graft may be passed through the humeral tunnels, and the reconstruction may be tensioned in the direction of the arrows: proximal traction being applied to the yoke tendon and distal traction to the longer limb of the graft. *(From Sanchez-Sotelo J: Lateral collateral ligament insufficiency. In Morrey BF, Sanchez-Sotelo J [eds]: The Elbow and Its Disorders, 4th ed. Philadelphia, Saunders Elsevier, 2009, p 676. Used by permission of the Mayo Foundation for Medical Education and Research. All rights reserved.)*

Anterior Elbow Pain

Distal Biceps Tendon Rupture

- The distal biceps tendon is most commonly injured at the radial tuberosity as either a complete or partial avulsion rather than a tear at the musculotendinous junction or within the tendon.

❑ Clinical Presentation
- Sudden tearing-type pain in the antecubital fossa with or without ecchymosis, usually in the dominant elbow in male patients.
- Proximal retraction of the biceps muscle is common. If there is no proximal retraction, the muscle is likely tethered to the lacertus fibrosus.
- Pain and weakness with supination, especially against resistance. Patient may have surprisingly strong elbow flexion despite rupture of the distal biceps tendon, a finding that is consistent with the role of the biceps muscle as a contributor to elbow flexion but, more importantly, as the predominant supinator of the forearm.

❑ Mechanism
- Eccentric loading on a contracting biceps.

❑ Risk Factors
- Anabolic steroid use.
- Hyperparathyroidism.
- Systemic lupus erythematosus.

❑ Diagnosis

Hook Test
- Performed with the patient's shoulder abducted 90°, elbow flexed to 90°, and forearm fully supinated with the patient facing the palm. The examiner's index finger is then used to "hook" the lateral side of the cordlike structure in the antecubital fossa, which is the biceps tendon. If the distal biceps tendon is ruptured, there is no cordlike structure in the fossa.
- In the hook test, the examiner's finger passes under the distal biceps tendon and above the brachialis muscle belly (Fig. 4–42).
- Original terminology for results, used by O'Driscoll in the original description of the test:
  - Normal: intact distal biceps tendon.
  - Abnormal: ruptured distal biceps tendon.
  - Highly sensitive and specific.
- Subsequently, it was discovered that in cases of a partial tear of the distal biceps, the hook test elicits a pain response despite a "normal" (i.e., intact distal biceps) result. A more descriptive and less confusing terminology is proposed below:
  - Painless intact: normal, intact distal biceps.

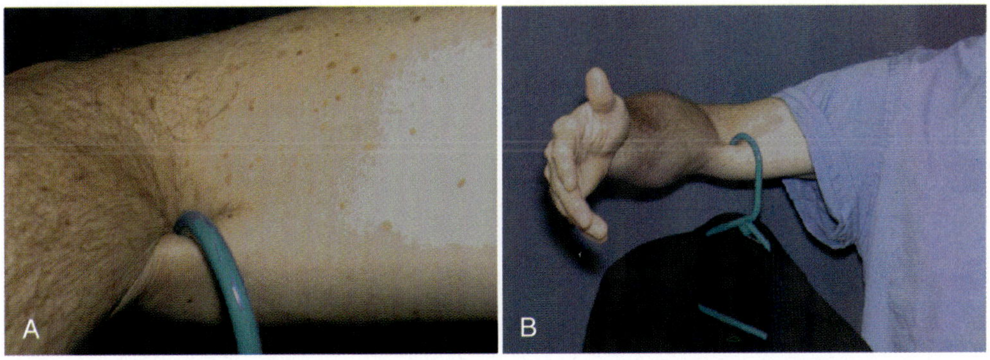

Figure 4–42 A and B, Photographs showing clearly the concept of the hook test. The intact biceps tendon is a cordlike structure spanning the antecubital fossa and behind which it is possible to pass an examining finger or a hooklike structure (a plastic blunt coat hanger in these photographs). One must hook the *lateral* edge of the tendon so as not to confuse the lacertus fibrosus, which can be intact in some cases of distal biceps tendon avulsions, with the biceps tendon itself. *(From O'Driscoll SW, Goncalves LBJ, Dietz P: The hook test for distal biceps avulsion. Am J Sports Med 2007;35:1865-1869.)*

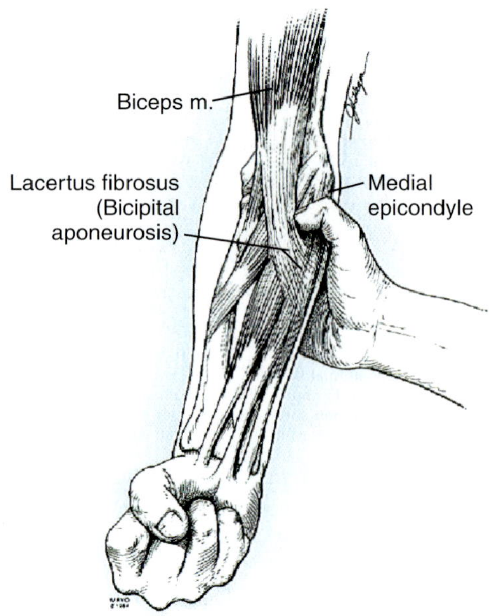

Figure 4–43 The lacertus fibrosus is easily palpable at its medial margin; It covers the brachial artery and median nerve and becomes attenuated with distal biceps tendon disruption. *(From Regan WD, Morrey BF: Physical examination of the elbow. In Morrey BF, Sanchez-Sotelo J [eds]: The Elbow and Its Disorders, 4th ed. Philadelphia, Saunders Elsevier, 2009, p 73. Used by permission of the Mayo Foundation for Medical Education and Research. All rights reserved.)*

- Painful intact: partial tear of the distal biceps.
- Disrupted: complete tear of the distal biceps.

- False-negative hook test result:
  - If the distal biceps tendon is completely avulsed but is tethered to the lacertus fibrosus, it is possible for the examiner to "hook" the lacertus fibrosus and mistakenly conclude that the tendon is intact (Fig. 4–43). Comparison with the contralateral elbow, if not injured, is recommended.
  - In the patient who has chronic complete rupture of the distal biceps tendon or has undergone surgery in the antecubital fossa previously, there may be a significant amount of scar tissue in the antecubital fossa region that may make interpretation of the hook test difficult. Merely being able to "palpate" an area of taut tissue in the antecubital fossa is not sufficient to conclude that there is an intact distal biceps tendon; one must be able to "hook" a cordlike structure (Fig. 4–44).

❑ Imaging Studies
- For evaluation of the distal biceps tendon, MRI is the study of choice because findings of plain radiographs are usually normal. Plain radiographs may demonstrate spurring of the bicipital tuberosity.
- For patients with a disrupted result on the hook test who are considering surgical repair of the distal biceps, MRI is useful to differentiate between an avulsion of the distal biceps tendon and a tear at the musculotendinous junction (uncommon), which is not easily repairable.

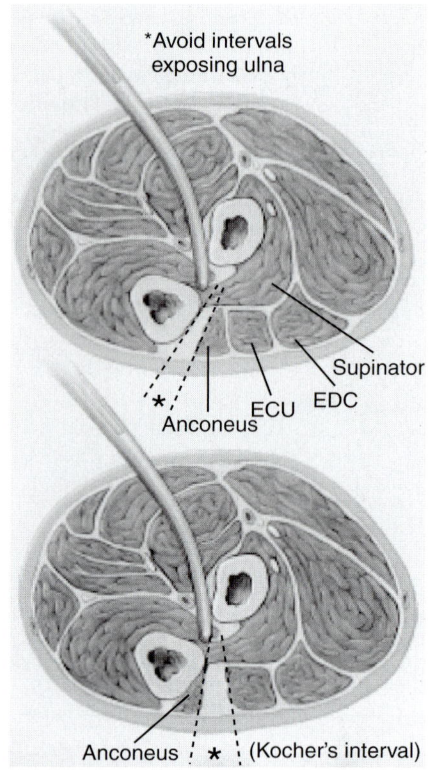

Figure 4–44 Two diagrams demonstrating the incorrect path for exposure of the radial tuberosity with the posterior incision. It is important to avoid exposing the ulna either subperiosteally or through Kocher' interval. ECU, extensor carpi ulnaris; EDC, extensor digitorum communis. *(From Hughes JS, Morrey BF: Injury of the flexors of the elbow: Biceps tendon injury. In Morrey BF, Sanchez-Sotelo J [eds]: The Elbow and Its Disorders, 4th ed. Philadelphia, Saunders Elsevier, 2009, p 529. Used by permission of the Mayo Foundation for Medical Education and Research. All rights reserved.)*

- For patients with a painful intact hook test result, who likely have a partial tear of the distal biceps, MRI rarely provides additional information.
- For patients with a painless intact hook test result, various imaging studies may be indicated to look for pathology in the elbow other than the distal biceps tendon.

❑ Treatment
- For an acute rupture of the distal biceps tendon, the recommendation is prompt surgical repair.
- For a partial tear of the distal biceps, the patient may initially be treated conservatively with the recognition that many of these patients may ultimately require surgical repair because of persistent pain and/or functional loss.
- Contraindications to surgery:
  - Distal biceps tear at the musculotendinous junction, which is uncommon.
  - Absence of functional impairment (seen in sedentary individuals, but rarely do they sustain this type of injury).

Surgical Approach

TWO-INCISION TECHNIQUE

- Advantage: decreases the risk of iatrogenic radial nerve injury.
- The risk of heterotopic ossification is markedly diminished if the forearm incision is not through Kocher' interval and the periosteum of the ulna is not elevated or violated.
  - The original Boyd-Anderson two-incision approach did expose the ulna and was associated with formation of ectopic bone.
  - The Mayo modification of the Boyd-Anderson technique does not expose the ulna and is therefore associated with a markedly lower rate of heterotopic ossification (Figs. 4–44 and 4–45).

SINGLE-INCISION TECHNIQUE

- Advantages:
  - Lower risk of heterotopic ossification.
  - Avoidance of a second incision.
- Disadvantages:
  - Higher risk of iatrogenic injury to neurovascular structures in the antecubital fossa.
  - If there has been a delay of more than 2 weeks from injury to surgery, the tract of the biceps tendon may have scarred and may no longer be easily identified.
- A Henry or modified Henry approach to the anterior elbow is used.

❑ Fixation Techniques

- Docking into the bone tunnel:

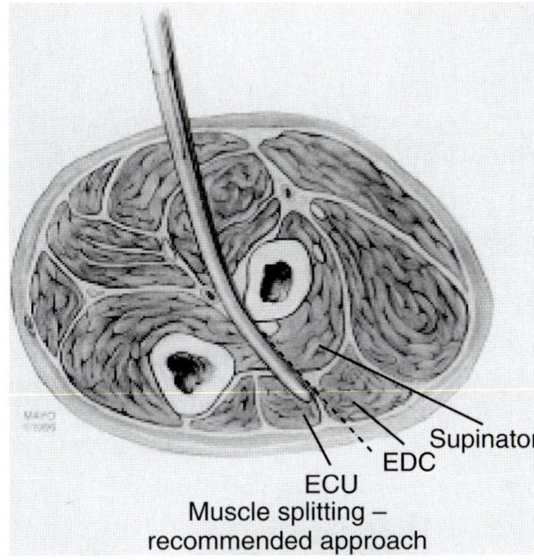

Figure 4–45 Diagram demonstrating the correct path for exposure of the radial tuberosity through a posterior incision. The preferred path utilizes a muscle-splitting approach through the extensor carpi ulnaris (ECU) and avoids exposure of the ulna. EDC, extensor digitorum communis. *(From Hughes JS, Morrey BF: Injury of the flexors of the elbow: Biceps tendon injury. In Morrey BF, Sanchez-Sotelo J [eds]: The Elbow and Its Disorders, 4th ed. Philadelphia, Saunders Elsevier, 2009, p 529. Used by permission of the Mayo Foundation for Medical Education and Research. All rights reserved.)*

  - Commonly employed when the two-incision technique is used (Fig. 4–46).
- EndoButton (Smith & Nephew, Memphis, TN):
  - Allows preparation of the biceps tendon fixation construct outside the wound rather than requiring application of fixation deep within the surgical field (Fig. 4–47).

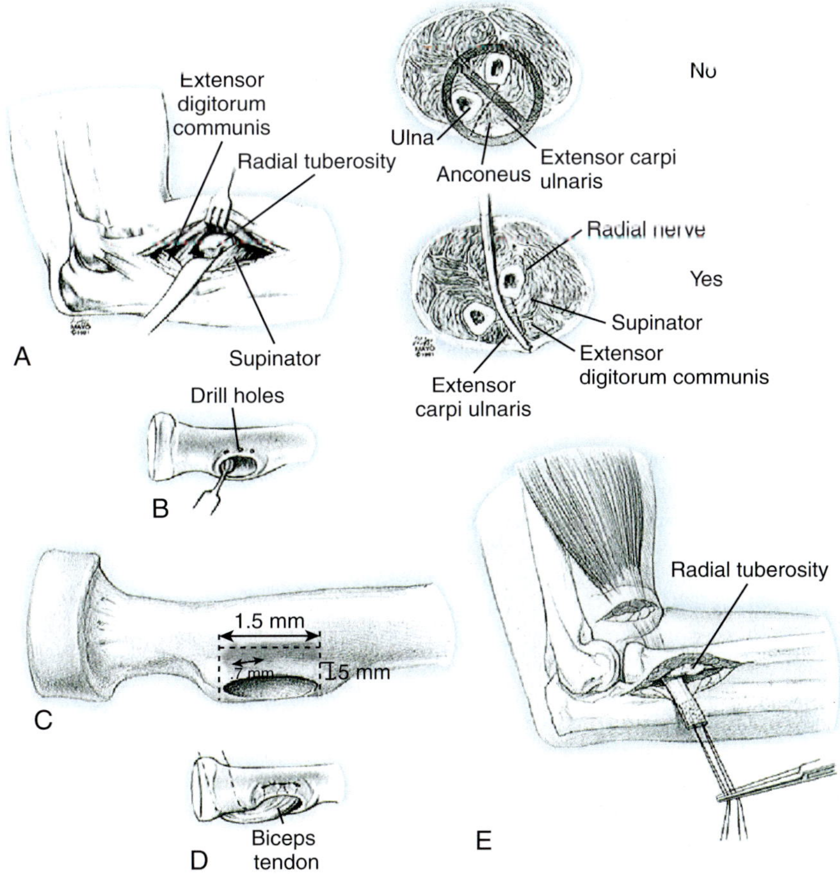

Figure 4–46 **A,** The common extensor and supinator muscles are then split to expose the radial tuberosity. The ulna is not exposed. Full pronation of the forearm brings the tuberosity into the field. **B,** The radial tuberosity is excavated with a high-speed bur. **C,** Osseous bridges 5 to 7 mm from the edge with 7 mm between the holes are ideal, and the biceps tendon is then brought through its previous tract (**D**) and re-inserted into the radial tuberosity with two nonabsorbable sutures (**E**). *(From Hughes JS, Morrey BF: Injury of the flexors of the elbow: Biceps tendon injury. In Morrey BF, Sanchez-Sotelo J [eds]: The Elbow and Its Disorders, 2009, 4th ed. Philadelphia, Saunders Elsevier, 2009, p 518. Used by permission of the Mayo Foundation for Medical Education and Research. All rights reserved.)*

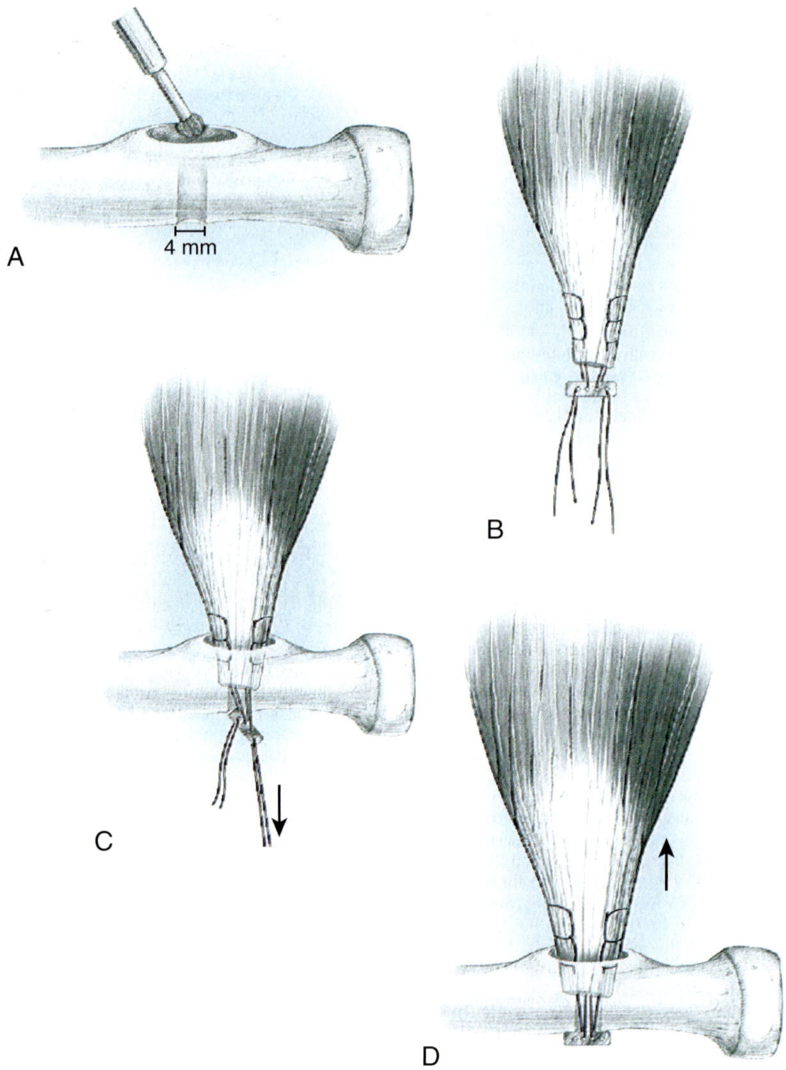

Figure 4–47 **A,** The radius is prepared by using a 2-mm drill through the tuberosity and through the opposite cortex. The proximal hole is enlarged with the bur, and the distal hole is enlarged with the 4-mm drill bit to allow the passage of the Endobutton (Smith & Nephew, Memphis, TN). **B,** A heavy, usually No. 5, nonabsorbable suture is placed in the distal biceps tendon and tied to the EndoButton. Two sutures are then passed through either hole of the EndoButton and inserted through the eye of a Keith needle. **C,** The Keith needle is passed retrograde through the tuberosity and out the hole in the opposite cortex, taking care not to touch the ulna. The suture is then grasped, and the leading edge of one of the sutures is differentially tensioned, allowing the EndoButton to slide through the hole in the opposite cortex. **D,** Once the EndoButton has been completely deployed, it is tightened against the opposite cortex by the application of opposite tension on the biceps tendon. The leading and trailing sutures are then removed. *(Modified from Bain GI, Prem H, Heptinstall RJ, et al: Repair of distal biceps tendon rupture: A new technique using the EndoButton. J Shoulder Elbow Surg 2000;9:120.)*

- Suture anchors:
  - Commonly employed when the single-incision technique is used.

❑ Surgical Complications
- The graph in Figure 4–48 summarizes the type of common complications as well as the timing of their postoperative occurrences. For example, for patients presenting with decreased range of motion after a distal biceps tendon repair, plain radiographs must be taken at least up to the sixth week after surgery to check for possible formation of heterotopic ossification.
- Of note, the rate of complications increases (nearly doubles) if there is a delay of more than 3 weeks from injury to surgery, likely owing to the greater dissection required to identify and repair the tendon.

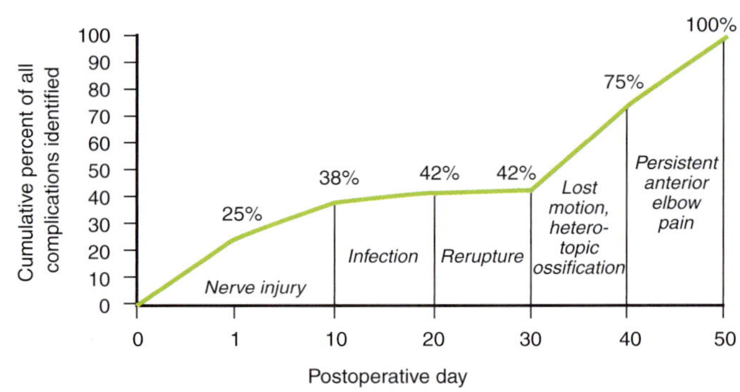

Figure 4–48 Graph showing the types of complications after repair of distal biceps tendon rupture and when they developed. All 24 complications were present by 7 weeks after surgery. *(From Morrey BF: Complications of Elbow Arthroscopy. In Morrey BF, Sanchez-Sotelo J [eds]: The Elbow and Its Disorders, 4th ed. Philadelphia, Saunders Elsevier, 2009.)*

Pronator Teres Syndrome

❑ Clinical Presentation
- Diffuse anterior elbow pain that radiates distally into the forearm because of compression of the median nerve.
- Thenar muscles may be weak, but muscles innervated by the anterior interosseus nerve (flexor pollicis longus [FPL], flexor digitorum profundus [FDP], and pronator quadratus) may not be affected.

- Negative results of tests for carpal tunnel syndrome.

❑ Potential Sites of Compression
- Two heads of pronator teres.
- Lacertus fibrosus.
- Ligament of Struthers.

❑ Diagnosis and Treatment
- Differential diagnosis includes C6-C7 cervical radiculopathy.
- Results of EMG and nerve conduction studies may or may not be diagnostic.
- If nonoperative treatment that includes activity modification does not alleviate symptoms, surgical decompression may be indicated.

Posterior Elbow Pain

Un-united Fractured Olecranon Osteophytes

- Classic presentation is sharp posterior pain with elbow at full extension.
- Examination maneuver: Forced extension or passive "bouncing" of the elbow at full extension recreates the posterior impingement pain caused by the un-united fractured osteophyte (Fig. 4–49).
- Fractured osteophytes at the posterior tip of the olecranon can be quite small and are often not detected on plain radiographs or MRI. CT may be required to confirm the diagnosis as well as to determine the precise location of osteophytes in order to allow ease of localization during arthroscopy (Fig. 4–50).
- Recommended treatment is arthroscopic excision and removal of an un-united fractured osteophyte (Fig. 4–51).

Triceps Tendon Rupture

- Rare but may be seen with various athletic activities, such as power-lifting, as well as in patients who have a systemic disease such as renal osteodystrophy or secondary hyperparathyroidism.
- Clinical presentation:
  - Pain and weakness with elbow extension.
  - Palpable defect may be present at insertion of triceps.
  - Location of pain may be proximal to the olecranon process if the injury is at the musculotendinous junction.
- Mechanism of injury: Eccentric loading on a contracting triceps.
- Imaging studies:
  - Plain radiographs are not generally useful unless a bony avulsion is present.
  - MRI is useful to delineate size and location of tear (avulsion vs. musculotendinous junction).
    - Usually, the central third of the tendon is involved.
- Treatment:
  - For complete ruptures, early surgical repair via crossed bone tunnels is recommended (Fig. 4–52).
  - For partial tears, nonoperative treatment may be initiated. Triceps tendinitis likely will resolve over time, but partial tears often do not heal and usually require surgical intervention.

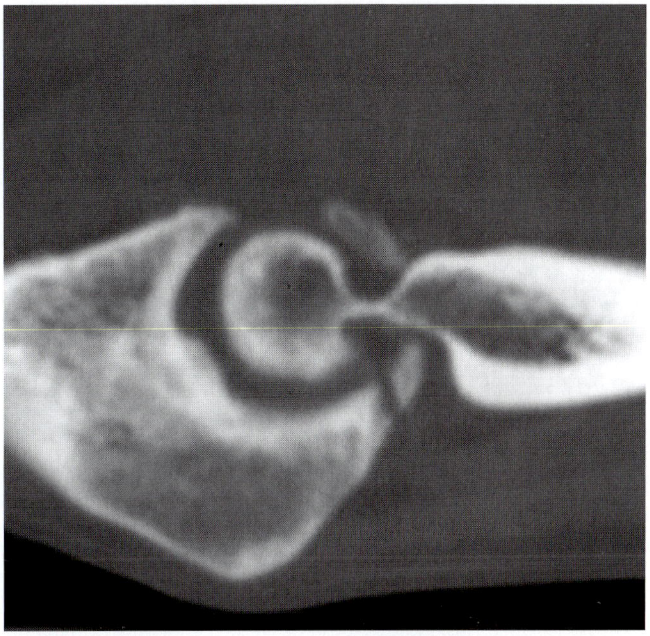

Figure 4–50 CT scan of a professional baseball pitcher's elbow demonstrating an ununited fractured olecranon osteophyte. This pitcher also has a large loose body in the coronoid fossa. *(© Luke S. Oh, MD.)*

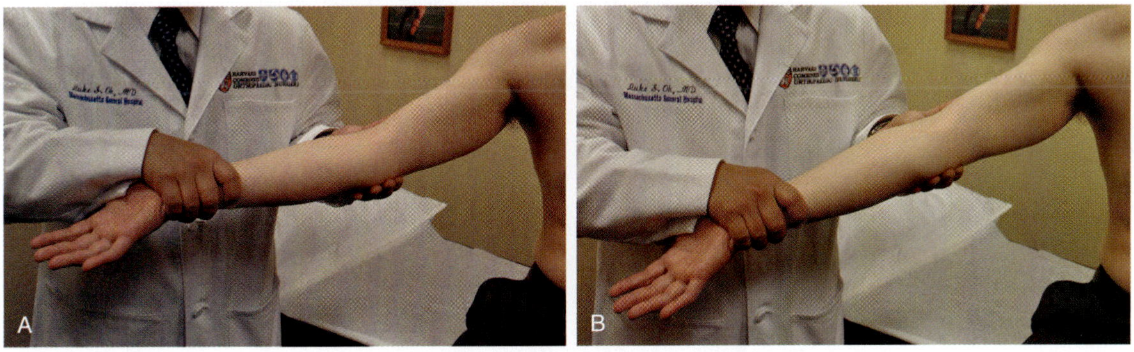

Figure 4–49 A and B, Forced terminal extension or passive "bouncing" of the elbow at full extension recreates posterior impingement pain caused by the ununited fractured olecranon osteophyte. *(© Luke S. Oh, MD.)*

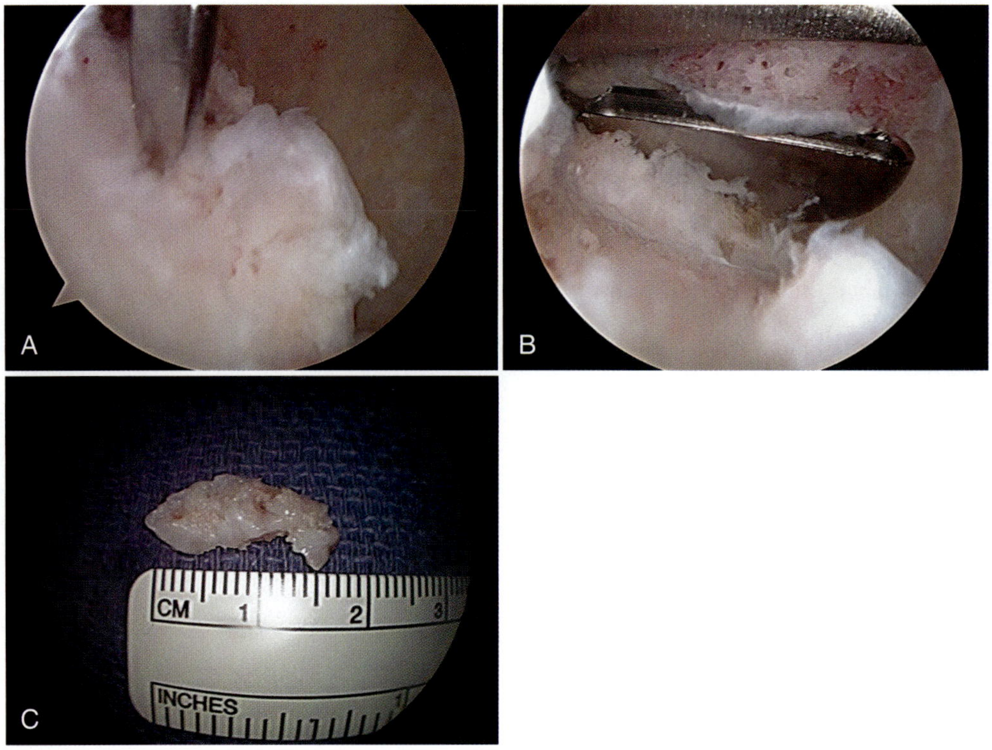

Figure 4–51 **A**, Arthroscopic view of the ununited fractured olecranon osteophyte seen in Figure 4–51. The free elevator is being used to separate the fractured osteophyte at the site of fibrous nonunion. **B**, A pituitary rongeur has grasped the ununited fractured olecranon osteophyte. **C**, This photograph demonstrates the size of the fractured olecranon osteophyte to be greater than 15 mm x 5 mm. *(© Luke S. Oh, MD.)*

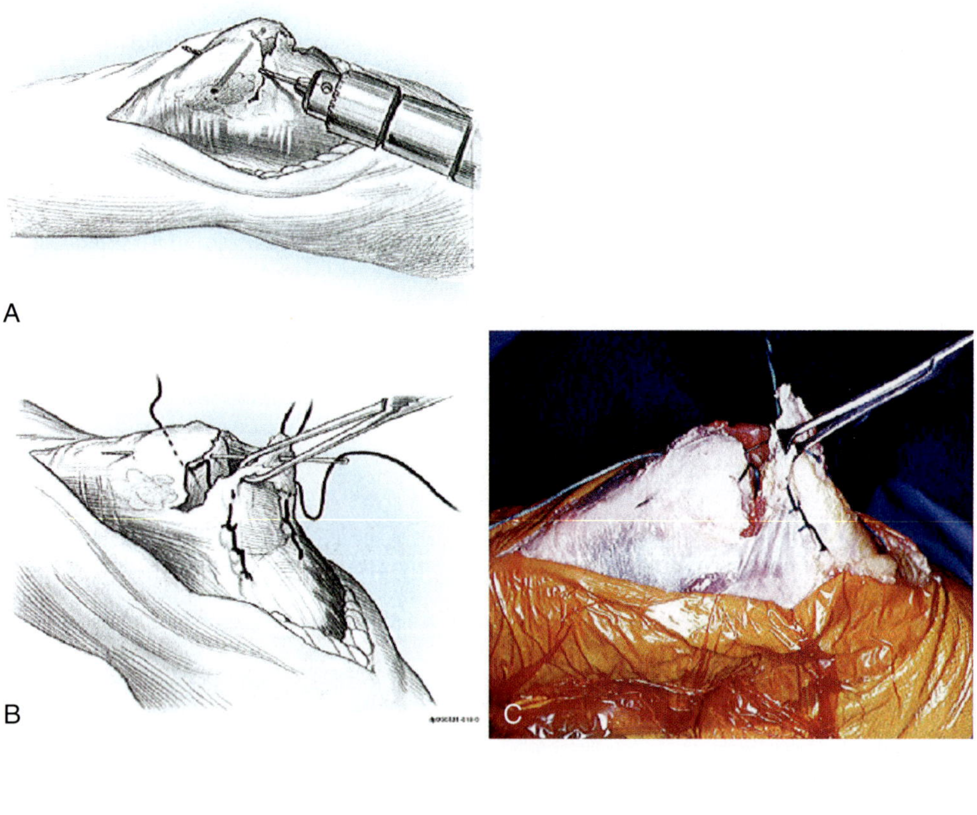

Figure 4–52 For acute triceps tendon avulsion, No. 5 nonabsorbable suture is passed through crossed bone tunnels (**A**) and into the avulsed tendon with a running locked stitch (**B**). *(From Morrey BF: Rupture of the Triceps Tendon. In Morrey BF, Sanchez-Sotelo J [eds]: The Elbow and Its Disorders, 4th ed. Philadelphia, Saunders Elsevier, 2009, p 539.)*

Olecranon Bursitis

- Most common type of superficial bursitis.

❑ Clinical Presentation
- Distended olecranon bursa.
- Painless or painful.
  - 80% of cases of septic bursitis and 20% of cases of aseptic bursitis are painful.
  - Traumatic bursitis is surprisingly painless in most cases.
- The bursa may rupture and dissect proximally to create swelling over the triceps.

❑ Etiology

Traumatic
- Repetitive trauma is twice as common as a single direct traumatic event in causing olecranon bursitis.

Inflammatory
- Rheumatoid arthritis.
- Gout.
- Chondrocalcinosis.
- Diffuse pigmented villonodular synovitis.

Infectious
- 20% of cases of olecranon bursitis are of infectious origin.
- Approximately one third of patients with septic bursitis report a history of previous noninfected olecranon bursitis.
- Septic bursitis is not necessarily associated with a septic elbow joint because the bursa and joint usually do not communicate.
  - The bursa and joint may indeed communicate in patients with rheumatoid arthritis and after total elbow arthroplasty.
- Rare in children because the olecranon bursa develops between 7 and 10 years of age.

Noninfectious
- 80% of cases of olecranon bursitis are of noninfectious origin.

❑ Risk Factors for Septic Bursitis

Immunocompromise
- Diabetes mellitus.
- Alcoholism.
- Human immunodeficiency virus (HIV).

Hemodialysis
- Up to 7% of patients undergoing hemodialysis may experience olecranon bursitis on the extremity with dialysis port.
- Approximately 25% of cases are septic bursitis.
- Pathophysiology is unclear; direct pressure from frequent dialysis treatments?

Artificial Turf
- Traumatic contact during a football tackle has been associated with olecranon bursitis.

❑ Evaluation
- Aspiration:
  - Septic bursitis is characterized by a high leukocyte count and predominance of polymorphonuclear cells in an aspirate from the bursa.
  - A separate elbow joint aspiration may also be needed in patients in whom a septic joint may be present in addition to a septic bursitis (immunocompromised hosts) or in whom there is an increased likelihood that the bursa communicates with the joint (rheumatoid arthritis).

❑ Treatment
- If bursitis is painful, aspiration is recommended.
- If bursitis is painless, initial treatment consists of compression and a resting splint.
- If bursitis does not rapidly improve with compression and a resting splint, erythema develops, or pain persists, septic bursitis is likely.
  - Perform either a second aspiration or consider operative treatment if clinically indicated.
- Corticosteroid injection:
  - May be considered in the setting of a noninfected olecranon bursitis.
  - Decreases the recurrence rate but increases the complication rate (infection, subdermal atrophy).

Surgery
- Arthroscopic synovectomy has been described but lacks long-term follow-up results.
- Open bursectomy:
  - Longitudinal incision medial to the midline.
  - Bursectomy may devitalize the skin over the olecranon process.
  - Postoperatively, the arm should be immobilized for 2 weeks in a compressive dressing with the elbow flexed approximately 45° in order to reduce tension over the incision and decrease risk of wound healing problems.

Elbow Arthroscopy

Patient Positioning

❑ Supine
- Advantages:
  - Allows easy access to patient's airway for the anesthesiologist.
  - Allows easier conversion to positioning of the elbow on a hand table for an open procedure.
- Disadvantages:
  - Assistant needed to hold the elbow to prevent swinging and/or rotation.
  - Awkward for working in posterior compartment.

❑ Prone
- Advantages:
  - Stabilizes the shoulder and therefore the elbow.

- Disadvantages:
  - Makes access to patient's airway more difficult for the anesthesiologist.
  - Elbow flexion and hyperflexion during arthroscopic procedure are difficult.
  - Access to anterior compartment with various instruments may be limited by the operating room table.
  - Does not allow repositioning the elbow to a hand table for conversion to an open procedure (Fig. 4–53).

❑ Lateral Decubitus
- Advantages:
  - Maintains access to patient's airway.
  - Extremity is stabilized but allows for flexion/hyperflexion if needed.
- Disadvantage:
  - Does not allow repositioning the elbow to a hand table for conversion to an open procedure.

Nerve Anatomy

❑ Ulnar Nerve
- Palpate the ulnar nerve to evaluate for subluxating ulnar nerve.
- If no prior ulnar nerve transposition has been performed, create anteromedial portal *anterior* to the intermuscular septum.
- In cases of prior transposition of the ulnar nerve, create a mini-open incision to locate, identify, and protect the nerve prior to creating the anteromedial portal. It is important to minimize traffic through this portal to avoid injury to the nerve.
- During visualization of the medial elbow with the arthroscope, one must appreciate that the ulnar nerve is within millimeters of the medial capsule. Therefore, access to some of the posteromedial olecranon osteophytes may be more safely achieved via a small arthrotomy posterior to the ulnar nerve rather than an arthroscopic ostectomy with a bur, especially early in a surgeon's learning curve.

❑ Radial/Posterior Interosseus Nerve
- Understanding the exact location of the radial/posterior interosseus nerve as visualized from the arthroscope is critical:
  - The radial nerve runs longitudinally across the anterior aspect of the elbow at the 12-o'clock position of the radial head.
  - At this location, the radial nerve is located approximately 2 to 3 mm anterior to the capsule. In fact, the fat pad surrounding the radial nerve is usually juxtaposed to the capsule (Table 4-1).

❑ Median Nerve
- The median nerve is at risk during creation of the anteromedial portal.

❑ Cutaneous Nerves
- To avoid injury to cutaneous nerves, cut only the skin with the scalpel, and then dissect bluntly down to the capsule to enter the joint.
- Cutaneous nerves are within 4 to 7 mm of the direct lateral portal and both the anteromedial and anterolateral portals.

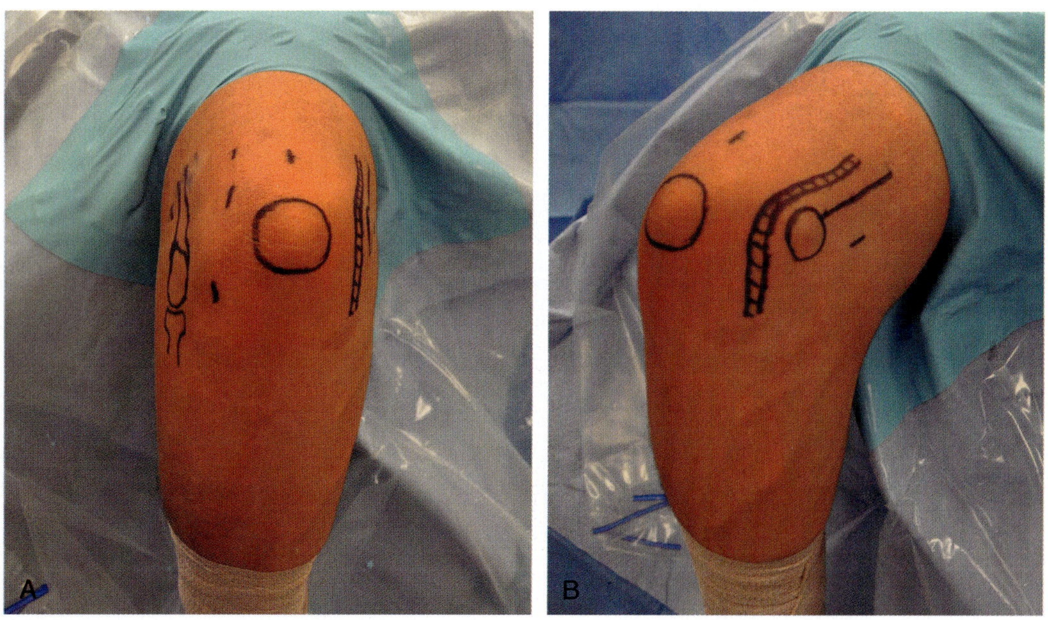

Figure 4–53 A, Direct posterior view of a left elbow in the lateral decubitus position demonstrating the locations of various posterior portals. The large central circle is the olecranon. Approximately 2 cm directly superior to the proximal tip of the olecranon is the location of the posterocentral portal. Left of the posterocentral portal is the location of the proximal posterolateral accessory portal for placement of an arthroscopic retractor. The other two portals appearing below it are the posterolateral portal and the direct lateral soft-spot portal. B, The hash lines depict the course of the ulnar nerve. The smaller circle is the medial epicondyle with the intermuscular septum outlined. The anteromedial portal location is shown anterior to the intermuscular septum. *(© Luke S. Oh, MD.)*

Table 4–1 Nerve Distances to Capsule and Portals

Nerve	Portal Site	Distance, mm (Range)		
		Portal		Capsule
		Flaccid	*Distended*	
Radial	Anterolateral	5	10 (1-13)	9 (6-16)
Median	Anteromedial	10	15	14 (6-24)
Ulnar	Anteromedial	1-22	1-22	1-2 (?)

From Morrey BF: Anatomy of the elbow joint. In Morrey BF, Sanchez-Sotelo J [eds]: The Elbow and Its Disorders, 4th ed. Philadelphia, Saunders Elsevier, 2009.

Arthroscopic Portals (Fig. 4–54)

❑ For Posterior Compartment Access

Posterocentral Portal

- The posterocentral portal is created approximately 2 to 3 cm proximal to the proximal tip of the olecranon when the elbow is flexed to 90°. If the portal is too distal, then access to the olecranon fossa for the arthroscope and/or instruments may be limited or blocked by the olecranon.
- Use a scalpel with a No. 15 blade to create a portal through the skin and triceps in one stab incision, down to the olecranon fossa.

Posterolateral Portal

- Created at the posterolateral corner of olecranon.
- A useful guideline is to find the midpoint between the olecranon tip and the lateral epicondyle, then move 1 cm proximal and perpendicular to the midpoint.
- Use a scalpel with a No. 15 blade to make a skin incision.
- Use a Steinmann pin to puncture the posterolateral capsule by aiming toward the olecranon fossa. Extend the elbow to approximately 45° so that the olecranon covers the articular surface of the posterolateral trochlea, in order to reduce the potential for inadvertent articular cartilage injury by the Steinmann pin during the creation of the portal.
- Slide the arthroscope sheath over the Steinmann pin, remove the Steinmann pin, and insert the arthroscope.
- If the point of entry in the capsule is not lateral enough, visualization of the posterolateral gutter will be diminished (Fig. 4–55).

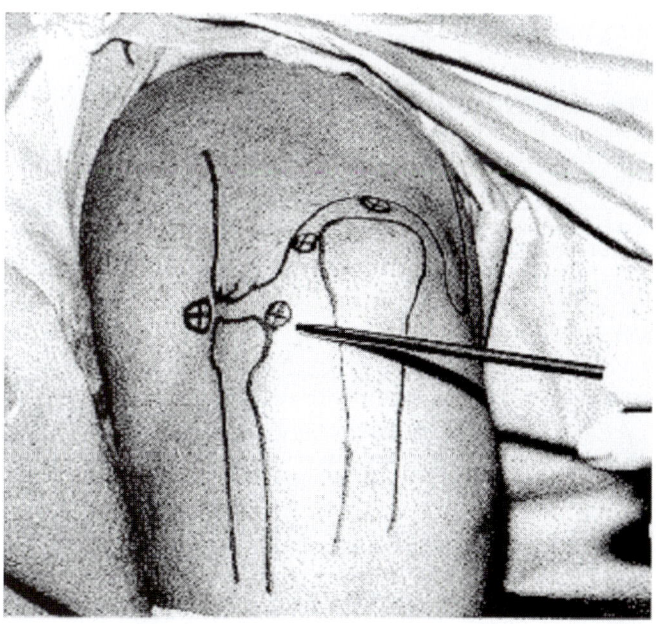

Figure 4–54 Posterolateral view of the elbow with the bones outlined and portals marked. The portals from left to right are: anterolateral, direct mid-lateral "soft spot" portal (pointer), posterolateral, and posterocentral. The anteromedial portal is not visible on this photo. *(From O'Driscoll S: Arthroscopic Treatment for Osteoarthritis of the Elbow. Ortho Clin N Am 1995;26(4):694.)*

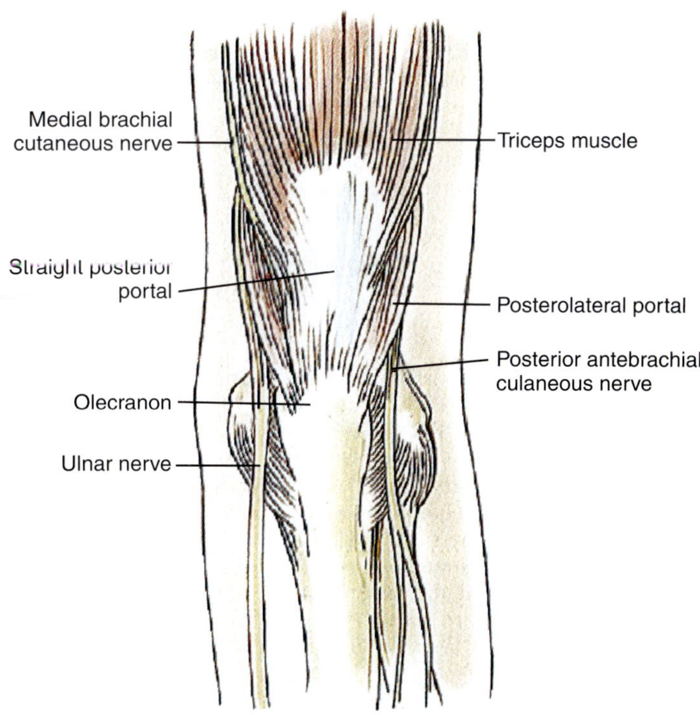

Figure 4–55 The two standard posterior portals most commonly used in the elbow: Posterocentral portal (labeled Straight posterior portal in this diagram) and Posterolateral portal. *(From McClung G, Field L, Savoie F: Diagnostic arthroscopy: Indications, portals, and techniques. In Morrey BF, Sanchez-Sotelo J [eds]: The Elbow and Its Disorders, 4th ed. Philadelphia, Saunders Elsevier, 2009, p 570.)*

Proximal Posterolateral Portal

- The proximal posterolateral portal is an accessory portal used to insert a retractor to improve visualization in the posterior compartment.
- The skin incision is created in line with the posterolateral portal and approximately 5 to 6 cm proximal to the posterolateral portal. Use a scalpel to incise the skin only, and then use blunt dissection to enter the posterior compartment.

Direct Lateral "Soft Spot" Portal

- The direct lateral "soft spot" portal is at the triangular soft spot between the radial head, capitellum, and ulna.
- With the arthroscope in the posterolateral portal, guide the arthroscope into the lateral gutter. Place a spinal needle through the triangular soft spot and visualize the tip of the needle as a method to determine the anticipated position of the direct lateral soft spot portal.
- Make a diagonal skin incision in line with the fibers of the deeper important structures such as the LCL complex in order to minimize disruption of these structures.

❑ For Anterior Compartment Access

- Entry to the anterior compartment of the elbow may be initiated from either the anteromedial or anterolateral side. The description here starts with the anteromedial portal (Fig. 4–56).

Anteromedial Portal

- Palpate the ulnar nerve and then the intermuscular septum. Ensure that the ulnar nerve has not been previously transposed and is not currently subluxating.
- Create a skin incision 1 cm anterior to the intermuscular septum and 2 cm proximal to the ulnotrochlear joint articulation.
- Use a Steinmann pin to bluntly enter the capsule. Aim the pin toward the center of the joint. Make sure that the joint is distended to increase safety as well as to make it easier to puncture through the capsule.
- Ensure that the bony architecture within the joint is palpable with the tip of the Steinmann pin. If the joint is not distended or if there is scarring from prior surgery, it is not uncommon for the tip of the Steinmann pin to remain anterior to the capsule. In this situation, there is a palpable sensation of a thin layer of tissue at the tip of the Steinmann pin.
- Once the Steinmann pin has punctured through the capsule, slide the arthroscope sheath over the Steinmann pin and insert the arthroscope (Fig. 4–57).

Anterolateral Portal

- After visualization of the lateral aspect of the anterior compartment, either an inside-out technique or outside-in technique may be used to create the anterolateral portal:
  - An outside-in technique uses a spinal needle to localize the desired position of the anterolateral portal.

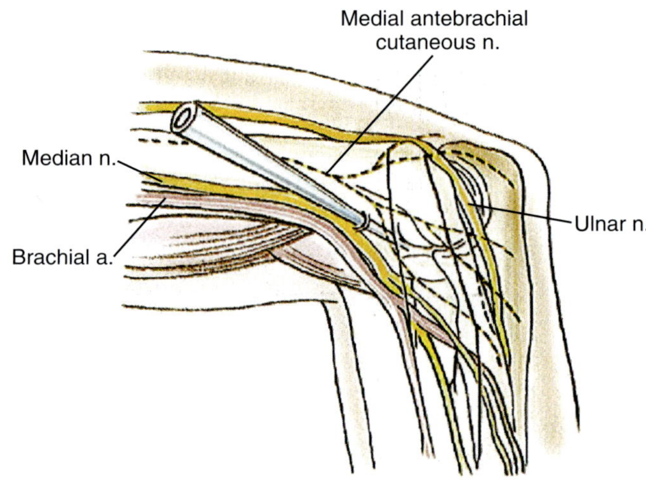

Figure 4–57 The proximal anteromedial portal located approximately 2 cm superior and 2 cm anterior to the medial epicondyle is shown, along with relevant neurovascular structures. *(From McClung G, Field L, Savoie F: Diagnostic arthroscopy: Indications, portals, and techniques. In Morrey BF, Sanchez-Sotelo J [eds]: The Elbow and Its Disorders, 4th ed. Philadelphia, Saunders Elsevier, 2009, p 571.)*

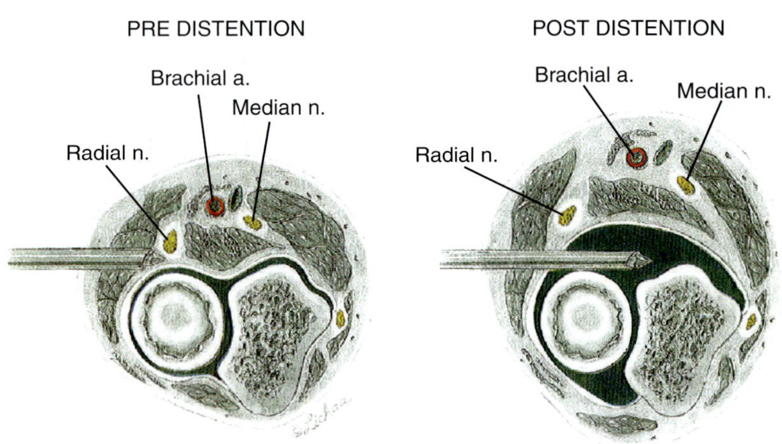

Figure 4–56 Importance of capsular distention. The anterior neurovascular structures are very close to the instruments placed in the anterior portals. The radial nerve, which can lie right on the capsule, is an average of only 4 mm from the arthroscope sheath and trocar as it enters the undistended joint. With joint distention and the elbow in 90° of flexion, the neurovascular structures are displaced anteriorly and protected. The distance between the radial nerve and the scope increases to about 11 mm with joint distention, making portal establishment much safer. *(Courtesy of Chantal Lichaa.)*

- An inside-out technique uses the arthroscope to point to the desired position of the portal and a switching stick technique to create the portal.
- Fine-tuning the position of the anterolateral portal depends on the procedure to be performed. In order to safely and effectively perform the procedure, it is important to anticipate the angle of entry for various instruments through each portal.

Proximal Anterolateral Portal

- The proximal anterolateral portal is created approximately 3 cm superior to the anterolateral portal.
- It is used for insertion of an arthroscopic retractor.
- Many writers regard the use of an arthroscopic retractor as the most important step in improving visualization and reducing nerve injury, particularly in cases that require a capsulectomy or capsulotomy.

Indications for Elbow Arthroscopy

- Various indications exist for elbow arthroscopy, and a review of the steps required for its execution for various procedures is beyond the scope of this chapter.
- Often, removal of a loose body is considered a simple procedure. However, if the loose body is truly loose and not tethered to the soft tissues, considerable skill is required to visualize all corners of the elbow with the arthroscope in both the anterior and posterior compartments to ensure that all loose bodies have been removed.
- The most technically challenging elbow arthroscopy procedure is an arthroscopic osteocapsular arthroplasty for elbow arthritis. This procedure should be reserved for surgeons formally trained in elbow arthroscopy.

Complications

❑ Elbow Swelling

- Elbow swelling is not a complication per se; it is, however, an important troubleshooting issue, because moderate elbow swelling causes the tissues to become edematous and may compromise visualization enough to preclude safe completion of elbow arthroscopy.
- Attention to arthroscopic fluid management to minimize elbow swelling is critical.

❑ Nerve Injury

- Published rates of neurologic complications after elbow arthroscopy range from 0% to 14%.
- Steps to avoid nerve injury:
  - The surgeon must know where the nerves are with certainty at all times.
  - Avoid using suction while using the motorized shaver. Detach the suction hose and allow arthroscopic fluid to drain out of the outflow onto the floor.
  - Do not use a shaver in an area where visualization is compromised.
  - Use retractors. Judicious placement of retractors via accessory portals significantly decreases the risk of inadvertent nerve injury, especially in the elbow with a contracture, in which capsular distension is limited or not possible. Many writers consider the use of retractors during elbow arthroscopy to be the single most important factor in reducing iatrogenic nerve injury and improving visualization and safety.
- Factors significantly associated with the development of transient nerve palsy after elbow arthroscopy performed by experienced surgeons:
  - A diagnosis of rheumatoid arthritis.
  - Presence of an elbow contracture.
  - Performance of a capsulectomy or capsular release.

❑ Delayed Ulnar Nerve Palsy

- Delayed ulnar nerve palsy may be encountered after an arthroscopic contracture release. This nerve may be injured as a result of the marked improvement in postoperative elbow range of motion and subsequent increased traction on or tethering of the ulnar nerve.
- If a postoperative continuous passive motion (CPM) machine is used, delayed ulnar nerve palsy may result from shear forces acting on the nerve.
- Open in situ ulnar nerve decompression decreases this risk.
- Some writers suggested performing an ulnar nerve decompression only if the contracture release will allow a stiff elbow that flexed to less than 90° preoperatively to achieve a flexion angle greater than 90° postoperatively.
  - Review of cases at the Mayo Clinic 'revealed an unpredictable nature of ulnar nerve behavior based on either preoperative or postoperative range of motion or gains in range of motion (2009; personal communication with Shawn W. O'Driscoll, PhD, MD). Therefore, an in situ nerve decompression may perhaps be considered in all cases of contracture release regardless of the degree of contracture.
  - Open in situ ulnar nerve decompression may be performed with the patient's upper extremity prepared for arthroscopy in the lateral decubitus position. A limited open decompression may be performed via a 2- to 4-cm incision with the patient in the lateral decubitus position and the arm in a tourniquet. The in situ ulnar nerve decompression is best performed prior to arthroscopy in order to minimize distortion of anatomy from swelling and arthroscopy fluid.

❑ Infection

- An 0.8% incidence of septic arthritis was noted in a Mayo Clinic series of 473 consecutive elbow arthroscopy procedures (Kelly et al, 2001).

- Deep infection was more common in patients who received intra-articular corticosteroids at the end of the procedure (4 of 117 procedures) than in those to whom steroids were not administered (0 of 356 procedures).
- Superficial infection was noted in 2% of the cases in this series; in all cases, the infection was treated and subsequently resolved with a course of oral antibiotics.

❑ Persistent Drainage

- Serous drainage from arthroscopic portal sites for more than 5 days was the most frequent complication (5%) in the Mayo report (Kelly et al, 2001).
- Direct lateral soft spot portal and anterolateral portals are at highest risk because of the thin subcutaneous tissues at these locations.
- Drainage was most commonly encountered if no sutures were placed and the arthroscopic portal was reapproximated with adhesive skins closures (Steri-Strips) only. However, persistent drainage occurred even with simple interrupted nylon suture or subcuticular polyglactin (Vicryl) sutures. Therefore, nylon sutures placed in locked horizontal mattress fashion are recommended (Kelly et al, 2001).

❑ Loss of Motion

- Heterotopic ossification is uncommon but may develop after extensive bony work has been performed in the elbow. Meticulous lavage and removal of bony debris at the end of the procedure and the use of indomethacin postoperatively are techniques used to reduce the risk of heterotopic ossification.
- Loss of motion may be observed during the immediate postoperative period even without the presence of heterotopic ossification. In such cases, the loss of motion is usually minor (5 to 15°) and persists in only a small number of patients.

References and Resources

Antuna, S.A., O'Driscoll, S.W., 2001. Snapping plicae associated with radiocapitellar chondromalacia. Arthroscopy 17, 491–495.

Azar, F., 2002. The elbow. In: Miller, M. (Ed.), Review of Sports Medicine and Arthroscopy. Saunders Elsevier, Philadelphia.

Azar, F.M., Andrews, J.R., Wilk, K.E., Groh, D., 2000. Operative treatment of ulnar collateral ligament injuries of the elbow in athletes. Am. J. Sports Med. 28, 16–23.

Callaway, G.H., Field, L.D., Deng, X.H., et al., 1997. Biomechanical evaluation of the medial collateral ligament of the elbow. J. Bone Joint Surg. Am. 79, 1223–1231.

DiGiovine, N.M., Jobe, F.W., Pink, M., Perry, J., 1992. An electromyographic analysis of the upper extremity in pitching. J. Shoulder Elbow Surg. 1, 15–25.

Dines, J.S., ElAttrache, N.S., Conway, J.E., et al., 2007. Clinical outcomes of the DANE TJ technique to treat ulnar collateral ligament insufficiency of the elbow. Am. J. Sports Med. 35, 2039–2044.

Fealy, S., Rohrbough, J.T., Allen, A.A., et al., 2002. Athletic injuries and the throwing athlete: Elbow. In: Norris, T.R. (Ed.), Orthopaedic Knowledge Update: Shoulder and Elbow 2. American Academy of Orthopaedic Surgeons, Rosemont, IL.

Jobe, F.W., Stark, H., Lombardo, S.J., 1986. Reconstruction of the ulnar collateral ligament in athletes. J. Bone Joint Surg. Am. 68, 1158–1163.

Kamineni, S., Ankem, H., Patten, D.K., 2009. Anatomic relationship of the radial nerve to the elbow joint: clinical implications of safe pin placement. Clin. Anat. 22 (6), 684–688.

Kelly, E.W., Morrey, B.F., O'Driscoll, S.W., 2001. Complications of elbow arthroscopy. J. Bone Joint Surg. Am. 83-A, 25–34.

Kraushaar, B.S., Nirschl, R.P., 1999. Tendinosis of the elbow (tennis elbow): Clinical features and findings of histological, immunohistochemical, and electron microscopy. J. Bone Joint Surg. Am. 81, 259–278.

Morrey, B.F., 2009. In: Sanchez-Sotelo, J. (Ed.), The Elbow and Its Disorders. fourth ed. Saunders Elsevier, Philadelphia.

O'Driscoll, S.W., 2002. Acute, recurrent, and chronic elbow instabilities. In: Norris, T.R. (Ed.), Orthopaedic Knowledge Update: Shoulder and Elbow 2. American Academy of Orthopaedic Surgeons, Rosemont, IL.

O'Driscoll, S.W., Morrey, B.F., 1992. Arthroscopy of the elbow: Diagnostic and therapeutic benefits and hazards. J. Bone Joint Surg. Am. 74, 84–94.

O'Driscoll, S.W., Bell, D.F., Morrey, B.F., 1991. Posterolateral rotatory instability of the elbow. J. Bone Joint Surg. Am. 73, 440–446.

O'Driscoll, S.W., Lawton, R.L., Smith, A.M., 2005. The "moving valgus stress test" for medial collateral ligament tears of the elbow. Am. J. Sports Med. 33, 231–239.

O'Driscoll, S.W., Goncalves, L.B.J., Dietz, P., 2007. The hook test for distal biceps avulsion. Am. J. Sports Med. 35, 1865–1869.

Rohrbough, J.T., Altchek, D.W., Hyman, J., et al., 2002. Medial collateral ligament reconstruction of the elbow using the docking technique. Am. J. Sports Med. 30, 541–548.

Smith, A.M., O'Driscoll, S.W., 2005. Diagnosing medial elbow pain in throwers. J. Musculoskeletal Med. 22, 305–316.

Smith, G.R., Altchek, D.W., Pagnani, M.J., Keeley, J.R., 1996. A muscle-splitting approach to the ulnar collateral ligament of the elbow. Neuroanatomy and operative technique. Am. J. Sports Med. 24, 575–580.

Spinner, R.J., Goldner, R.D., 1998. Snapping of the medial head of the triceps and recurrent dislocation of the ulnar nerve: Anatomical and dynamic factors. J. Bone Joint Surg. Am. 80, 239–247.

CHAPTER 5

Wrist and Hand

John V. Ingari and Angelo R. Dacus

Anatomy

- The wrist and hand comprise a complex of bony, articular, ligamentous, vascular, tendinous, muscular, and neuroanatomic structures that allow its seemingly effortless motion and function in virtually unlimited planes.

Bones

- ❑ Wrist
  - Radius.
    - The distal aspect functions as the articular platform for the carpal bones.
    - The hand and radius move as a unit and articulate with the ulna at the sigmoid notch.
  - Ulna.
    - Anatomically placed on the medial side of the forearm.
    - In broad proximally and narrows distally with the distal most end being the styloid process.
    - Maintains its relationship with the radius via the triangular fibrocartilage complex.
  - Proximal carpal row.
    - Scaphoid, lunate and triquetrum (radial to ulnar).
    - Articulate with the radius via the scaphoid and lunate fossa.
    - Move as a unit due to intercarpal ligaments.
- ❑ Hand
  - There are 14 phalanges, 2 for the thumb and 3 for each digit:
    - Each phalanx is considered a long bone, with proximal and distal metaphyseal regions and a narrower diaphyseal region.
    - Each phalanx has a cam-shaped head distally, and a convex base proximally to articulate with the head of the bone immediately proximal to it.
    - Phalangeal flexion and extension are accomplished by the hinge, or ginglymus, joints at the metacarpophalangeal (MCP), the proximal interphalangeal (PIP), and the distal interphalangeal (DIP) levels.
  - There are 5 metacarpals:
    - The index and middle finger metacarpals have little motion at the carpometacarpal (CMC) joints and are known as the "immobile rays."
    - The ring and small finger metacarpals allow moderate motion at the CMC joints and are known as the "mobile rays."
  - There are 8 carpal bones:
    - Carpal bones are actually part of the wrist and are discussed further in that section.
    - The scaphoid, lunate, and triquetrum make up the proximal carpal row.
    - The trapezium, trapezoid, capitate, and hamate make up the distal carpal row.
    - The pisiform is actually a sesamoid bone contained within the flexor carpi ulnaris tendon; it articulates with the triquetrum.

Joints

- ❑ Radiocarpal Joint
- ❑ Distal Radioulnar Joint (DRUJ)
- ❑ The Wrist Has Both Static and Dynamic Stabilizers:
  - Static stabilizers:
    - Volar ligaments.
      - Radioscaphocapitate.
      - Long radiolunate.
      - Radioscapholunate (Ligament of Testut).
      - Ulnolunate.
      - Ulnotriquetral.
    - Dorsal ligaments.
      - Dorsal intercarpal.
      - Dorsal radiocarpal.

    - TFCC.
        - functions to extend the articular surface to cover the lunate, transmit axial force, allow forearm rotation and support the carpus on the ulnar side of the wrist.
        - palmar and dorsal radioulnar ligaments.
        - ulnolunate, ulnotriquetral and ulnocapitate ligaments.
- Dynamic or secondary stabilizers:
    - ECU.
    - Pronator quadratus.
    - Interosseous membrane.
    - Sigmoid notch.

❑ Carpometacarpal Joint
- Where the wrist "meets" the hand.
- Thumb CMC joint is particularly prone to osteoarthritis in middle age owing to its motion in multiple planes:
    - It is considered a biconcave, or saddle, joint and the thumb metacarpal and distal trapezium "fit" together much like two processed potato chips do.
    - Allows flexion, extension, radial, and ulnar deviation as well as rotation.
- Index and middle finger CMC joints are relatively immobile.
- Ring and small finger CMC joints allow flexion, extension, and slight rotation.
- A *CMC boss* is an arthritic change at the CMC joints (Hunt, 2006):
    - The dorsal bony prominence may or may not be symptomatic.
    - If symptomatic, the boss can be surgically excised.

❑ Metacarpophalangeal Joints
- Cam-shaped metacarpal heads articulate with the concave bases of the proximal phalanges.
- Collateral ligaments are tight in flexion, lax in extension.
- The volar plate forms the palmar ligamentous connection.
- Sagittal bands "lift" the joint into extension.
- MCP flexion occurs primarily via the interossei, and secondarily by the flexor tendons (Smith, 1975).

❑ Proximal Interphalangeal Joints
- Flexion occurs via the flexor digitorum superficialis (FDS).
- Extension is due to the *central slip*—insertion of extensor tendon on middle phalanx dorsally.
- Lumbrical muscle action also extends the PIP joints.

❑ Distal Interphalangeal Joints
- Flexion occurs via the flexor digitorum profundus (FDP).
- Extension occurs via the terminal tendon insertion on the dorsal base of distal phalanx.

Bone and Joint Questions

1. Which of the following best describes the metacarpophalangeal (MCP) joint?
A. The collateral ligaments are tight in flexion and extension.
B. The collateral ligaments are tight in flexion and lax in extension.
C. The collateral ligaments are lax in flexion and extension.
D. The volar plate is tight in flexion and lax in extension.
E. Extension of the MCP joint occurs via the central slip.

2. A 40-year-old man, an ex-boxer, has gradually increasing pain and swelling at the middle finger CMC joint. Radiographs demonstrate osteophytes at the base of the metacarpal and distal capitate. The most likely diagnosis is:
A. Fracture of the middle phalanx.
B. CMC boss.
C. Rheumatoid arthritis.
D. CMC dislocation.
E. Extensor tendon rupture.

3. Which of the following describes flexion and extension of the DIP joint?
A. Flexion occurs via the central slip, and extension via the terminal tendon.
B. Flexion occurs via the flexor digitorum profundus, and extension via the central slip.
C. Flexion occurs via the flexor digitorum profundus, and extension via the terminal tendon.
D. Both flexion and extension occur via the terminal tendon.
E. Flexion occurs via the terminal tendon, and extension via the sagittal bands.

4. Which of the following carpal bones is a sesamoid?
A. The scaphoid.
B. The trapezium.
C. The capitate.
D. The pisiform.
E. The hamate.

■

Tendons and Muscles of the Hand

Volar

- Flexor carpi radialis (FCR).
- Flexor pollicic longus (FPL).
- Flexor digitorum superficialis (FDS).
- Flexor digitorum profundus (FDP).
- Palmaris longus.
- Flexor carpi ulnaris (FCU).

Dorsal (6 compartment)

- 1st compartment – Abductor pollicis longus (APL), extensor pollicis brevis (EPB).
- 2nd compartment – Extensor carpi radialis longus and brevis (ECRL/ECRB).

- 3rd compartment – Extensor pollicis longus (EPL).
- 4th compartment – Extensor digitorum comminus (EDC), extensor indicis proprius (EIP).
- 5th compartment – Extensor digiti quinti (EDQ).
- 6th compartment – Extensor carpi ulnaris (ECU).

Muscles

- The extrinsic muscles of the hand originate in the forearm and tendons and insert in the hand.
  - Flexor digitorum superficialis (FDS).
  - Flexor digitorum profundus (FDP).
  - Flexor pollicis longus (FPL).
  - Abductor pollicis longus (APL).
  - Extensor pollicis brevis (EPB).
  - Extensor indicis proprius (EIP).
  - Extensor digitorum communis (EDC).
  - Extensor digiti minimi (EDM).
- Intrinsic muscles of the hand originate and insert in the hand.
- Lumbricals:
  - Originate on FDP tendons (antagonist muscles).
  - When lumbricals contract, FDP muscles relax.
- Interossei:
  - Four dorsal interossei abduct the digits (*d*orsal *ab*duct = DAB).
  - Three palmar interossei adduct the digits (*p*almar *ad*duct = PAD).
  - The middle finger is considered the central ray of the hand; movement away from the middle finger is abduction, and movement toward the middle is adduction.
- Opponens pollicis.
- Abductor pollicis brevis.
- Flexor pollicis brevis.
- Adductor pollicis.
- Opponens digiti minimi.
- Abductor digiti minimi.
- Flexor digiti minimi.

Tendons

- Tendons connect muscle to bone to facilitate joint motion.
- Tendons are susceptible to ruptures, lacerations, and inflammation.
- Tendons are named by their associated muscle; for example FDS tendon, FDP tendon.
- The ring finger FDP tendon is most common deep flexor tendon ruptured in sports (75%); this rupture is also known as a Jersey finger (Tuttle et al, 2006) (Fig. 5–1).

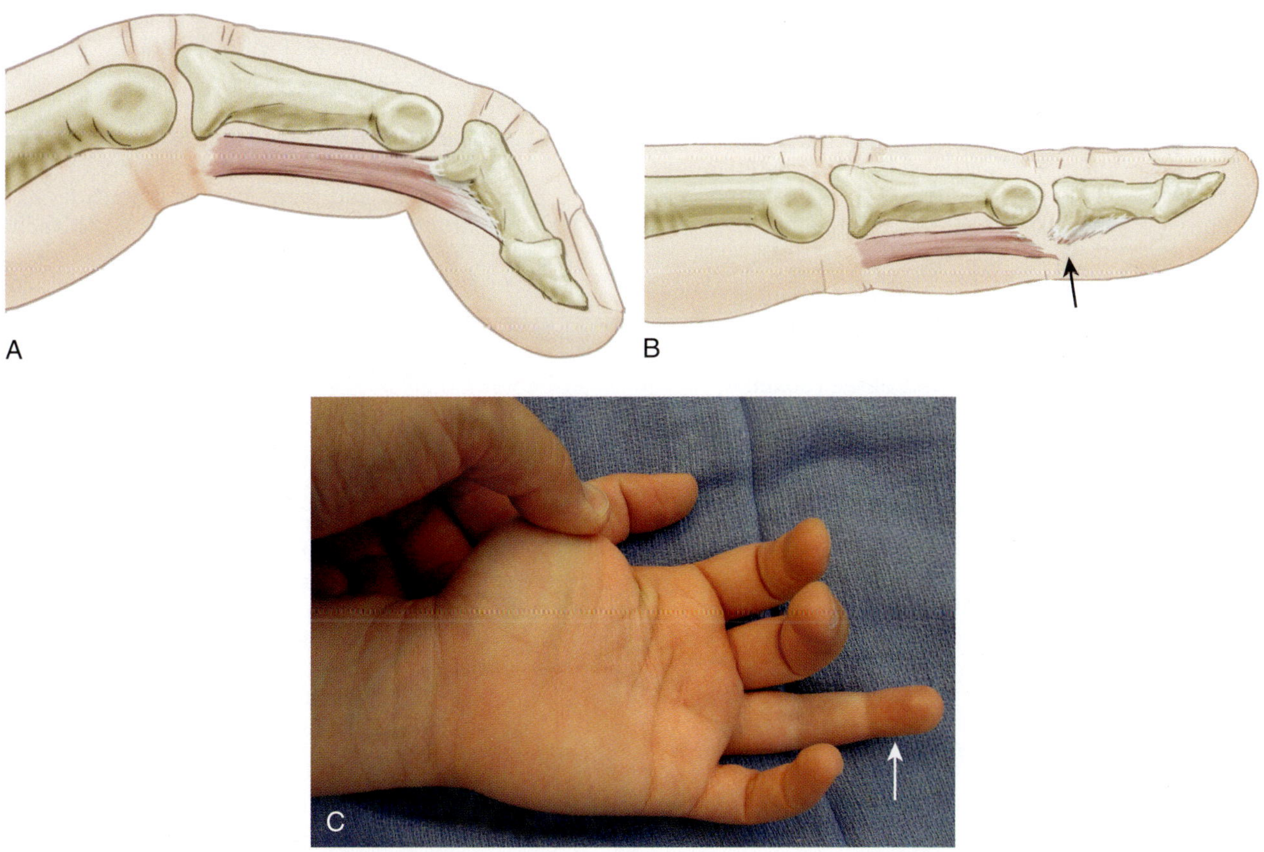

Figure 5–1 A, The deep flexor tendon attaches to the distal phalanx. B, With rapid extension the flexor tendon can rupture, resulting in Jersey finger injury. C, The normal resting flexion position of the finger is lost with a Jersey finger injury.

- Thickenings of the retinacular flexor sheath called pulleys keep the flexor tendons close to the bones and optimize digital joint motion (Doyle, 2001):
  - The A2 and A4 pulleys are the most clinically important flexor pulleys.
  - The A2 pulley overlies the proximal aspect of the proximal phalanx.
  - The A4 pulley overlies the middle aspect of the middle phalanx.
  - Disruption of the A2 or A4 pulley can lead to "bowstringing" of a tendon.

Tendon/Muscle Questions

1. A 17-year-old football player feels a pop with subsequent pain after grabbing another player's jersey during a tackle. He is unable to flex the distal phalanx of one digit. The structure most likely to be injured is:
   A. FDS tendon of the middle finger.
   B. FDP tendon of the ring finger.
   C. FDP tendon of the index finger.
   D. FDP tendon of the small finger.
   E. FDS tendon of the ring finger.
2. The only intrinsic muscle to relax its own antagonist in the hand is the:
   A. Flexor digitorum manus brevis.
   B. Lumbrical muscle.
   C. Dorsal interosseous muscle.
   D. Palmar interosseous muscle.
   E. Opponens pollicis.
3. All of the following are true except:
   A. Palmar interosseous muscles adduct the digits.
   B. Dorsal interosseous muscles abduct the digits.
   C. The flexor digitorum superficialis flexes the PIP joint.
   D. The flexor digitorum profundus flexes the DIP joint.
   E. Lumbrical muscles extend the MP joint.
4. Disruption of the A2 pulley:
   A. Can lead to bowstringing of the flexor tendon.
   B. Occurs at the middle aspect of the middle phalanx.
   C. Occurs at the proximal aspect of the proximal phalanx.
   D. Is of little clinical relevance.
   E. Both A and C are correct.

Neurovascular Anatomy

Arteries

- Radial and ulnar arteries provide the major blood supply to the hand (Fig. 5–2).
- The radial artery has a palpable pulse at volar radial wrist:
  - Continues into hand as deep palmar arch, anastomosing with ulnar artery branches.
  - The deep palmar arch is proximal to the superficial arch.

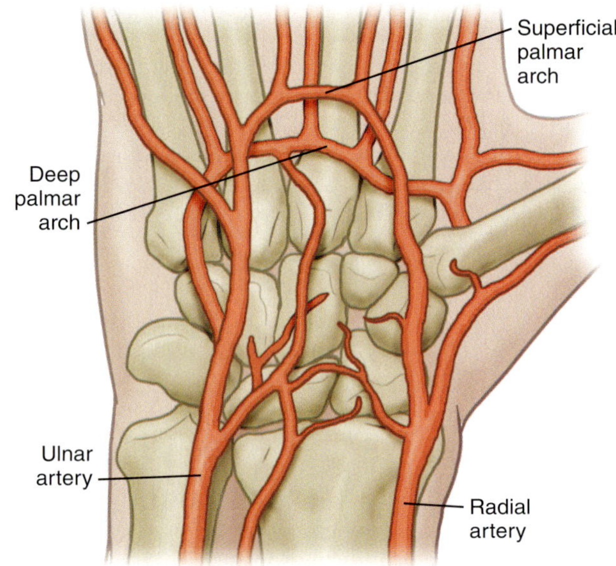

Figure 5–2 The rich arterial anatomy supplying the hand and wrist.

- The ulnar artery lies deep to the FCU tendon, and its pulse is difficult to palpate.
  - Continues into palm as superficial palmar arch, anastomosing with radial artery branches.
  - The superficial palmar arch is distal to the deep palmar arch.
  - The superficial palmar arch is complete in 84% of hands (Gellman et al, 2001).

❑ Allen Test

Procedure

- The patient makes a tight fist.
- The examiner puts digital pressure over both the radial and ulnar arteries at wrist level.
- The patient opens the fist, which is blanched (Fig. 5–3A).
- The examiner lifts his/her finger off the radial artery to watch hand "pink up" as blood flows into the palm (Fig. 5–3B).
- The above steps, with examiner lifting his/her finger off the ulnar artery.

Results

- A normal Allen test result means that the hand "pinks up" when either finger is lifted, indicating flow through both radial and ulnar arteries into the hand.
- An abnormal result is seen with an incomplete arch (anatomic variant) or pathologic occlusion (i.e., thrombus) of artery.
  - Visibly, the hand remains blanched when the examiner's finger is removed from one artery.

Nerves

- Radial, median, and ulnar nerves are major nerves into the hand.
  - Median nerve:

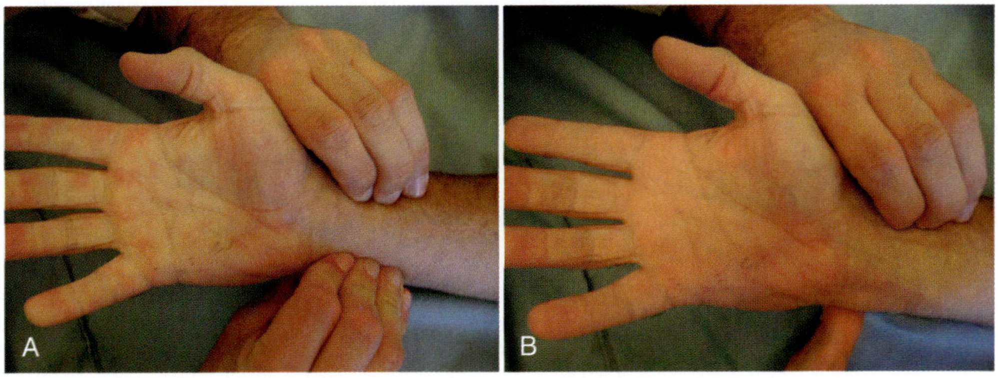

Figure 5–3 A, The examiner occludes both radial and ulnar arteries. B, The examiner lifts pressure off the ulnar artery to assess flow into the hand.

- Crosses the wrist between the FDS and FDP just anterior to the Palmaris longus prior to entering the carpal tunnel.
- Supplies the following intrinsic hand muscles: *l*umbrical muscles to index and middle, *o*pponens pollicis, *a*bductor pollicis brevis, and *f*lexor pollicis brevis (LOAF muscles).

- Ulnar nerve:
  - Crosses the wrist beneath the FCU and ulnar to the ulnar artery prior to entering Guyon's canal.
  - Supplies all other hand intrinsic muscles.
- Radial nerve:
  - The superficial branch crosses the wrist dorsally after exiting the volar compartment beneath brachioradialis between it and ECRL.
  - Does not normally supply hand intrinsic muscles.

❑ Sensory Patterns for Nerves

- "Classic" patterns:
  - Median nerve: Palmar aspect of thumb, index finger, middle finger, and radial half of ring finger.
  - Ulnar nerve: Dorsal and palmar aspect of small finger, ulnar half of ring finger.
  - Radial nerve: Dorsal aspect of thumb, index finger, middle finger, and radial half of ring finger.
- Sensory patterns can vary from these "classic" patterns.
- Each digit has radial and ulnar digital nerves both palmarly and dorsally.
  - The dorsal digital nerves end distally at the DIP joint level.
  - Fingertip sensation is provided by the palmar digital nerves.
- Normal two-point discrimination distance is 5 mm in the fingertips.
  - Two-point discrimination distance greater than 15 mm indicates complete nerve injury/laceration.
  - Two-point discrimination distance between 5 and 15 mm indicates incomplete nerve injury.

Neurovascular Questions

1. An abnormal Allen test result would be found in the following clinical scenario:
A. A thrombus in the ulnar artery at the level of the wrist.
B. A laceration of the anterior interosseous artery in the forearm.
C. Median nerve injury in the index finger.
D. Radial nerve injury at the base of the thumb.
E. Ulnar nerve compression at the elbow.

2. A patient is seen in the emergency department following an accidental laceration to his nondominant index finger at the level of the PIP joint. He complains of numbness along the radial side of the index fingertip, although he can flex the DIP joint actively. Two-point discrimination distance is greater than 15 mm on the radial aspect of the fingertip and is 5 mm on the ulnar aspect of the fingertip. The most likely diagnosis is:
A. Partial injury to the dorsal digital nerve to the index finger.
B. Complete laceration of the palmar radial digital nerve to the index finger, with intact flexor tendon.
C. Complete laceration of the palmar radial and palmar ulnar digital nerve to the index finger.
D. Partial flexor tendon laceration and partial palmar radial digital nerve to the index finger.
E. Nerve status cannot be assessed on the basis of the clinical findings.

History and Physical Examination of the Hand

History

- Hand dominance.
- Patient age.
- Occupation, hobbies.
- Time of injury.
- Location of pain ("Point to where it hurts").
  - Radial.

    - Snuffbox.
    - Ulnar.
- Mechanism of injury:
    - Wrist hyperflexion or hyperextension.
    - Twisting.
    - Laceration.
    - "Jamming" injury (e.g., struck by a ball at the tip of the finger).
    - Sports injury (e.g., grabbing a jersey, felt a "pop").
    - Crush.
    - Compression.
- Comorbidities (diabetes, hypertension, etc.).
- Medications.
- History of prior injury.

Physical Examination

- ❑ Inspection
    - Resting posture (i.e., is one digit straight, while others are flexed?) (see Fig. 5–1C).
    - Color (erythema).
    - Swelling.
    - Ecchymosis.
        - Indicates bleeding secondary to underlying injury
    - Deformity:
        - Rotational deformity of the digits is best assessed by observing the fingernails, especially with the digits flexed (Freeland & Lindley, 2006).
        - The index finger is normally slightly supinated compared to the other digits.
    - Lacerations:
        - May indicate injury to underlying structures, including nerves, vessels, tendons, and joint capsules.
        - Open joints proximal to the DIP should undergo irrigation and débridement in the operating room.
- ❑ Palpation
    - Point of maximal tenderness often indicates the anatomic structure injured.
        - Snuffbox.
        - Ulnocarpal joint.
        - 1st dorsal compartment/radial styloid
        - Distal radius.
        - Metacarpals.
        - Phalanges.
    - Suspected tendon ruptures are typically tender at their insertion sites.
    - Assess mass/swelling for firmness, mobility, fluctuance.
- ❑ Vascular Assessment
    - Allen test.
    - Chronic ulcers.
- ❑ Neural Assessment
    - Two-point discrimination:
        - Normal is 5 mm (Marx et al, 1998).
        - Complete anesthesia = greater than 15 mm.
    - Tinel sign, or tingling that occurs when nerves are tapped, may indicate nerve compression or partial injury.
- ❑ Functional Assessment
    - Grip strength:
        - Jamar dynamometer is a reliable grip strength tool (Peolsson et al, 2001).
        - Compare right and left sides.
        - Dominant hand is typically stronger.
    - Tendon function:
        - Test each finger and each joint independently.
        - Keep other digits fully extended when testing individual FDS tendon function (to prevent the FDP from causing flexion at the PIP joint).
        - Special tests
            - Finkelstein's—pain with forced ulnar deviation of the thumb/wrist.
            - Watson's—pain or clunk with scaphoid pressure while taking the wrist from ulnar to radial deviation.
            - DRUJ ballotment.

Imaging

- Plain radiographs of the hand in at least two orthogonal planes (posteroanterior and lateral).
- For suspected digital injury, a radiograph of the individual digit is needed to prevent missing a subtle fracture.
- Special views for specific injuries:
    - scaphoid fracture—scaphoid view (ulnar deviated AP).
    - Pisotriquetral joint injury—supinated lateral view.
    - Hook of the hamate fracture—carpal tunnel view
    - Metacarpal fracture—(30 degree supinated view to see lateral view of individual metacarpals).
    - suspected ligament injury—(stress views).
- Adjunctive studies as needed:
    - Magnetic resonance imaging (MRI) to view soft tissue structures, including tendons, ligaments, and cartilaginous structures (triangular fibrocartilage), may help if indicated.
    - MRI may also demonstrate "occult" fractures not seen on plain film (Fig. 5–4).
    - Arthrogram can be a useful adjunct to MRI.
    - Bone scintigraphy (bone scan) is very sensitive but not specific for delineating the location of an injury.
    - CT scan can aid in the evaluation of DRUJ injuries, scaphoid nonunion, and intra-articular distal radius fractures.
    - Selective radiocarpal/ulnocarpal injections can also aid in diagnosis.

History and Physical Examination Questions

1. All of the following are important issues in obtaining a history for a hand injury except:
A. Age of the patient.

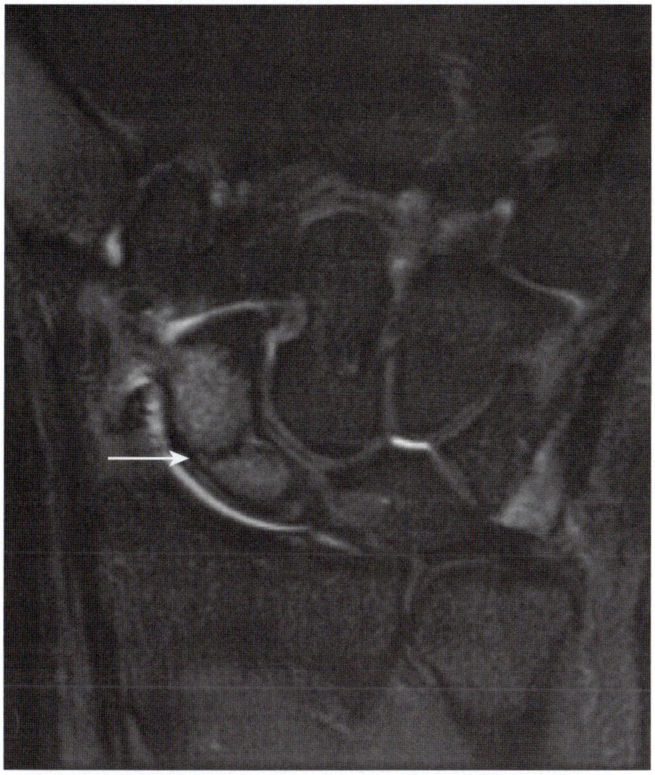

Figure 5–4 Magnetic resonance imaging can detect an occult fracture of the scaphoid not seen on plain radiography. *Arrow* denotes MCP joint.

B. Hobbies enjoyed/sports involvement.
C. Hand dominance.
D. Time of injury.
E. Favorite subject in school.

2. The FDP is prevented from flexing the PIP joint of a finger being examined by:
   A. Having the patient flex all digits simultaneously to maximize tendon excursion.
   B. Holding the thumb in maximal extension while flexion of the digit is attempted.
   C. Holding the remaining digits in full extension, thereby preventing FDP excursion.
   D. Extending the MCP joint fully to place maximal tension on the FDP tendon.
   E. None of the above.
3. A patient is suspected of having a scaphoid fracture because of tenderness in the anatomic snuffbox (overlies the scaphoid) from an injury 4 days ago, but his radiographs are read as "negative." A helpful adjunctive study would be:
   A. Bone scan.
   B. C-reactive protein measurement.
   C. MRI.
   D. PET scan.
   E. Both A and C.
4. During the Allen test, a patient's hand remains blanched when the examiner's finger is lifted off the palmar ulnar side of the wrist. This indicates:
   A. Ulnar nerve injury.
   B. Absence or incompleteness of filling from the ulnar artery.
   C. Fracture of the hook of the hamate.
   D. TFC tear.
   E. Injury to the lunotriquetral ligament.

Common Sports Hand Injuries

Tendon Injuries

- ❑ "Jersey Finger"
  - FDP rupture (see Fig. 5–1).
  - 75% of such ruptures occur in the ring finger.
  - Often results when a flexed fist is rapidly jerked into extension.
  - Requires surgical repair.
- ❑ Mallet Injury
  - "Bony mallet": Dorsal avulsion fracture of distal phalanx (Jablecki & Syrko, 2007) (Fig. 5–5).
  - "Nonbony mallet": Disruption of terminal (extensor) tendon.
  - Both bony and nonbony mallet injuries result in extensor lag or droop of distal phalanx.
  - Rarely requires surgery (Jablecki & Syrko, 2007).
  - Treatment consists of immobilization in an extension splint for 6 weeks (Stack splint).
  - Can be treated as late as 3 months after injury with good results.
  - Patients are cautioned that some extensor lag/droop may persist despite treatment, but function should be fine.
  - Symptomatic, chronic mallet injury can be fused in extension (0–15 degrees of flexion at the DIP joint).
- ❑ Central Slip Injury (Boutonnière Deformity) (Fig. 5–6)
  - "Jammed" finger.
  - Results *from* disruption of the central slip of the extensor tendon at the dorsal lip of the middle phalanx.
  - Untreated, leads to boutonnière (buttonhole) deformity.

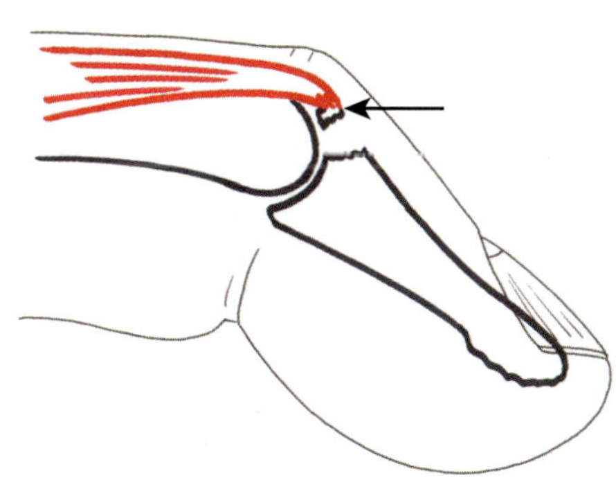

Figure 5–5 A bony mallet injury. Notice the avulsion fracture and the extensor lag or "droop." *(Courtesy of Dr. Steve Henry.)*

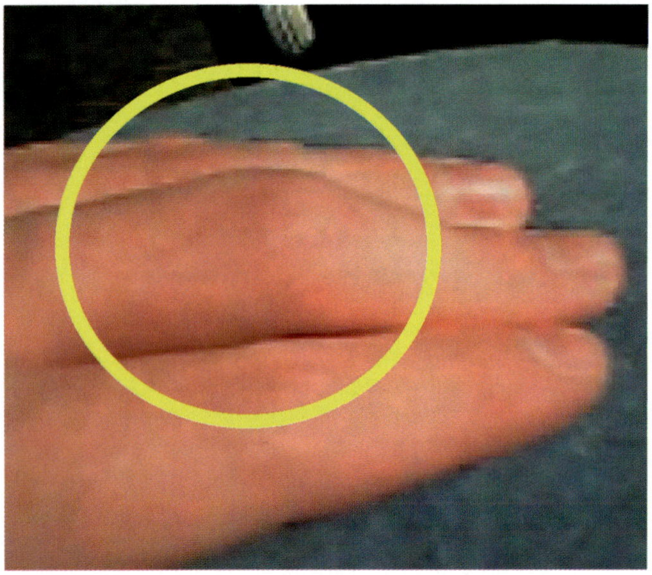

Figure 5–6 A boutonnière deformity at the PIP joint. Notice the chronic-type swelling.

- Diagnosis aided by the finding of maximal tenderness dorsally at the central slip insertion.
- Treatment is immobilization in a PIP extension splint, full time, for 4 weeks followed by night-time splinting if needed.
  - The DIP is left free to allow active flexion, avoiding scarring of the lateral bands.
- Chronic boutonnière deformity may require surgical treatment to restore central slip function (Urbaniak & Hayes, 1981).

Tendon Injury Questions

1. A 35-year-old man who suffered a nonbony mallet injury 6 months ago has a persistent 30-degree extensor lag at the DIP joint of his middle finger, despite 6 weeks of Stack splinting and 6 additional weeks of night-time splinting. He complains of pain and catching of the finger when he puts his hands in his pockets. Appropriate treatment would be:
A. Surgical reconstruction of the extensor mechanism using a pullout suture technique.
B. Pinning of the DIP joint in 30 degrees of flexion.
C. Arthrodesis (fusion) of the DIP joint in 0 to 15 degrees of flexion.
D. Observation and buddy taping to the adjacent digit.
E. Amputation at the base of nail plate level.

2. A 19-year-old softball player jammed her right finger when it was struck by a ball on the tip. The finger is most tender dorsally at the base of middle phalanx. She is unable to actively extend the PIP joint. Radiographs show no evidence of fracture. Initial treatment should include:
A. An ulnar gutter cast with the ring and small fingers flexed at the MCP, PIP, and DIP joints.
B. Buddy taping of the ring finger to the middle finger for 4 weeks.
C. Arthrodesis of the PIP joint as soon as swelling subsides.
D. Extension splinting of the PIP joint full time for 4 weeks, leaving the DIP joint free to flex.
E. No treatment is required; the injury will heal with no deformity or functional deficit.

3. A 16-year-old football player felt a pop in his left ring finger when he grabbed the jersey of an opposing player during a tackle 2 days ago. He is now unable to actively flex the DIP joint of the involved digit. Radiographs show no evidence of fracture. He and his parents should be counseled that:
A. He has a finger sprain that will resolve with ice, rest, and elevation.
B. He likely has ruptured his deep flexor (FDP) tendon ("Jersey finger"), and surgery to reattach the tendon will give the most satisfactory functional recovery.
C. No surgery is needed, and when the ecchymosis resolves, range-of-motion exercises must be started under the direction of a hand therapist.
D. A steroid injection into the joint will decrease pain and allow flexion to resume.
E. Buddy taping of the ring finger to the middle finger will be adequate to allow the tendon to heal in the proper position.

Ligament Injuries

- Dislocations, hyperextension, and lateral bending can result in ligament injuries.

❑ TFCC
- Arthroscopic treatment.
  - Central tears are treated with debridement to a stable rim.
  - Peripheral tears are repaired
    - Inside-out or outside-in technique.
    - Suture tied over the capsule.

❑ Carpal Instability
- Wrist kinematics:
  - Active wrist motion is dependent on the tendons that cross the joint, the muscle function and its distance from the center of rotation.
    - The distal carpal row is rigid and moves as a unit.
    - The proximal row moves synergistically but in a less rigid manner.
    - The proximal row moves from extension to flexion as the wrist moves in ulnar to radial deviation.
  - DISI (dorsal intercalated segment instability).
    - Results from scapholunate ligament disruption.
    - The scaphoid is no longer tethered by the proximal row and falls into flexion.
    - The lunate and triquetrum now fall into extension due to the now unrestrained force on the triquetrum.

- VISI (volar intercalated segment instability).
  - Results from lunotriquetral ligament disruption.
  - The extension moment of the triquetrum can no longer counterbalance the flexion moment of the scaphoid.
  - The lunate follows the scaphoid into flexion.

❑ Scapholunate
- Mechanism of injury.
  - Wrist hyperextension, ulnar deviation and midcarpal supination.
  - Dorsal portion of the ligament is the strongest.
  - Permanent malalignment results from failure of the scaphocapitate ligament as well.
- Diagnosis.
  - Wrist pain, typically radial sided.
  - Positive Watson's test
    - Palmar pressure over scaphoid causes pain with radial deviation of the wrist.
  - MRI to evaluate the ligament.
  - Wrist arthroscopy
    - Best evaluated in the midcarpal joint.
- Treatment.
  - Partial tear can be treated in a cast for 6 weeks.
  - Ligament repair/reconstruction with capusolodesis.
  - Salvage procedure when chronic or arthritis present.

❑ Gamekeeper's Thumb (Fig. 5–7)
- Tear of the ulnar collateral ligament at the MP joint.
- Also known as skier's thumb.
- A Stener lesion occurs when the adductor aponeurosis is interposed between a ligament and its bony insertion; prevents ligament healing (Carlsen & Moran, 2009).
- The tear can be partial or complete.
- Complete tears are best addressed surgically to reattach ligament to bone (Carlsen & Moran, 2009).
- May also take the form of an avulsion fracture instead of pure ligament injury: bony gamekeeper's thumb (Fig. 5–8).
- Bony gamekeeper's thumb requires surgery if the fragment is displaced more than 2 mm or is rotated.
- Nondisplaced bony gamekeeper's thumb or partial ligament tear can be treated in a thumb spica cast for 4 weeks, followed by protective splinting for sports (typically 3 months for contact sports) (Carlsen & Moran, 2009) (Fig. 5–9).

❑ Dislocations
- Dorsal PIP dislocations are common (Fig. 5–10).
  - They typically reduce easily with traction ("coach's finger").
  - Once reduced, treatment is buddy taping.
  - Rarely, rotatory dislocation does not reduce.
- MP joint dislocations, including in the thumb, are less common.
  - May be irreducible because of an entrapped volar plate.
  - If irreducible, surgery is needed to dislodge the volar plate.

❑ Fracture-Dislocations
- Fracture-dislocations are more serious than dislocations.
- Extension block splinting may reduce the joint effectively.
- Referral to a hand surgeon is required.

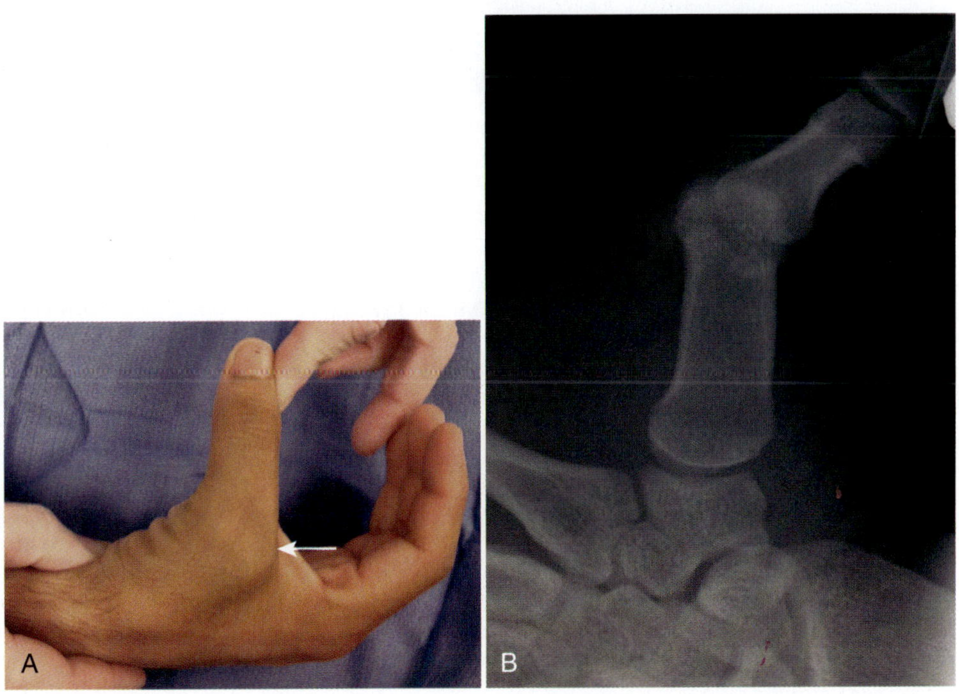

Figure 5–7 **A,** Gamekeeper's injury of the thumb showing instability at the MCP joint with radial stress. **B,** Radiograph of gamekeeper's injury showing the MP joint instability.

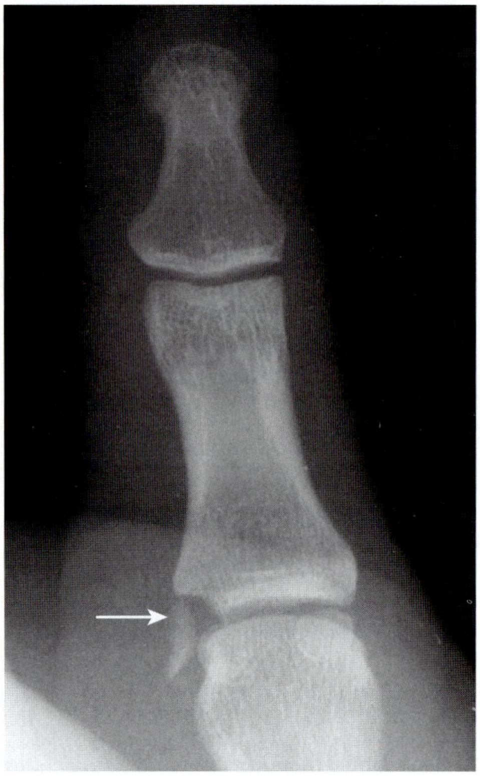

Figure 5–8 A bony gamekeeper's injury with a displaced, rotated fragment. This should be surgically repaired.

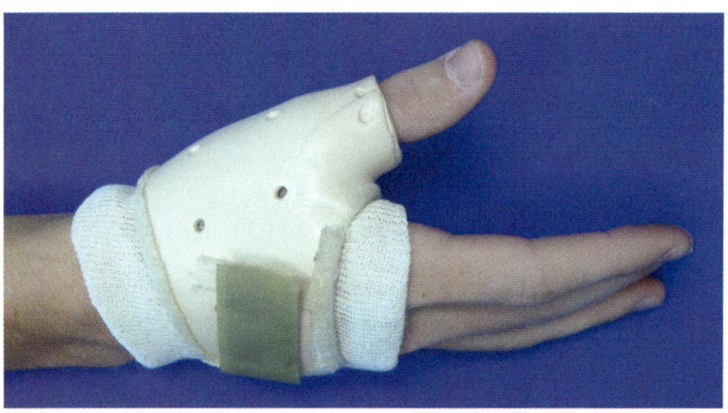

Figure 5–9 A custom thumb spica splint to protect a healing gamekeeper's injury during sports.

- ❑ Collateral Ligament Injury
  - Collateral ligaments are injured with lateral bending of the digits.
  - Injury commonly occurs at the MP or PIP joint level.
  - May be associated with dislocation.
  - Buddy taping to the adjacent finger is acceptable treatment, except for an injury to the thumb (Fig. 5–11).
  - It may take as long as 12 months for pain to subside.
  - Patients should be counseled that PIP joints will likely have residual swelling after full healing.
  - Ulnar collateral ligament injury of thumb is gamekeeper's thumb (see previous discussion).

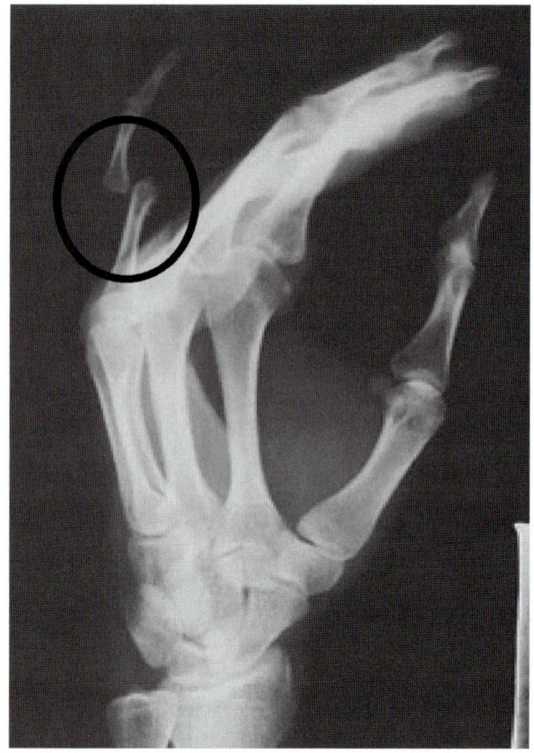

Figure 5–10 A dorsal PIP dislocation (coach's finger), which usually reduces easily with distal traction.

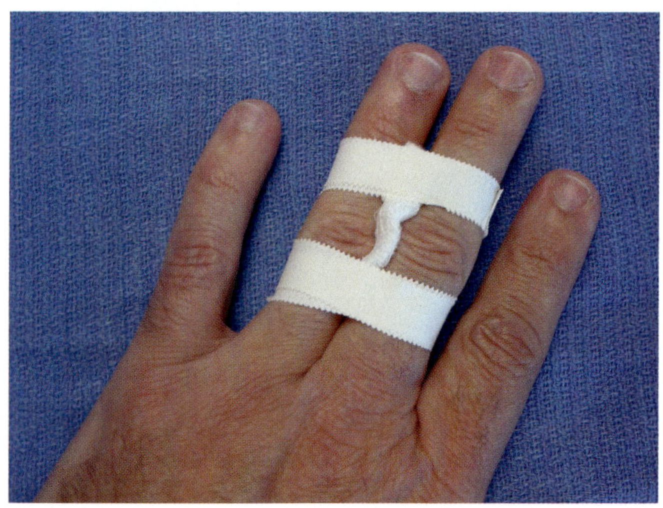

Figure 5–11 Buddy taping to allow protection and mobility.

Ligament Injury Questions

1. A 17-year-old baseball catcher sustained a hyperextension and radial deviation injury to his left thumb. Radiographs demonstrate a fragment avulsed from the ulnar side of the base of the proximal phalanx that is displaced 3 mm and rotated. Appropriate treatment for the injury should be:

A. Surgical fixation of the avulsed ulnar collateral ligament, typically with a small bone anchor.

B. Thumb spica casting for 4 weeks, followed by protective bracing for 3 months.
C. Taping of the thumb to prevent hyperextension and radial deviation for the remainder of the baseball season.
D. Fusion of the MP joint of the thumb to prevent future injury and allow return to sports.
E. Ice, elevation, and rest. The bone fragment will heal uneventfully, resulting in complete restoration of stability.

2. A 12-year-old football player dislocated the MP joint of the left index finger from a hyperextension injury incurred while making a tackle. The family practitioner was unable to reduce the joint with traction. The structure most likely preventing successful reduction is:
A. The collateral ligament.
B. The extensor tendon.
C. The volar plate.
D. The digital nerve.
E. The flexor tendon.

3. A trainer performed a successful reduction of a dorsal dislocation of a player's middle finger PIP joint during volleyball practice. Subsequent radiographs show no fracture, and there is no tenderness at the insertion of the central slip. Treatment should now consist of:
A. An ulnar gutter cast for 6 weeks to restore stability.
B. Buddy taping to the adjacent digit to provide stability and early motion.
C. Extension splinting of the digit for 6 weeks.
D. A radial gutter cast for 6 weeks to restore stability.
E. An external fixator for the digit to allow optimal healing.

4. Two weeks ago a 22- year-old college athlete sustained a lateral bending injury to her nondominant ring finger PIP joint. The finger is maximally tender over the ulnar collateral ligament of the joint and minimally tender over the volar plate. The patient is able to fully extend the finger, and the flexor tendons are intact. Radiographs are read as "negative." The athlete should be counseled that:
A. Surgery is needed to reconstruct the ulnar collateral ligament within 3 weeks of injury.
B. There will be residual swelling of the PIP joint, and symptoms (pain) may last as long as a year.
C. Arthrodesis (fusion) of the joint will be required to restore stability to the joint.
D. She will have to discontinue sports for the remainder of her college career because of the nature of the injury.
E. Buddy taping is ineffective for collateral ligament sprains, and casting will be required for 6 weeks.

Fractures

- Hand and wrist fractures are common in sports, in the following locations:

❑ Distal Radius Fractures.
- Metaphyseal fractures are common.
- Physis or growth plate can be involved in skeletally immature patients.
- Most common fracture in the upper extremity.
- Normal alignment:
  - Radial inclination of 22 degrees.
  - Volar tilt of 11 degrees.
  - Neutral ulnar deviation.
- Common eponyms:
  - Colles' fracture—dorsal angulation, comminution, and displacement.
  - Smith's fracture—volar displacement.
  - Barton's fracture—volar or dorsal articular fragment subluxation.
  - Chauffeur's fracture—radial styloid fracture.
  - Die-punch fracture—depression in the lunate articular surface.
- Treatment:
  - Acceptable alignment.
    - <2 mm articular displacement.
    - <20 degrees metaphyseal angulation.
    - <3 mm metaphyseal shortening.
  - Closed fractures.
    - Splint and casting for stable extra-articular fractures with good alignment.
    - Closed reduction percutaneous pinning (CRPP).
    - Open reduction internal fixation (ORIF).
    - External fixation with or without additional fixation.
  - Open fractures
    - Thorough irrigation and debridement.
    - External fixation for complex wounds with poor tissue coverage.
    - ORIF.

❑ Galeazzi Fracture
- Fracture of the radial shaft between the middle and distal third with associated dislocation of DRUJ.
  - May be purely ligamentous or involve the ulnar styloid.
- Treatment:
  - Compression plating to obtain anatomic reduction.
  - Then re-evaluate DRUJ.
  - If unstable, use K wire fixation from the ulna to radius.
  - May require ORIF of ulnar styloid or repair of TFCC.
- Carpal fractures, the most common being a scaphoid fracture (Rizzo & Shin, 2006).
- Metacarpal fractures.
- Phalangeal fractures.
- Avulsion fractures may accompany ligament or tendon injuries in the hand and provide clues to the injured tendon or ligament.
- The hand and wrist contain 14 phalanges, 5 metacarpals, and 8 carpal bones; in all, 27 bones distal to the radius and ulna can be fractured.

- The point of maximal tenderness often leads to the diagnosis:
  - Anatomic snuffbox tenderness suggests scaphoid fracture.
  - Metacarpal and phalangeal fractures are tender directly at the fracture site.

❑ Metacarpal Fractures

- Metacarpal shaft fractures tend to have apex dorsal angulation.
- Metacarpal neck fractures, especially involving the small finger, can occur from a fist striking a solid object ("boxer's fracture").
- Single metacarpal fractures usually do well with splint or cast immobilization.
- Multiple metacarpal fractures are more likely to need surgical fixation (Fig. 5–12).

❑ Phalangeal Fractures

- Avulsion fractures may indicate associated tendon or ligament injury.
- Phalangeal shaft fractures tend to have apex volar angulation.
- Fractures involving joints need anatomic restoration of the joint surface and may require surgery.

Fracture Questions

1. The fracture listed here that is most likely to need surgical fixation is:
A. Spiral fracture of the middle finger metacarpal shaft.
B. Collateral ligament avulsion fracture of the proximal phalanx.
C. Displaced intra-articular fracture of the metacarpal head.
D. Metacarpal neck fracture with apex dorsal angulation of 30 degrees.
E. Dorsal avulsion fracture of the distal phalanx (bony mallet).

2. The most commonly fractured carpal bone is the:
A. Triquetrum.
B. Capitate.
C. Hamate.
D. Lunate.
E. Scaphoid.

3. All of the following are true except:
A. Proximal phalangeal shaft fractures tend to angulate with the apex volar.
B. Metacarpal shaft fractures tend to angulate with the apex dorsal.
C. Avulsion fractures often represent ligamentous or tendinous injury.
D. Distal radius fractures are uncommon in sports because of the size of the bone.
E. Tenderness to palpation in the anatomic snuff box should lead to suspicion of a scaphoid fracture.

Wrist Arthroscopy

Positioning

- Patient supine with arm on a hand table.
- Traction table to allow for 10-15 lbs with the elbow at 90 degrees flexion.
- Tourniquet applied to upper arm.
- Finger traps utilized for distraction.

Portals

- Based on dorsal wrist compartments
  - 3-4 portal.
    - 1 cm distal to Lister's tubercle.
    - Primary arthroscopy portal.
  - 4-5 portal.
    - Working portal.

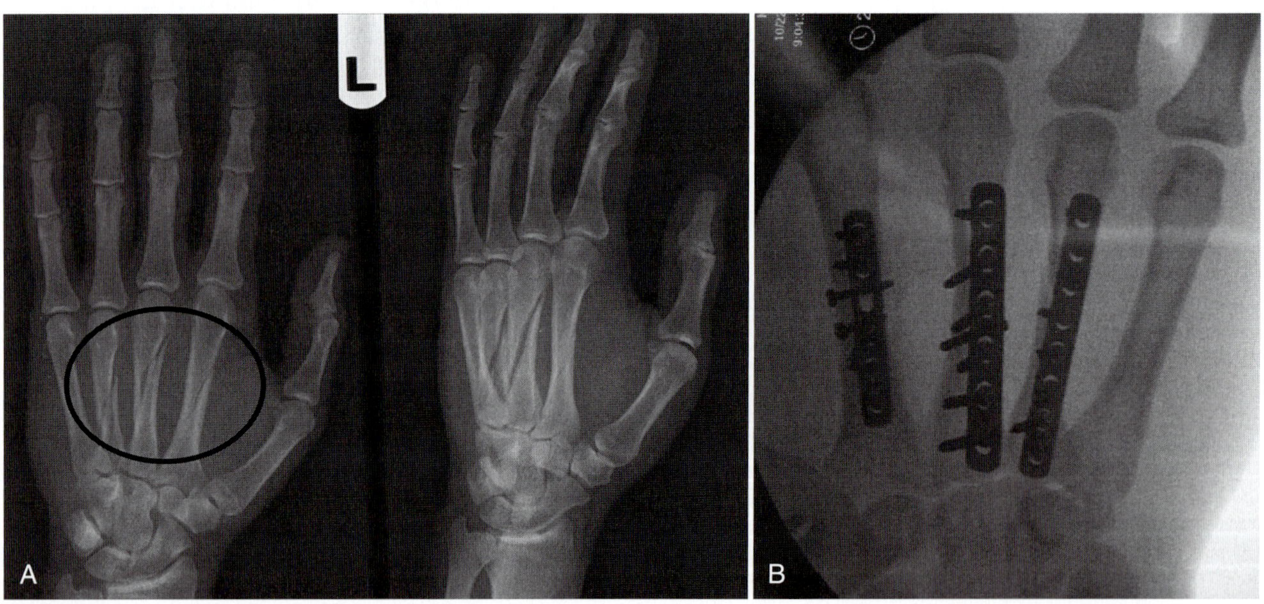

Figure 5–12 A, Multiple metacarpal fractures (black circle delineates fractures). B, Open reduction and internal fixation of the metacarpal fractures.

- 6U portal.
  - Just ulnar to ECU.
  - May be an outflow portal.
- Midcarpal portals (radial and ulnar).
  - 1cm distal to radiocarpal portals.
  - Allows for assessment of scapholunate and lunotriquetral stability.
- 1-2 portal.
  - May serve as inflow portal.
  - Care must be taken to protect radial artery.

Diagnostic

- Insufflate joint with 10 cc sterile saline.
- Enter 3-4 portal with a blunt trocar followed by the arthroscope.
- Establish an outflow portal.
- A pump is rarely needed for fluid management.
- Identify to working 4-5 portal with a needle and then enter with a probe.
- Begin radially and assess the chondral and ligamentous integrity.
- Palpate the TFCC and evaluate for tears.
- Insert a arthroscopic shaver to debride loose or frayed tissue.
- Remove the scope and identify the midcarpal portal with a needle.
- Access the midcarpal joint with a blunt trocar followed by the arthroscope.
- Establish a working portal using a needle followed by a probe.
- Evaluate the scapholunate and lunotriquetral intervals.
- Return to the radiocarpal joint and perform repairs/debridement as needed.

References and Resources

Carlsen, B.T., Moran, S.L., 2009. Thumb trauma: Bennett fractures, Rolando fractures, and ulnar collateral ligament injuries. J. Hand Surg. Am. 34, 945–952.

Doyle, J.R., 2001. Palmar and digital flexor tendon pulleys. Clin. Orthop. Relat. Res. 383, 84–96.

Freeland, A.E., Lindley, S.G., 2006. Malunions of the finger metacarpals and phalanges. Hand Clin. 22, 341–355.

Gellman, H., Botte, M.J., Shankwiler, J., Gelberman, R.H., 2001. Arterial patterns of the deep and superficial palmar arches. Clin. Orthop. Relat. Res. 383, 41–46.

Hunt 3rd, T.R., 2006. Degenerative and post-traumatic arthritis affecting the carpometacarpal joints of the fingers. Hand Clin. 22, 221–228.

Jablecki, J., Syrko, M., 2007. Zone 1 extensor tendon lesions: Current treatment methods and a review of literature. Ortop. Traumatol. Rehabil. 9, 52–62.

Marx, R.G., Hudak, P.L., Bombardier, C., et al., 1998. The reliability of physical examination for carpal tunnel syndrome. J. Hand Surg. Br. 23, 499–502.

Peolsson, A., Hedlund, R., Oberg, B., 2001. Intra- and inter-tester reliability and reference values for hand strength. J. Rehabil. Med. 33, 36–41.

Rizzo, M., Shin, A.Y., 2006. Treatment of acute scaphoid fractures in the athlete. Curr. Sports Med. Rep. 5, 242–248.

Smith, R.J., 1975. Intrinsic muscles of the fingers: Function, dysfunction and surgical reconstruction. In: AAOS Instructional Course Lectures. Vol. 24. Mosby, St. Louis, pp. 200–220.

Tuttle, H.G., Olvey, S.P., Stern, P.J., 2006. Tendon avulsion injuries of the distal phalanx. Clin. Orthop. Relat. Res. 445, 157–168.

Urbaniak, J.R., Hayes, M.G., 1981. Chronic boutonniere deformity—an anatomic reconstruction. J. Hand Surg. Am. 6, 379–383.

CHAPTER 6

Knee

MARK D. MILLER

Anatomy and Biomechanics

- The knee is a ginglymus (hinge) joint that also allows gliding and rolling (Fig. 6–1).

Bones

❑ Distal Femur
- Lateral femoral condyle is longer (in anteroposterior [AP] dimension) and straight.
  - Grooved by the sulcus terminalis.
- Medial femoral condyle is wider and curved.

❑ Proximal Tibia
- Lateral plateau—smaller and convex.
- Medial plateau—larger and concave.

❑ Proximal Fibula
- Does not actually articulate with the femur, but serves as an attachment for lateral structures.

❑ Patella
- Sesamoid bone in quadriceps tendon.
- Smaller medial and larger lateral facets.

Ligaments

- Four major ligaments (mostly of type I collagen) stabilize the knee.

❑ Anterior Cruciate Ligament (ACL)
- Origin: Tibia, just anterior to area between eminences.
- Insertion: Lateral femoral condyle; broad insertion.
- Size: 11 × 33 mm.
- Two bundles: Anteromedial (AM) (tight in flexion) and posterolateral (PL) (tight in extension).
- Blood supply: Middle geniculate artery.

❑ Posterior Cruciate Ligament (PCL)
- Origin: Tibia, posterior, below articular surface.
- Insertion: Medial femoral condyle; broad insertion.
- Size: 13 × 38 mm.
- Two bundles: Anterolateral (AL) (tight in flexion; *most important*) and posteromedial (PM) (tight in extension).
- Blood supply: Middle geniculate artery.

❑ Medial Collateral Ligament (MCL)
- Origin: Medial femoral epicondyle.
- Insertion: Medial tibia; extended insertion.
- Size: 2.5 × 10 cm.
- Two components: Superficial and deep (capsular thickening).
- Anterior fibers tight in flexion; posterior fibers tight in extension.

❑ Lateral Collateral Ligament (LCL)
- Origin: Lateral femoral epicondyle.
- Insertion: Anterolateral aspect of fibular head.
- Size: 8 × 30 mm.
- Tight in extension and lax in flexion.

❑ "Corners"
- There are two "corners" that help provide rotational stability to the knee.
- Posteromedial corner (PMC):
  - Deep and posterior to superficial MCL.
  - Includes posterior oblique ligament (capsular thickening contiguous with the semimembranosus insertion).
- Posterolateral corner (PLC):
  - Biceps, iliotibial band, popliteus, popliteofibular ligament, and capsular thickenings.
    - Popliteus inserts medial (deep), anterior, and distal to LCL insertion on the femur.
  - Prevents excessive external rotation.
  - Often injured in multiple knee ligament injuries.

Menisci

- Crescent shaped; triangular in cross section:
  - Medial: "C" shaped.
  - Lateral: More circular.
- Type I collagen.

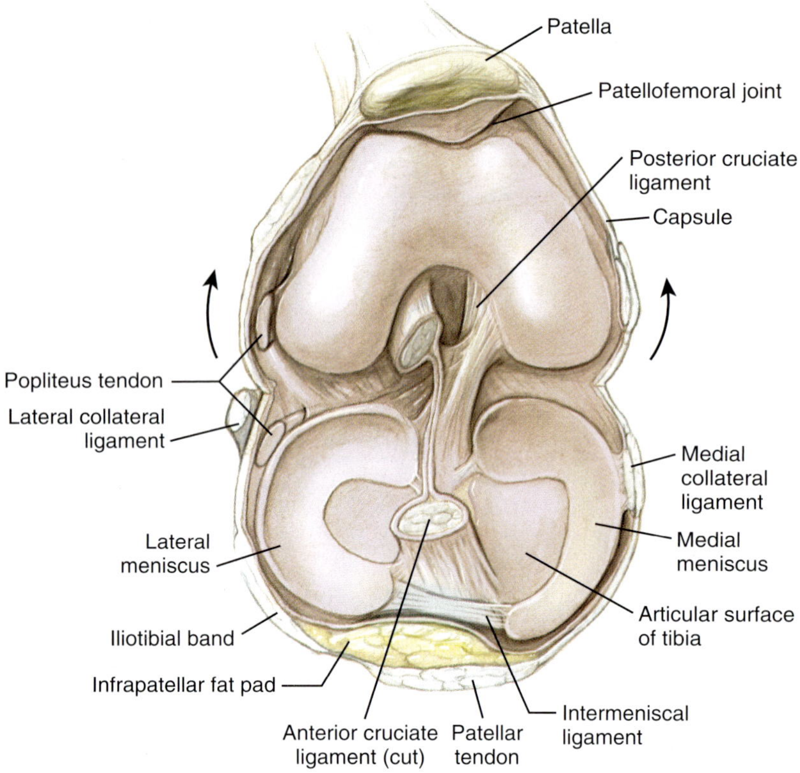

Figure 6–1 Anatomy of the knee joint. *(From Miller MD, Chhabra AB, Hurwitz SR, et al [eds]: Orthopaedic Surgical Approaches. Philadelphia, Saunders, 2008, p 429.)*

- Peripheral 25% vascularized (medial and lateral geniculate arteries).
- Attachments: Anterior and posterior horns, coronary ligaments.
- Function: Protection of articular cartilage, stability, lubrication, nutrition.

Biomechanics

- Tensile strength of ligaments:
  - ACL: 2500 Newtons (N).
  - PCL: 3000 N.
  - MCL: 5000 N.
  - LCL: 750 N.
- Role of ligaments:
  - ACL: Prevents anterior displacement (functions near full extension).
  - PCL: Prevents posterior displacement (functions in flexion).
  - MCL: Prevents valgus opening.
  - LCL: Prevents varus opening.
  - Corners: Prevent excessive rotation.

❑ Patellofemoral Joint

- Engages femur in 20 to 60 degrees of knee flexion.
  - Contact point moves proximally and laterally with flexion.
  - Maximum contact pressure at 60 degrees of flexion.
- Thickest articular cartilage in the body.
- Stabilized by muscles and the medial patellofemoral ligament (MPFL), which prevents lateral displacement.

Anatomy and Biomechanics Questions

1. Which of the following statements best describes the tension in the different components of the posterior cruciate ligament as the knee is taken from full extension to 90 degrees of flexion?

A. Both the AL and PM bands are isometric and do not change.
B. AL band is lax and becomes tight; PM band is tight and becomes lax.
C. AL band is tight and becomes lax; PM band is lax and becomes tight.
D. Both the AL and PM bands are lax and become tight.
E. Both the AL and PM bands are tight and become lax.

2. What is the relationship of the insertions of the LCL and the popliteus tendon on the femur?

A. The popliteus insertion is more distal, anterior, and deep.
B. The popliteus insertion is more proximal, anterior, and deep.
C. The popliteus insertion is more distal, inferior, and deep.
D. The popliteus insertion is more proximal, inferior, and deep.
E. The popliteus insertion is more distal, anterior, and superficial.

3. List the four major knee ligaments in order of biomechanical strength (load to failure) from weakest to strongest:
   A. ACL, PCL, LCL, MCL.
   B. LCL, MCL, ACL, PCL.
   C. LCL, ACL, PCL, MCL.
   D. MCL, ACL, PCL, LCL.
   E. PCL, ACL, LCL, MCL.
4. Which of the following structures is the main restraint to lateral translation of the patella at 20 degrees of knee flexion?
   A. Lateral retinaculum.
   B. Medial patellofemoral ligament.
   C. Medial patellotibial ligament.
   D. Patellar tendon.
   E. Quadriceps tendon.

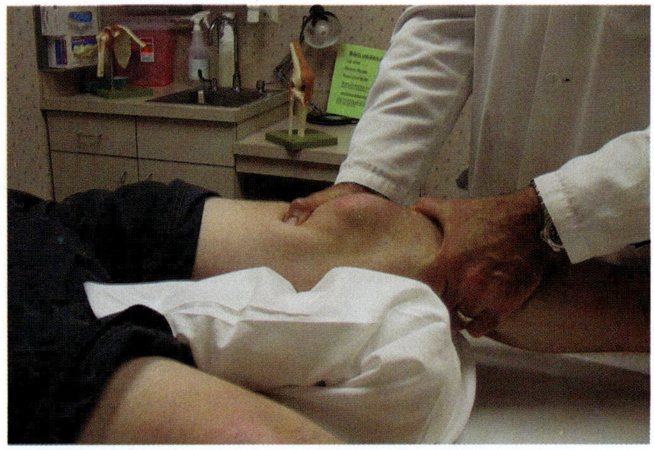

Figure 6–2 The Lachman test. *(From Miller MD, Hart J, MacKnight JM [eds]: Essential Orthopaedics. Philadelphia, Saunders Elsevier, 2010, p 605.)*

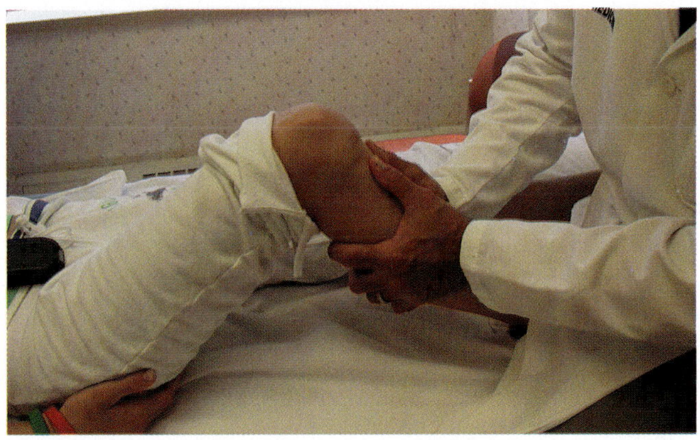

Figure 6–3 The posterior drawer examination. *(From Miller MD, Hart J, MacKnight JM [eds]: Essential Orthopaedics. Philadelphia, Saunders Elsevier, 2010, p 605.)*

History, Physical Examination, and Imaging

History

- ACL injury: Noncontact pivoting injury, "pop," immediate effusion; knee "gives way."
- PCL injury: Blow to proximal tibia (foot plantarflexed or dashboard injury); knee doesn't "feel right."
- MCL injury: Contact valgus force.
- LCL injury: Contact varus force (very unusual).
- PLC injury: Twisting injury, foot fixed; hyperextension.
- Meniscal tear: Squatting injury; pain with deep flexion; mechanical symptoms/locking/catching.
- Chondral injury: Remote injury; swelling, mechanical symptoms.
- Patellofemoral pain: Pain with stair climbing/sitting for long periods.
- Patella dislocation: Twisting injury in flexion; reduced with extension; knee "dislocated."

Physical Examination

- ❑ Anterior Cruciate Ligament Injury
  - Lachman test: anterior tibial translation at 30 degrees of flexion (Fig. 6–2).
  - Pivot shift/jerk test: Knee in valgus, external rotation axial load applied; tibia is subluxated anteriorly in 0, 20, and 30 degrees of flexion and reduced in higher degrees of knee flexion.
- ❑ Posterior Cruciate Ligament Injury
  - Posterior drawer test: Anterior tibial translation at 90 degrees of flexion; check tibia in relation to medial femoral condyle and compare against normal side (Fig. 6–3).
  - Quadriceps active test: Foot is fixed with knee at 90 degrees of flexion, and patient is asked to "kick" foot against resistance; tibia translates anteriorly from a posteriorly subluxated to a reduced position.
- ❑ Medial Collateral Ligament Injury
  - Valgus laxity:
    - Evaluated in 30 degrees of flexion (isolated injury) and in full extension (implies injury to other knee ligaments).
- ❑ Lateral Collateral Ligament Injury
  - Varus laxity:
    - Evaluated in 30 degrees of flexion (isolated injury) and in full extension (implies injury to other knee ligaments).
- ❑ Posterolateral Corner Injury
  - External rotation asymmetry (dial) test: With knees stabilized, external rotation of the foot will result in 15 degrees of additional rotation on the side of the PLC injury (Fig. 6–4).
    - Test is done in 30 and 90 degrees of knee flexion
      - Asymmetry in only 30 degrees of knee flexion suggests an isolated PLC injury (or combined ACL-PLC injury).

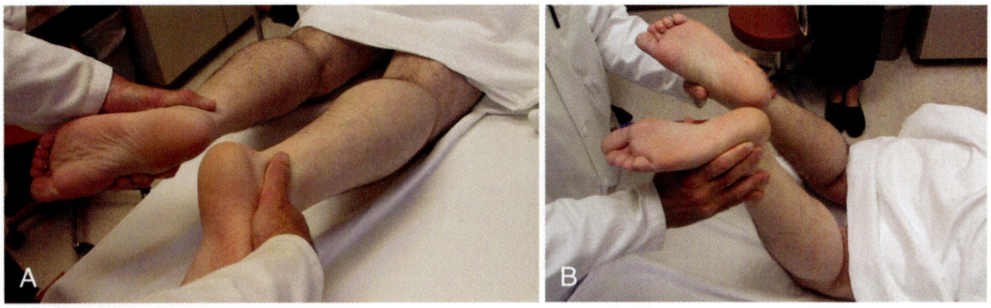

Figure 6–4 The dial test. **A**, 30 degrees; **B**, 90 degrees. *(From Miller MD, Hart J, MacKnight JM [eds]: Essential Orthopaedics. Philadelphia, Saunders Elsevier, 2010, p 606.)*

- Asymmetry in both 30 and 90 degrees of knee flexion implies injury to both the PLC and the PCL (PCL injury is confirmed with posterior drawer test).

❑ Posteromedial Corner Injury
- Slocum test:
  - Anterior drawer test with the foot in external rotation should result in less tibial translation than with the foot in neutral position.
  - Equal or greater translation with the foot externally rotated is consistent with a PMC injury.
  - Valgus laxity is also usually present.

❑ Meniscal Tear
- Joint line tenderness.
- Provocative testing: flexion McMurray test (Fig. 6–5), duck walk, Apley compression test.

❑ Patellar Instability
- Apprehension: Passive lateral patellar displacement results in asymmetrical displacement and apprehension.
- Q (quadriceps) angle: Measured using the anterior superior iliac spine (ASIS), patella, and tibial tubercle (Fig. 6–6); for chronic instability and patellar malalignment.

Imaging

❑ Plain Films
- Segond fracture (lateral capsular sign): Represents an avulsion of the lateral capsule that is highly associated with an ACL tear (Fig. 6–7A).
- Pellegrini-Stieda syndrome: Calcification near the medial femoral condyle associated with a chronic MCL injury (Fig. 6–7B).
- Patellar height: Seen best on lateral radiographs.

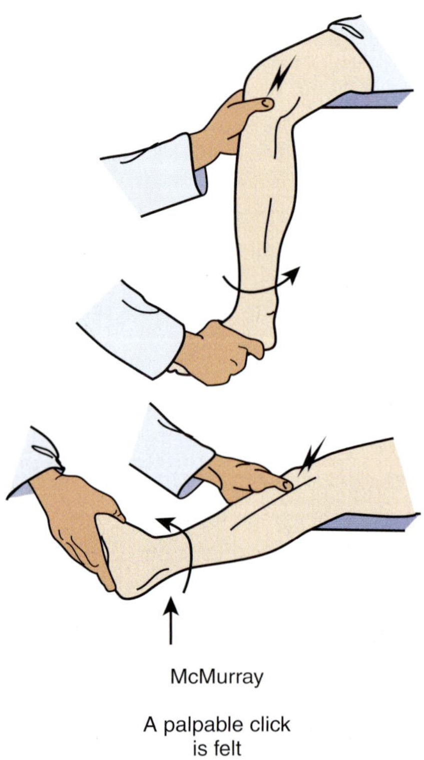

Figure 6–5 The McMurray test. *(Redrawn from Insall JN [ed]: Surgery of the Knee. New York, Churchill Livingstone, 1984.)*

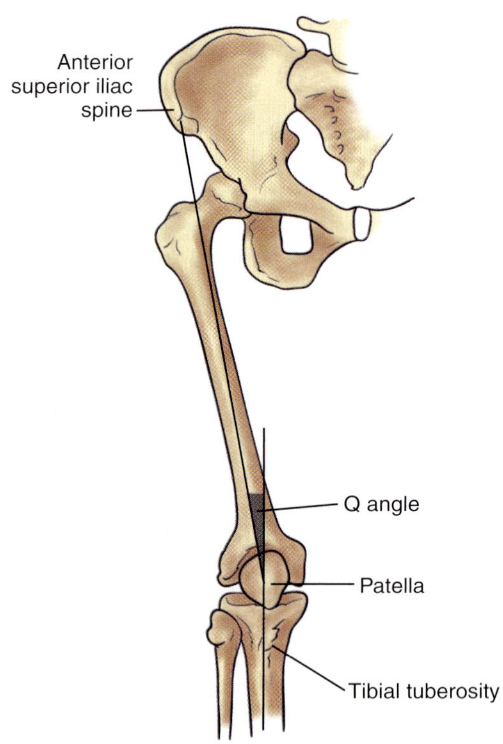

Figure 6–6 Q angle. *(From Miller MD, Hart J, MacKnight JM [eds]: Essential Orthopaedics. Philadelphia, Saunders Elsevier, 2010, p 661.)*

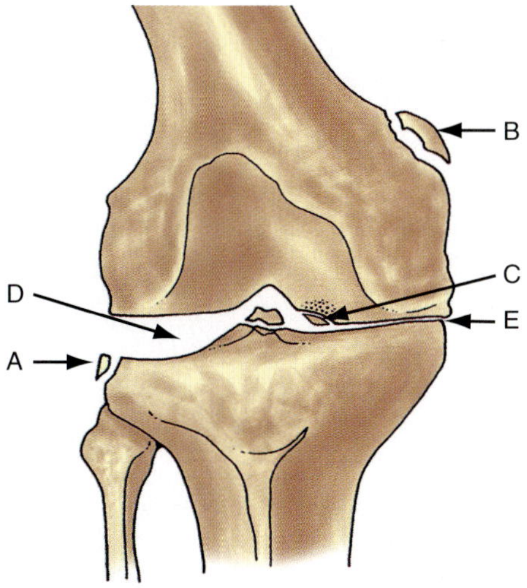

A. Segond fracture
B. Pellegrini-Stieda
C. OCD
D. Widened lateral compartment with discoid meniscus
E. Fairbanks changes

Figure 6–7 Findings on plain radiographs of the knee. *(From Miller MD, Hart J, MacKnight JM [eds]: Essential Orthopaedics. Philadelphia, Saunders Elsevier, 2010, p 607.)*

  - High-riding patella (patella alta): Associated with patellar instability.
  - Low-riding patella (patella baja): Associated with chronic loss of motion (arthrofibrosis).
- Osteochondritis dissecans (OCD): Classically located at the lateral aspect of the medial femoral condyle (Fig. 6–7C).
- Discoid meniscus may show widening and cupping of the lateral compartment (Fig. 6–7D).
- Fairbanks changes: Narrowing, squaring, and ridging (osteophytes) associated with degenerative joint disease; best seen on flexion weight-bearing radiographs (Fig. 6–7E).

❑ Stress Radiographs
- Physeal injuries: Stress radiographs may be helpful to determine whether there is a collateral ligament injury versus a physeal fracture in younger patients.
- PCL injuries: Stress radiography is becoming standard for reporting results of PCL injuries and reconstructions (Fig. 6–8).

❑ Nuclear Imaging
- Overuse injuries such as stress reactions/fractures.
- Early arthrosis.

❑ Computed Tomography
- Evaluation of bony fractures, tunnel osteolysis.

❑ Magnetic Resonance Imaging
- Magnetic resonance imaging (MRI) is very helpful for a variety of conditions (Fig. 6–9).

History, Physical Examination, and Imaging Questions

1. A college football player twists his knee while making a block. Examination reveals no medial or lateral laxity and no joint line tenderness. Anterior and posterior drawer test results are negative; however, the Lachman test result is positive. What is the most likely diagnosis?
   A. Minor knee sprain.
   B. Medial collateral ligament injury.
   C. Lateral collateral ligament injury.
   D. Anterior cruciate ligament injury.
   E. Posterior cruciate ligament injury.
2. Which of the following physical examination findings indicates isolated posterolateral instability of the knee?
   A. Reverse pivot shift.
   B. Positive quadriceps active test result.

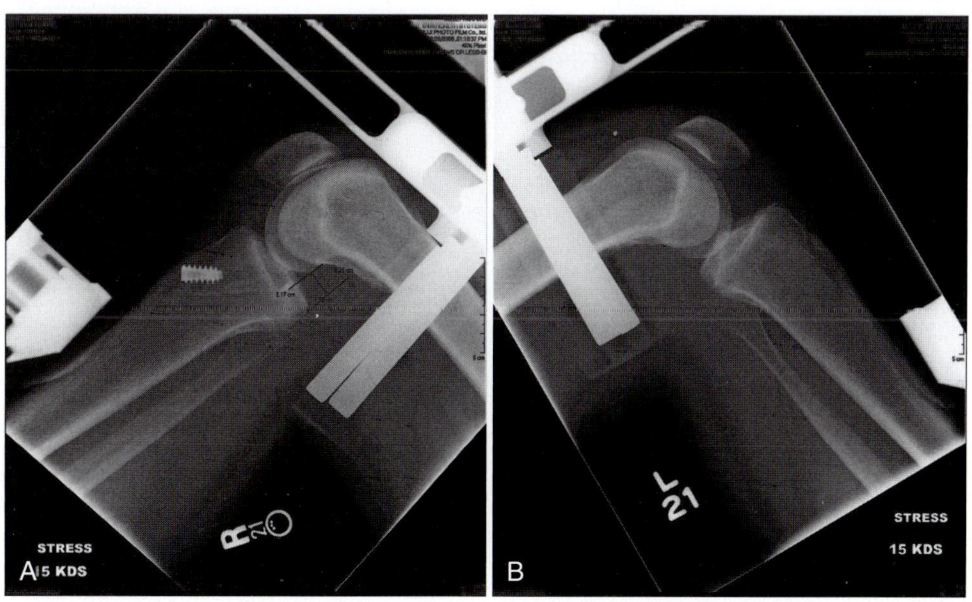

Figure 6–8 Stress radiographs of the knee demonstrating a posterior cruciate ligament (PCL)–deficient right knee after attempted reconstruction (**A**) and a normal knee (**B**). *(From Miller MD, Hart J, MacKnight JM [eds]: Essential Orthopaedics. Philadelphia, Saunders Elsevier, 2010, p 608.)*

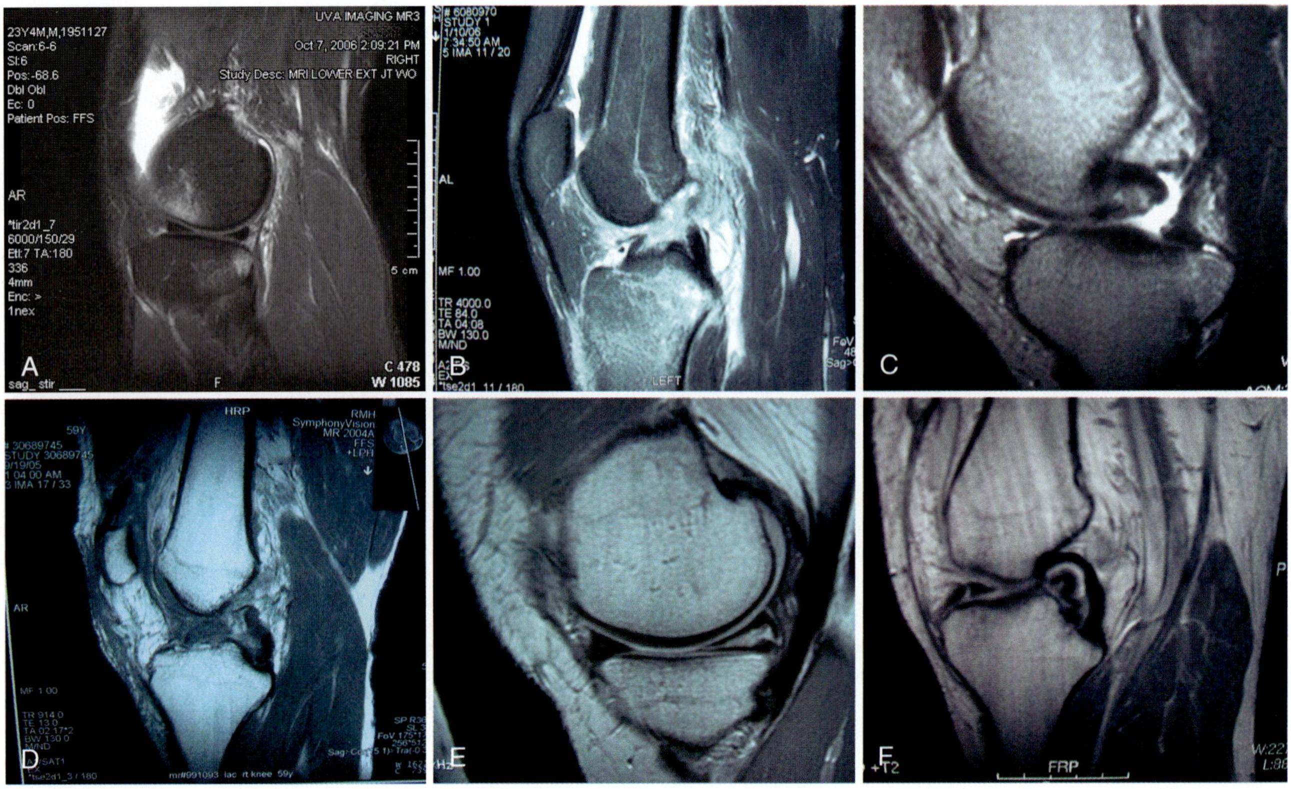

Figure 6–9 Magnetic resonance imaging of the knee. **A,** Bone bruise pattern associated with anterior cruciate ligament (ACL) deficiency. **B,** ACL injury with linear fracture. **C,** Posterior cruciate ligament (PCL) injury. **D,** Combined ACL and PCL injury. **E,** Complex tear of the posterior horn of the medial meniscus with a "picture frame" meniscus. **F,** Displaced bucket-handle tear of the medial meniscus with a double PCL sign. *(From Miller MD, Hart J, MacKnight JM [eds]: Essential Orthopaedics. Philadelphia, Saunders Elsevier, 2010, p 608.)*

C. Increased external rotation of the foot relative to the contralateral side at 90 degrees of flexion only.
D. Increased external rotation of the foot relative to the contralateral side at 30 degrees of knee flexion only.
E. Isolated external rotation of the foot relative to the contralateral side at both 30 and 90 degrees of knee flexion.

3. The lateral fragment of bone associated with an injury of the anterior cruciate ligament injury is a result of an avulsion of the:
A. Oblique popliteal ligament.
B. Lateral capsule.
C. Popliteal tendon.
D. Lateral collateral ligament.
E. Posterior oblique ligament.

4. Osteochondral bone bruises associated with ACL injuries most commonly are located at the:
A. Posterior third of the lateral femoral condyle (LFC) and middle third of the lateral tibial plateau (LTP).
B. Posterior third of the LFC and anterior third of the LTP.
C. Anterior third of the LFC and posterior third of the medial tibial plateau (MTP).
D. Middle third of the medial femoral condyle (MFC) and posterior third of the MTP.
E. Middle third of the LFC and posterior third of the LTP.

Knee Arthroscopy

- The knee was the first joint to be examined arthroscopically, and many of the fundamental principles for arthroscopy were originally developed for the knee.
- Knee arthroscopy quickly progressed from a diagnostic to a therapeutic modality.
- As for any joint, a systematic evaluation of the entire joint should precede treatment.
- Documentation, including images of all pathology and treatment thereof, should be kept in the patient's medical records.

Examination under Anesthesia

- Perform prior to placing the leg in a leg holder.
- Physical examination should be performed systematically with special attention to ligamentous stability.

Positioning (Fig. 6–10)

- Positioning is supine with a commercially available leg holder or post to support the operative extremity.
- The nonoperative leg should be padded and protected.
- Standard sterile preparation and draping should be used in every case.

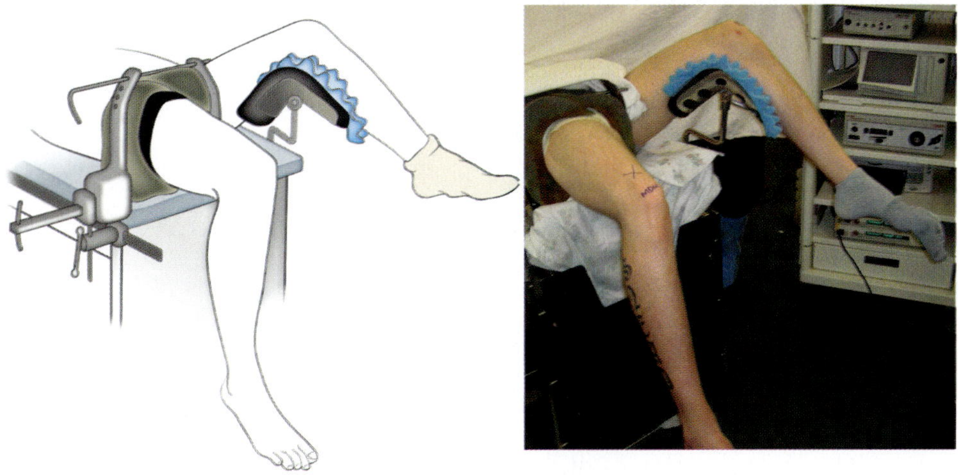

Figure 6–10 Positioning for knee arthroscopy. *(From Miller MD, Chhabra AB, Hurwitz SR, et al [eds]: Orthopaedic Surgical Approaches. Philadelphia, Saunders Elsevier, 2008, p 483.)*

Equipment

- Arthroscope:
  - 30-degree scope is used most commonly.
  - A 70-degree scope can be helpful for areas that may be otherwise difficult to access.
- Arthroscopic probe:
- Handheld instruments:
  - Medial compartment: "up-going" instruments are best.
  - Lateral compartment: straight instruments are best.
  - Meniscal contouring: right- and left-angled instruments are useful.
- Motorized instruments:
  - Remove debris and contour tissue.
  - Larger (5.5-mm) shavers best for synovium/central areas.
  - Smaller (4.5-mm) shavers best in the compartments to avoid iatrogenic cartilage damage.

Portal Placement (Fig. 6–11)

❑ Inferolateral Portal
- Just lateral to patellar tendon and just above the joint line.
- Primary viewing portal.

❑ Inferomedial Portal
- Just medial to the patellar tendon and just above the joint line.
- Usually easier to palpate, and lateral portal location can be based on this portal.
- Primary instrument portal.

❑ Superior Portals
- Created above the level of the patella.
- Lateral is favored because it avoids vastus medialis oblique (VMO) injury.
- Can be used to observe patellar tracking.

❑ Posteromedial Portal
- Just posterior to the MCL, above the joint line.
- Localized with a spinal needle.
- Avoid saphenous nerve/vein.
- Used for viewing the posterior horn of the medial meniscus, removing loose bodies, and complete synovectomy.

❑ Posterolateral Portal
- Just posterior to the LCL but anterior to the biceps, above the joint line.
- Localized with a spinal needle.
- Avoid the peroneal nerve (posterior to biceps).
- Used for viewing posterior horn of lateral meniscus, loose body removal, complete synovectomy.

Additional Portals

- As needed.
- Useful for extensive synovectomies and posterior loose body removal.

Diagnostic Arthroscopy (Fig. 6–12)

❑ Scope Insertion
- Through anterolateral portal.

❑ Suprapatellar Pouch
- Search for synovitis, loose bodies, plicae, and adhesions both medially and laterally.

❑ Patellofemoral Joint
- The undersurface of the patella can be visualized with withdrawal of the scope. Rotating the lens allows visualization of the entire patellar surface.
- The trochlea is also inspected, and the articulation with the patella is assessed. The patella should be full engaged in the trochlea at about 40 degrees of flexion.

❑ Lateral Gutter
- With the knee in extension, the lateral gutter may be visualized as the scope is taken over the lateral femoral condyle using care to avoid injury ("scuffing") to the articular cartilage.

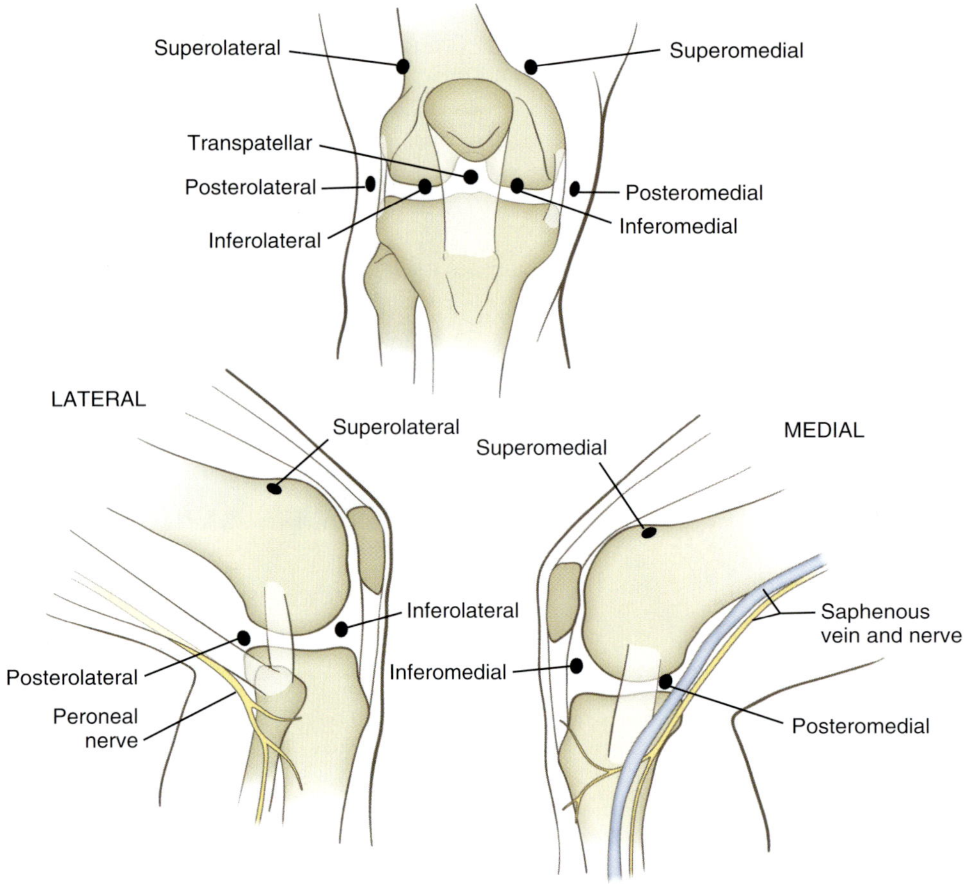

Figure 6–11 Knee arthroscopic portals. *(From Miller MD, Chhabra AB, Hurwitz SR, et al [eds]: Orthopaedic Surgical Approaches. Philadelphia, Saunders Elsevier, 2008, p 485.)*

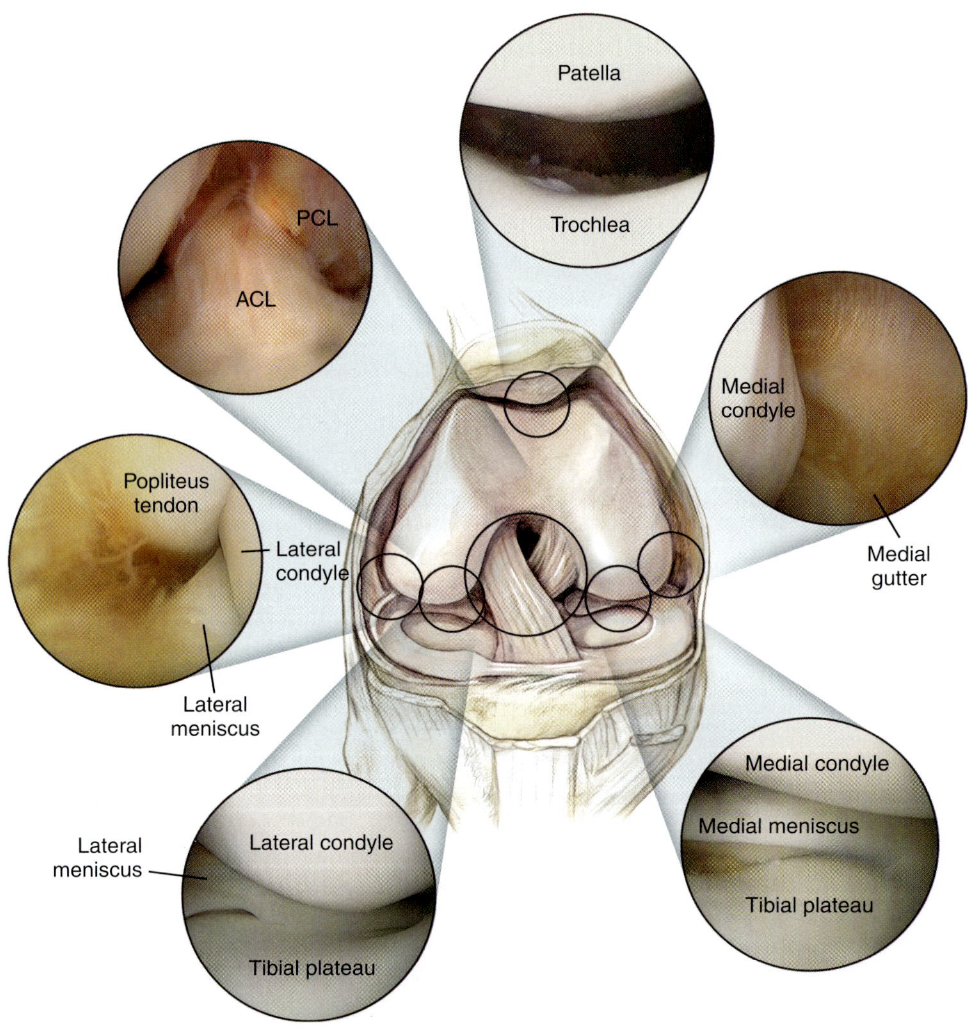

Figure 6–12 Arthroscopic portal visualization. *(From Miller MD, Chhabra AB, Hurwitz SR, et al [eds]: Orthopaedic Surgical Approaches. Philadelphia, Saunders Elsevier, 2008, p 486.)*

- The scope must also be retracted slightly to be directed below a constant reflection of the capsule in the gutter.

❑ Medial Gutter
- The scope is brought back up into the suprapatellar pouch and directed over the medial femoral condyle.
- Flexing the knee may improve visualization.

❑ Intercondylar Notch
- The scope is directed back up into the suprapatellar pouch and then down to the intercondylar notch as the knee is taken from extension to flexion.
- Both cruciate ligaments are inspected.

❑ Medial Compartment
- The medial meniscus is carefully inspected and probed.
  - It is helpful to consider the meniscus in zones as described by Cooper and associates (1990) (peripheral/middle/central and posterior/body/anterior).
  - If a medial meniscal tear is present, determine (by probing) its location, size, and stability.
- The articular surfaces are carefully examined for any chondral injuries. Any such injuries should be carefully characterized and documented to guide treatment decisions.

❑ Lateral Compartment
- The arthroscope is moved from the intercondylar notch laterally as the knee is placed in a figure-4 position (Fig. 6–13).
  - The scope is focused on the anterior edge of the lateral femoral condyle as the knee is positioned and then the scope is swept into the lateral compartment. This maneuver requires some practice to master.

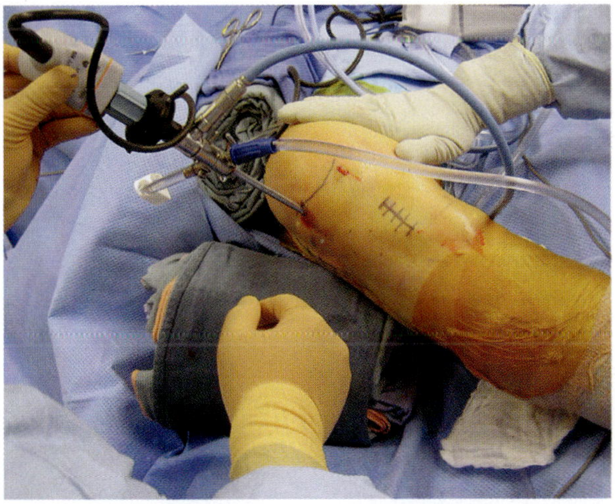

Figure 6–13 Figure-4 position for evaluating the lateral compartment of the knee during arthroscopy. ACL, anterior cruciate ligament; PCL, posterior cruciate ligament. *(From Miller MD, Sekiya JK [eds]: Core Knowledge in Orthopaedics: Sports Medicine. Philadelphia, Mosby/Elsevier, 2006, p 26.)*

- The lateral meniscus and articular cartilage is carefully inspected and probed.
  - Note that there is a normal hiatus, created by the traversing popliteus tendon, at the junction of the posterior horn and body of the lateral meniscus.

❑ Complications
- Iatrogenic chondromalacia.
  - More common that reported.
- Hemarthrosis.
  - May commonly follow lateral release—visualize after tourniquet released and consider a drain.
- Infection.
- Arthrofibrosis.
- Nerve injury.
  - Infrapatellar branches of the saphenous nerve commonly injured.
- Vascular injury.
  - Popliteal vessels can be injured with aggressive placement of cannulas and instruments posteriorly.
- Synovial cutaneous fistula.
  - Initial immobilization in extension often resolves symptoms.

Arthroscopy Questions

1. The primary viewing portal for knee arthroscopy is the:
A. Superolateral portal.
B. Superomedial portal.
C. Inferolateral portal.
D. Inferomedial portal.
E. Central portal.

2. The nerve most commonly injured during arthroscopy and related procedures is the:
A. Sural nerve.
B. Peroneal nerve.
C. Tibial nerve.
D. Sciatic nerve.
E. Saphenous nerve.

3. A 30-year-old woman complains of persistent clear drainage for several days following routine arthroscopy. She has no erythema, fevers, chills, or constitutional symptoms. Results of laboratory tests, including white blood cell count, erythrocyte sedimentation rate, and C-reactive protein level, are all within normal limits. Initial treatment for this condition should include:
A. Physical therapy.
B. Daily dressing changes.
C. Immobilization in full extension.
D. Emergency irrigation and débridement.
E. Operative excision of the fistula and layered closure.

The Meniscus

Meniscal Tears

- Meniscal tear is the most common injury to the knee requiring surgery.
- The medial meniscus is torn much more commonly than the lateral meniscus.
- Symptoms include pain and mechanical symptoms (catching, locking).
- Examination findings include joint line tenderness and pain with flexion and twisting (McMurray test or duck walk).
- Classification is based on location, appearance, and orientation (Fig. 6–14).

❑ Treatment

Observation

- For small tears without mechanical symptoms or in arthritic knees.

Partial Meniscectomy

- When repair is not possible; typically complex and radial tears.
- Complex/degenerative tears typically occur in the posterior horn of the medial meniscus.

Meniscal Repair

- A variety of techniques has been described.
- Placement of inside-out sutures in a vertical mattress fashion is the "gold standard" (Fig. 6–15).
- Newer "tensionable" all-inside devices are also popular and have been judged efficacious in short-term studies.
  - Saphenous nerve and vein at risk medially.
  - Common peroneal nerve at risk laterally.
- Results are related to tear location (peripheral tears in the vascularized "red" zone are best) and ACL status:
  - 90% success rate with concurrent ACL reconstruction.
  - 60% success rate with isolated meniscal repair.
    - May be improved with rasping and fibrin clot.
  - 30% success rate in ACL-deficient knees.

Meniscal Cyst (Fig. 6–16)

- Most commonly associated with a horizontal tear of the lateral meniscus.
- Synovial fluid collects in a ganglia-like cyst.
- Arthroscopic decompression through the leaves of the tear is favored.

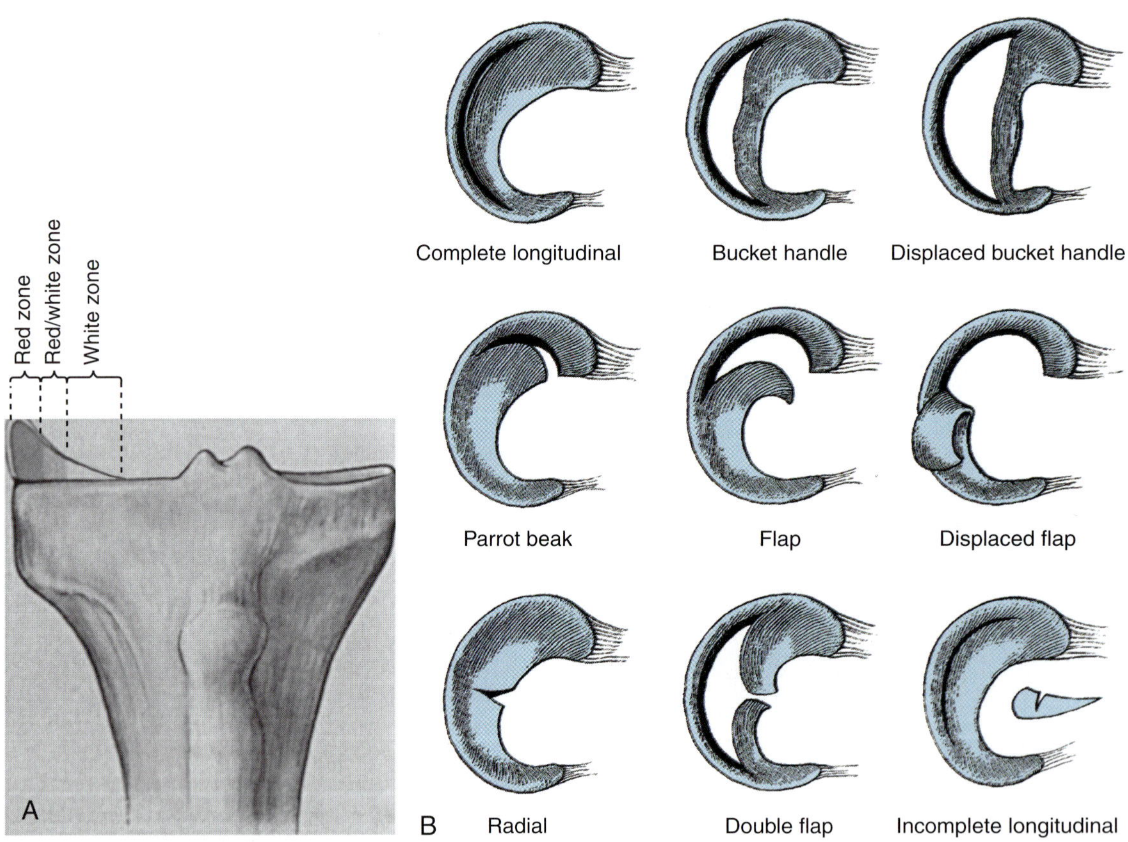

Figure 6–14 Classification of meniscal tears. A, Classification based on location. B, Classification based on appearance and orientation. *(From Miller MD: Review of Orthopaedics, 5th ed. Philadelphia, Saunders Elsevier, 2008, p 254.)*

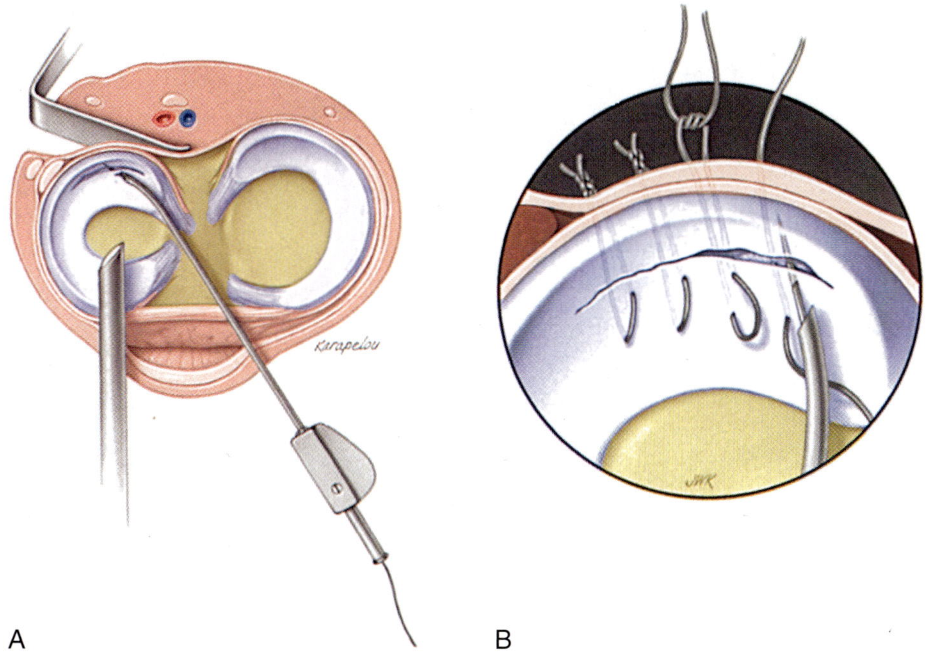

Figure 6–15 Inside-out meniscal repair technique. A, Passing the suture. B, Tying the knots and completing the repair. *(From Miller MD: Review of Orthopaedics, 5th ed. Philadelphia, Saunders Elsevier, 2008, pp 255-256.)*

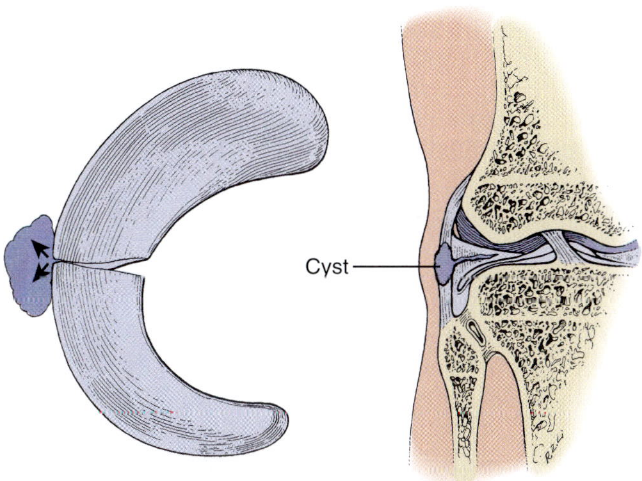

Figure 6–16 Meniscal cyst. *Arrows* show that the cyst occurring from fluid moves from tear to periphery of meniscus. *(From Miller MD: Review of Orthopaedics, 5th ed. Philadelphia, Saunders Elsevier, 2008, p 257.)*

- Popliteal (Baker) cyst represents synovial fluid expansion through a weak area in the knee capsule between the semimembranosus and the medial head of the gastrocnemius.
  - It is not pathologic in and of itself but is a manifestation of other knee pathology.
  - Cyst excision is not recommended because of high recurrence rates.

Discoid Meniscus

- Classification (Fig. 6–17):
  - Complete.
  - Incomplete.
  - Wrisberg variant (no coronary ligaments/attachment to the capsule).
- Treatment involves partial meniscectomy (saucerization) for torn discoid menisci and observation if there is no tear. Wrisberg variant should be treated with meniscal repair if possible.

Meniscal Transplantation

- Indications are unclear, but meniscal transplantation may be an option for symptomatic younger patients with absence of menisci and relatively minimal chondrosis.
- Sizing and surgical technique influence results.
- Surgical technique typically involves placement of plugs medially and a bony bridge laterally (Fig. 6–18).

Meniscus Questions

1. What part of the meniscus has the highest incidence of complex or degenerative tears?
A. Anterior horn of the medial meniscus.
B. Anterior horn of the lateral meniscus.
C. Posterior horn of the lateral meniscus.
D. Posterior horn of the medial meniscus.
E. Central third of the lateral meniscus.

2. Successful healing after meniscal repair is most likely associated with which of the following tear patterns?
A. Radial tear.
B. Parrot-beak tear.

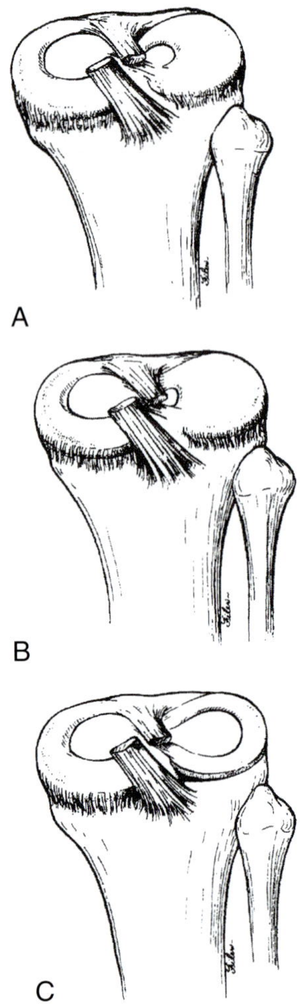

Figure 6–17 Classification of lateral discoid menisci. **A**, Incomplete. **B**, Complete. **C**, Wrisberg variant. *(From Miller MD: Review of Orthopaedics, 5th ed. Philadelphia, Saunders Elsevier, 2008, p 257.)*

C. Vertical tear in the red-red zone.
D. Vertical tear in the red-white zone.
E. Vertical tear in the white-white zone.

3. Palpable joint line cysts in the knee are most commonly associated with:
A. Baker cyst.
B. Medial meniscal tears.
C. Lateral meniscal tears.
D. Discoid lateral meniscus.
E. Anterior cruciate ligament and meniscal tears.

■

Ligament Injuries

Anterior Cruciate Ligament Injury

- Mechanism of injury: Noncontact pivoting injury, landing in extension, "pop." Female athlete risk.
- Physical examination findings: Acute effusion, instability (Lachman and pivot-shift tests).
- KT-1000/2000 instrumented Lachman (MEDMetric Corporation, San Diego, CA):
  - Greater than 3 to 5 mm of anterior displacement in comparison with normal side implies ACL deficiency.
- Radiographic findings
  - Segond fracture (lateral capsular sign; unusual) (Fig. 6–19).
  - Magnetic resonance imaging:
    - ACL fiber disruption.
    - Bone bruise pattern (lateral aspect of the middle third of the lateral femoral condyle and posterolateral tibia).

❑ Treatment
- Nonoperative: For patients with low activity levels and less laxity.
- Operative:
  - ACL reconstruction (Fig. 6–20) with a free graft (typically four-strand hamstring or central third of bone–patellar tendon–bone autograft, or allograft in some centers) placed through drill holes and fixed with interference screws or other implants.
  - Postoperative rehabilitation focuses on early weight-bearing and range-of-motion (ROM) exercises. Quadriceps rehabilitation with closed-chain exercises is favored.
  - Complications include aberrant tunnel placement (usually too anterior), arthrofibrosis, and graft harvest complications (numbness, fracture, etc.).

Posterior Cruciate Ligament Injury

- Mechanisms of injury: Blow to anterior tibia, fall with foot plantarflexed.
- Physical examination findings: Posterior drawer test (done in 70 to 90 degrees of knee flexion), posterior displacement of the tibia.
- Radiographic findings:
  - Stress radiographs (lateral with posterior drawer applied).
    - Greater than 12 mm side-to-side difference between posterior displacement of the tibia implies combined injuries.
  - MRI: Direct disruption of fibers.

❑ Treatment
- Nonoperative: For all isolated injuries.
  - Late sequelae may include medial femoral condyle and patellar chondrosis from altered contact pressures.
- Operative:
  - PCL reconstruction (Fig. 6–21):
    - For combined ligamentous injuries (typically PCL and posterolateral corner) and in patients with chronic PCL injuries for which nonoperative treatment failed.
    - Graft is either passed from front to back through the tibia or "inlayed" into a trough in the back of the tibia and

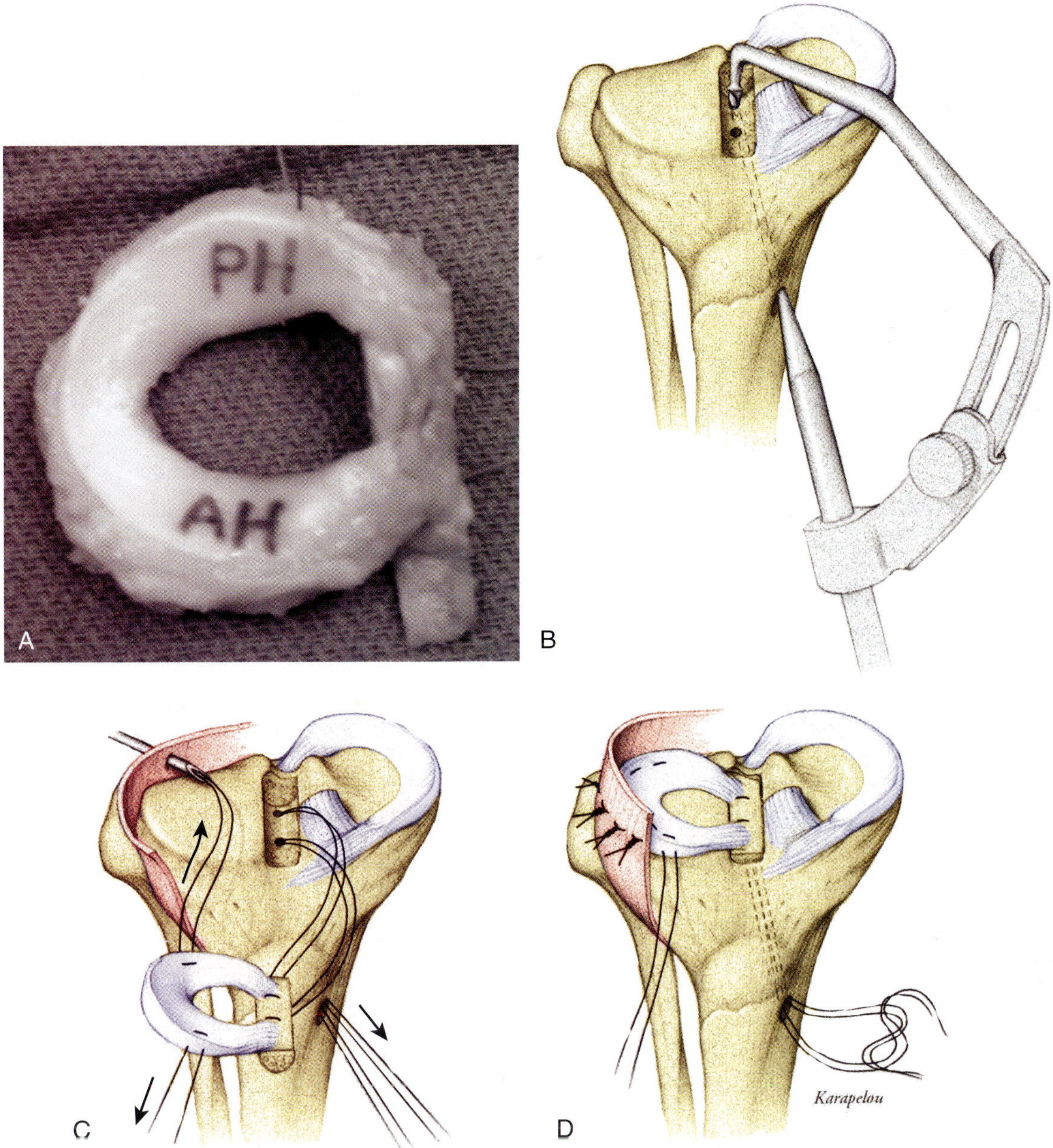

Figure 6–18 Lateral meniscus allograft with bone bridge. **A,** The allograft is labeled to ensure proper orientation. **B,** The bone trough is prepared. **C,** Sutures are passed to place the meniscal allograft. **D,** Sutures are tied to ensure fixation. *(From Miller MD, Sekiya JK [eds]: Core Knowledge in Orthopaedics: Sports Medicine. Philadelphia, Mosby/Elsevier, 2006, p 38.)*

brought up through femoral tunnel(s) and fixed with interference screws or other implants.
- The anterolateral bundle should be reconstructed for single-bundle constructs. Primary repair of bony avulsions (typically off the tibia) is favored.

- Postoperative rehabilitation emphasizes protected ROM (supported or prone) and quadriceps strengthening.
- Complications: Similar to those for ACL reconstruction but also may involve popliteal artery/vein risk.

Medial Collateral Ligament and Posteromedial Corner Injury

- Mechanism of injury typically involves a valgus contact force to the knee.
- Posteromedial injuries may have a combined rotational force.

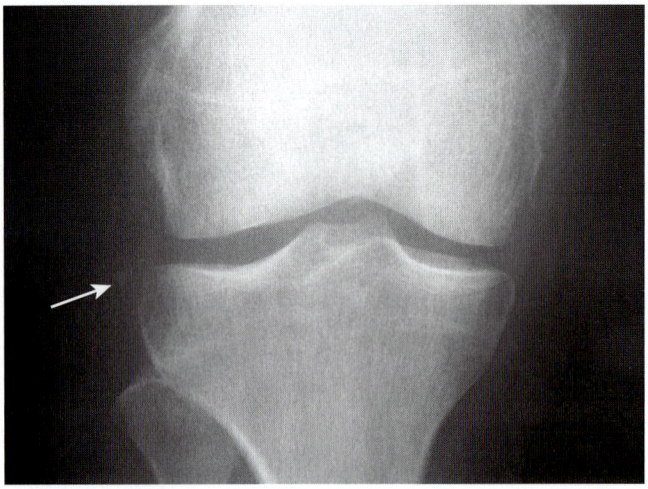

Figure 6–19 Segond fracture. *(From Miller MD, Sekiya JK [eds]: Core Knowledge in Orthopaedics: Sports Medicine. Philadelphia, Mosby/Elsevier, 2006, p 56.)*

- Physical Examination
  - Valgus stress test:
    - Opening in 30 degrees of knee extension only implies an isolated MCL tear and can be treated nonoperatively.
    - Opening in 0 degrees of knee extension implies a more significant injury and may require surgical stabilization.
  - Slocum test (Fig. 6–22): Anterior drawer test result with the foot in neutral rotation is compared with an anterior drawer test result with the foot in external rotation.
    - Normal result = reduced anterior translation with the foot in external rotation.
    - Abnormal = equal or increased translation with the foot in external rotation.
      - This implies a posteromedial corner injury and may require imbrication of the posterior capsule/posterior oblique ligament.
- Imaging
  - Plain film findings are typically normal.
    - Pellegrini-Stieda syndrome: Calcification near the medial femoral condyle may represent an old MCL injury.
  - Stress films can help diagnose medial versus lateral instability in patients with multiple knee ligament injuries.
  - MRI can be helpful in ruling out concurrent injuries (including other ligaments and meniscal tears).
- Treatment
  - Nonoperative: Recommended for all isolated MCL injuries and usually recommended for combined ACL-MCL injuries (in conjunction with staged ACL reconstruction).

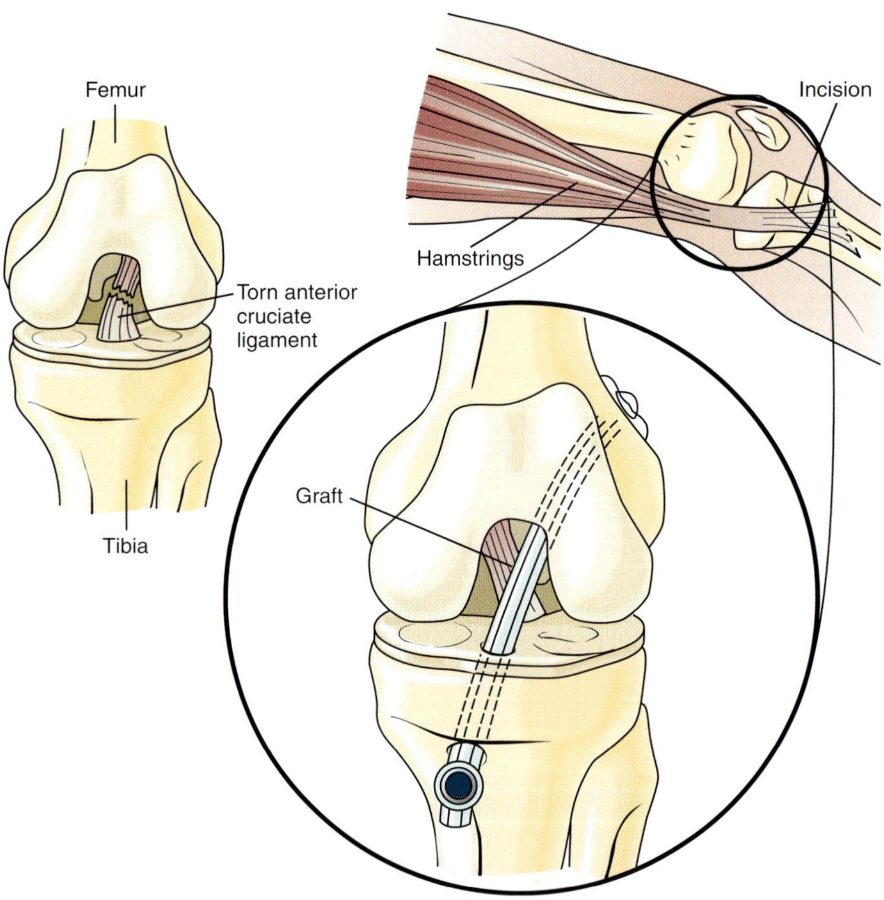

Figure 6–20 Anterior cruciate ligament reconstruction using a hamstring autograft. *(From Miller MD, Chhabra AB, Hurwitz SR, et al [eds]: Orthopaedic Surgical Approaches. Philadelphia, Saunders Elsevier, 2008, p 614.)*

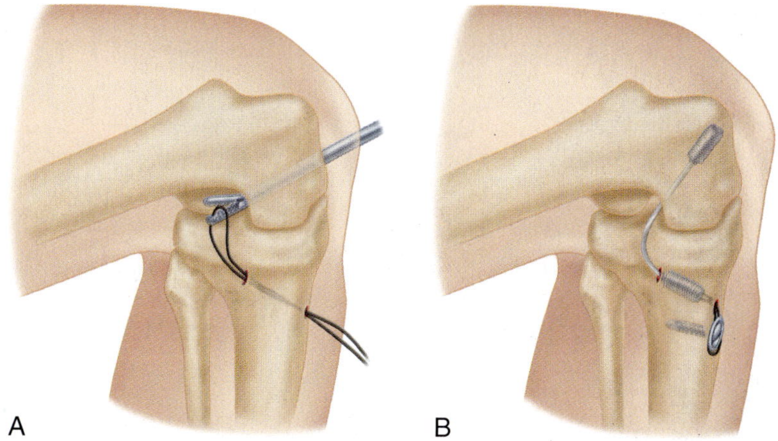

Figure 6–21 Posterior cruciate ligament reconstruction. A, The graft is passed from tibia to femur. B, Fixation is established with interference screws and back-up fixation may be used if desired. *(From Miller MD, Cole BJ, Cosgarea AJ, Sekiya JK [eds]: Operative Techniques: Sports Knee Surgery. Philadelphia, Saunders Elsevier, 2008, p 340.)*

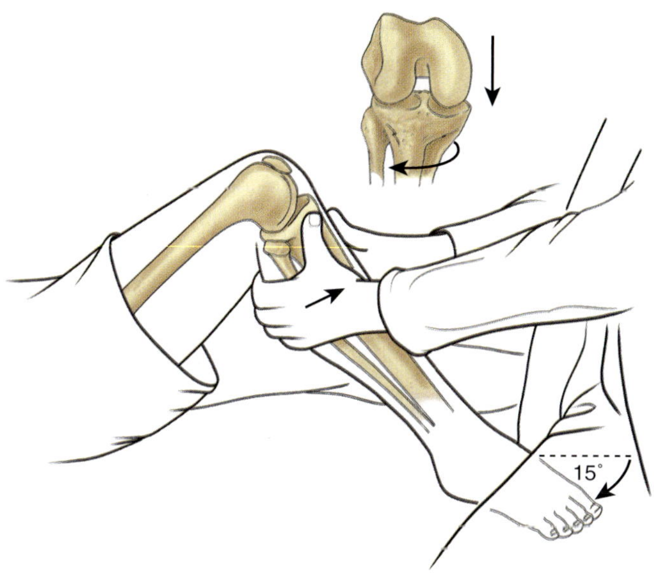

Figure 6–22 The Slocum test. *(From Miller MD, Chhabra AB, Hurwitz SR, et al [eds]: Orthopaedic Surgical Approaches. Philadelphia, Saunders Elsevier, 2008, p 607.)*

    - Hinged bracing for 6 to 8 weeks is typically recommended.
        - Some writers advocate limited motion in the brace, but recommendations are inconsistent.
- Operative: Usually recommended only for multiple ligament injuries involving the MCL.
    - Some surgeons consider MCL repair/reconstruction (and combined posteromedial imbrication) for patients with opening in full extension and/or with rotational instability.
        - Lesions on the tibial side (which, fortunately, are less common) typically heal less consistently because synovial fluid tracks distally with gravity.
    - Acute injuries can be repaired primarily.
    - Chronic injuries may need grafting:
        - Free grafts including allografts may be helpful.
        - Modified Bosworth technique (Fig. 6–23) uses semitendinosus tendon that is left attached distally, harvested, and placed over a post at the medial femoral condyle.

Lateral Collateral Ligament and Posterolateral Corner Injury

- Mechanism of injury typically involves a varus contact force to the knee.
- Posterolateral corner injuries may have a combined rotational force.

❑ Physical Examination
- Varus stress test:
    - Opening in 30 degrees of knee extension only implies an isolated LCL tear and can be treated nonoperatively.
    - Opening in 0 degrees of knee extension implies a more significant injury and may require surgical stabilization.
    - Isolated LCL injuries are uncommon and usually involve combined LCL and posterolateral corner injuries.
        - Both injuries more common with multiple knee ligament injuries.
- External rotation asymmetry (Fig. 6–24):
    - Dial test: Passive foot rotation with the knee flexed at both 30 and 90 degrees of knee flexion:
        - Asymmetry at 30 degrees of knee flexion only implies an isolated posterolateral corner injury.
        - Asymmetry at both 30 and 90 degrees of knee flexion implies and combined injury to the posterolateral corner and the PCL.
- Results of external rotation recurvatum test and posterolateral drawer test are positive for combined PCL and PLC injuries.

❑ Imaging
- Plain films are typically normal.
    - Arcuate sign = avulsion of fibular head.

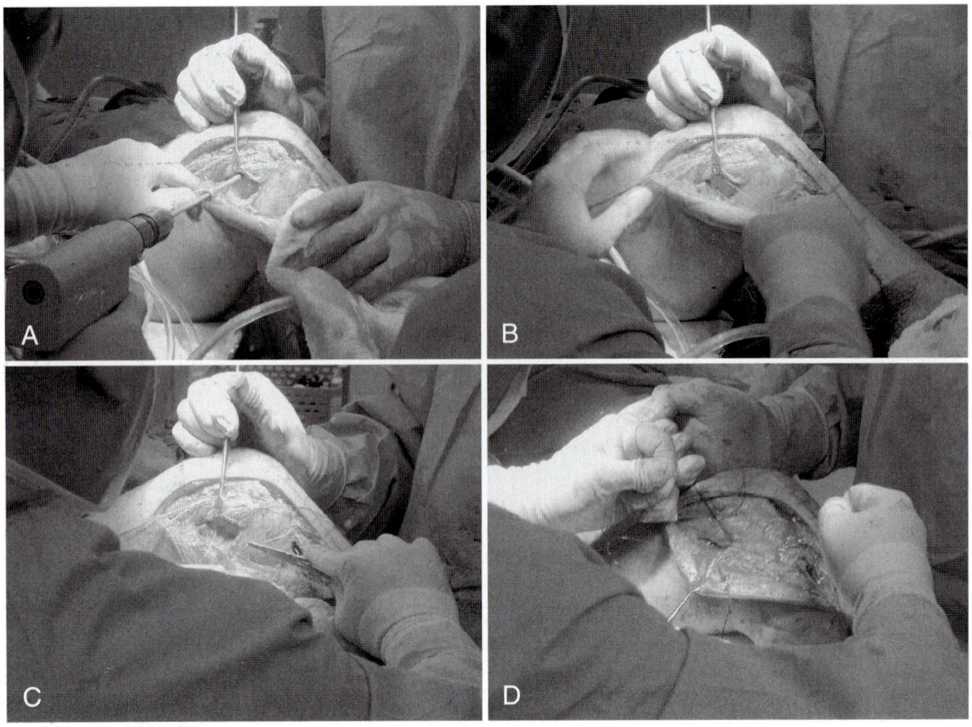

Figure 6–23 Medial collateral ligament (MCL) repair. **A**, Suture anchor placement. **B**, Two anchors are in place. **C**, Sutures are passed through the proximal MCL. **D**, Sutures are tied. *(From Miller MD, Sekiya JK [eds]: Core Knowledge in Orthopaedics: Sports Medicine. Philadelphia, Mosby/Elsevier, 2006, p 66.)*

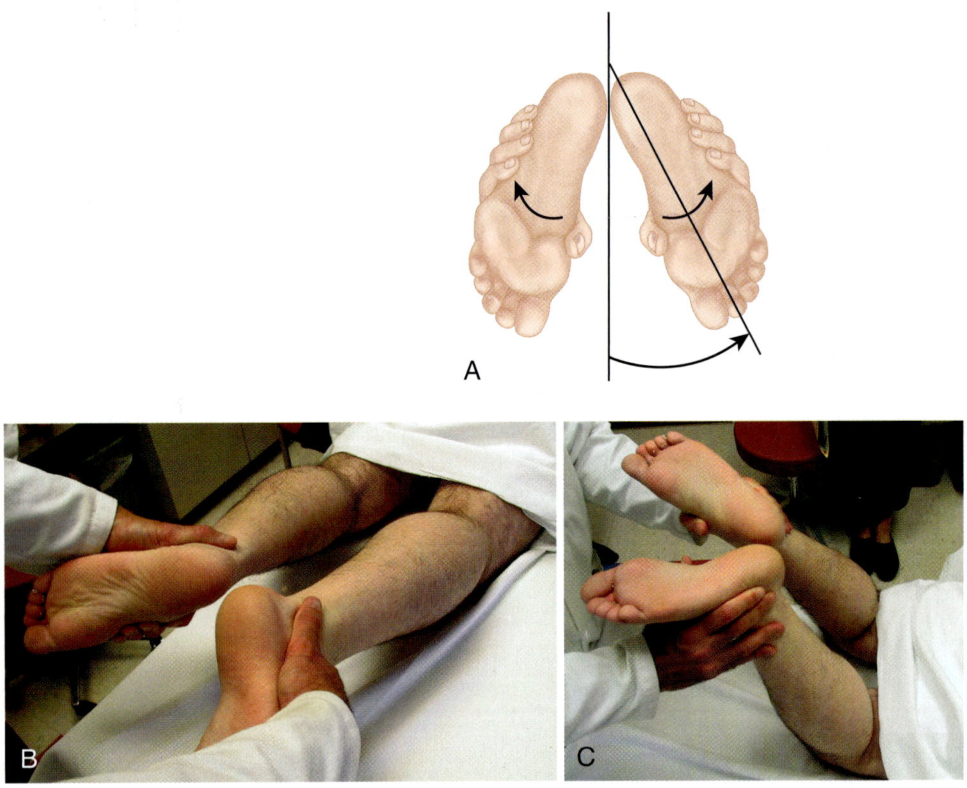

Figure 6–24 External rotation asymmetry. **A**, The thigh-foot angle is measured. **B**, At 0 degrees. **C**, At 90 degrees. *(From Miller MD, Cole BJ, Cosgarea AJ, Sekiya JK [eds]: Operative Techniques: Sports Knee Surgery. Philadelphia, Saunders Elsevier, 2008, p 363.)*

- Stress films can help diagnose lateral versus medial instability in patients with multiple knee ligament injuries.
- MRI can be helpful in ruling out concurrent injuries (including other ligaments and meniscal tears) and evaluating the extent of posterolateral structures involved.

❑ Treatment
- Nonoperative: Recommended for partial, isolated LCL injuries and usually recommended for combined ACL–partial LCL injuries (in conjunction with staged ACL reconstruction).
  - Hinged bracing for 6 to 8 weeks is typically recommended.

- Some writers advocate limited motion in the brace, but recommendations are inconsistent.
- Operative: Usually recommended for complete LCL and PLC injuries and multiple ligament injuries.
  - Acute injuries:
    - Primary repair is typically done, but free graft "back-up" is usually recommended.
  - Chronic injuries:
    - Free graft placement is accomplished to serve as a static restraint to external rotation.
    - A variety of techniques has been described (Fig. 6–25).

Ligament Injury Questions

1. An 18-year-old high school football running back injures his knee while trying to avoid a tackle. Swelling develops immediately. Examination demonstrates a large effusion, ROM of 15 to 90 degrees, and a 2+ Lachman test result. Treatment should consist of:

A. Acute ACL repair.
B. Acute ACL reconstruction using an autogenous graft.
C. Acute ACL reconstruction using an autogenous graft and an LAD.
D. ACL repair after ROM has returned to normal.
E. ACL reconstruction with an autogenous graft when ROM has returned to normal.

2. A 23-year-old man is injured in a motorcycle accident. Physical examination demonstrates an effusion, no varus or valgus laxity, a negative Lachman test result, and a positive posterior drawer test result. Radiographs show a bony avulsion off the posterior aspect of the tibia. Treatment should consist of:

A. Repair of the injured structures.
B. Posterior cruciate reconstruction with patellar tendon graft.
C. Immobilization for 4 weeks.
D. Physical therapy focusing on quadriceps rehabilitation and ROM.
E. Diagnostic arthroscopy followed by rehabilitation.

3. A 30-year-old woman is struck by a motor vehicle and sustains an injury to the left lower extremity. Radiographs show a posterior knee dislocation. The patient is neurologically intact. Initial management should consist of:

A. Application of an above-knee splint.
B. Application of an external fixator.
C. An arteriogram.
D. Closed reduction of the knee dislocation.
E. Open reduction of the knee dislocation.

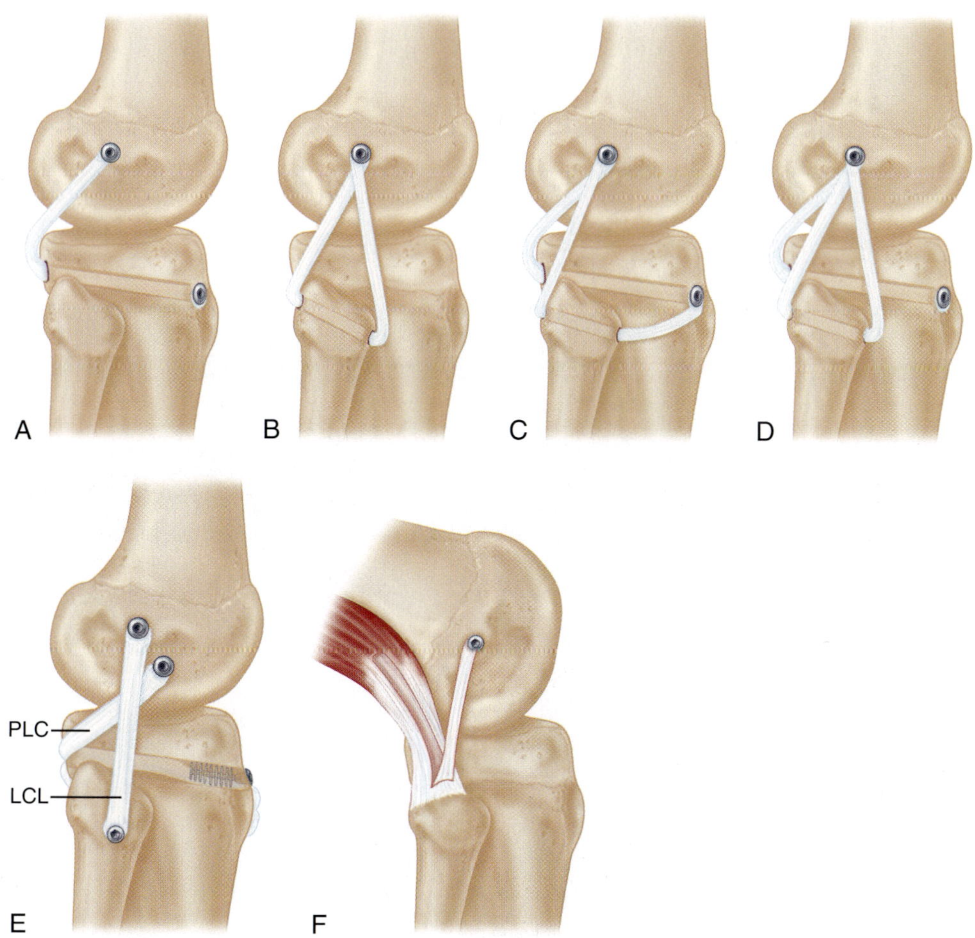

Figure 6–25 Posterolateral corner (PLC) reconstruction techniques. **A**, Muller popliteal bypass procedure. **B**, Larson figure-of-eight PLC reconstruction. **C**, Two-tail PLC reconstruction. **D**, Three-tail PLC reconstruction. **E**, Laprade PLC reconstruction. **F**, LCL reconstruction using a strip of the biceps tendon/fascia. *(From Miller MD, Cole BJ, Cosgarea AJ, Sekiya JK [eds]: Operative Techniques: Sports Knee Surgery. Philadelphia, Saunders Elsevier, 2008, p 371.)*

Osteochondral Lesions

Osteochondritis Dissecans

- OCD represents a separation of the subchondral bone and overlying articular cartilage from the underlying bone.
- The etiology is unclear but likely involves occult trauma and/or vascular insult.
- The lateral aspect of the medial femoral condyle is most commonly involved.
- Three types of OCD have been described on the basis of the status of the physis: juvenile (open), adolescent (closing), and adult (closed).

❑ Diagnosis
- OCD is often found incidentally because the patient has nonfocal findings (swelling, pain, etc).
- Radiographic and MRI findings are characteristic (Fig. 6–26).

❑ Treatment
- In general, prolonged conservative care (crutches, activity modification, etc.) should be favored until the physis is closed, because of the possibility of spontaneous healing.
- Operative treatment (including débridement of the base of the lesion, bone grafting, and fixation) is favored for adult OCD and for juvenile OCD for which nonoperative care has failed (and/or that involves displacement).
- Other forms of articular cartilage treatment (see later) may be necessary for OCD lesions that cannot be repaired.

Focal Articular Cartilage Injuries

- Chondral injuries typically do not involve bone and are likely shear injuries to the articular cartilage.
- Antecedent trauma (which may or may not be recalled) is likely the etiology. Delamination of the cartilage is not unusual.

❑ Diagnosis
- As with OCD, diagnosis of focal articular cartilage injury can often be difficult.
- Newer MRI machines and techniques have improved the accuracy of diagnosis (Fig. 6–27), but these lesions are still commonly found only during arthroscopy.

❑ Treatment
- Nonoperative: Initial treatment of focal cartilage lesions can be nonoperative, especially for well-contained smaller lesions and more diffuse lesions.
- Marrow stimulation (microfracture):
  - Following arthroscopic débridement of the edges of the lesions and removal of the calcified cartilage layer (usually with a curette), penetration of the subchondral plate releases pluripotent cells that "fill in" the defect.
  - This procedure results in healing with fibrocartilage that is sometimes less predictable and durable than with other techniques (Fig. 6–28).
- Osteochondral autograft transfer (OATS):
  - "Plugs" of cartilage and underlying bone are transferred from an area that has low contact pressures (such as the superolateral aspect of the lateral femoral condyle) into the defect.

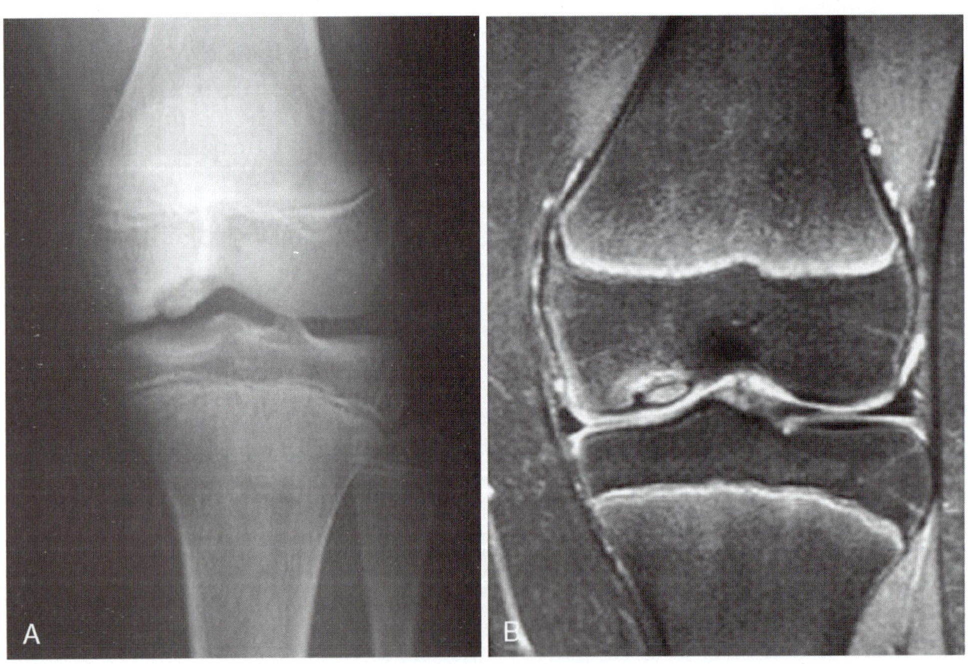

Figure 6–26 **A,** Appearance of osteochondrosis dissecans (OCD) on plain radiography. **B,** Magnetic resonance image demonstrating an OCD of the lateral aspect of the medial femoral condyle. *(From Miller MD, Chhabra AB, Hurwitz SR, et al [eds]: Orthopaedic Surgical Approaches. Philadelphia, Saunders Elsevier, 2008, p 920.)*

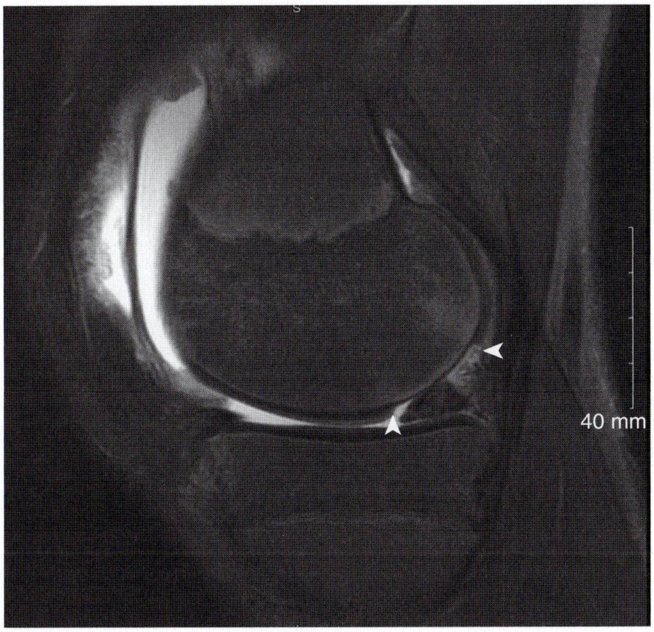

Figure 6–27 Sagittal magnetic resonance image demonstrating osteochondral injury (*arrowheads*). *(From Miller MD, Chhabra AB, Hurwitz SR, et al [eds]: Orthopaedic Surgical Approaches. Philadelphia, Saunders Elsevier, 2008, p 643.)*

- Several commercial devices are available to allow precise interference fit of the plugs. Perpendicularity is a key for both harvest and delivery of the plugs (Fig. 6–29).
- Autologous chondrocyte implantation (ACI):
  - In a two-stage procedure, articular cartilage is harvested and sent to a laboratory for processing and chondrocyte culture.
  - During the second stage, the chondrocytes are injected into the lesion under an autologous periosteal patch that is sewn in place over the defect (Fig. 6–30).
  - Newer techniques, not yet approved in the United States, include injection of the cells into a scaffold.
- Osteochondral allograft transfer:
  - Typically reserved for larger lesions, this technique involves transferring matched fresh osteochondral tissue from a donor into a prepared defect.
  - It typically uses techniques similar to osteochondral autograft transfer but with much larger "plugs" (Fig. 6–31).
- Newer techniques continue to be developed, including the use of growth factors, fetal tissue, and new matrices.

Degenerative Joint Disease

- Typically has more diffuse involvement. Symptoms consist of pain, swelling, crepitus, etc.
- Imaging:
  - Standing flexion weight-bearing radiographs are helpful to identify the extent of involvement (Fig. 6–32) and help guide treatment.
  - For unicompartment arthrosis, long-leg films may be required to measure the mechanical alignment (Fig. 6–33).
  - MRI is typically not helpful in this setting.

❑ Treatment

- Nonoperative: Consists of physical therapy, anti-inflammatory medications, nutritional supplements (glucosamine and chondroitin sulfate), activity modification, weight management, and injections (judicious use of steroids or hyaluronic acid).
- Arthroscopy: Several studies have confirmed that arthroscopic débridement is not appropriate for the treatment of knee osteoarthritis.
- Cartilage surgical procedures: These are reserved for focal chondral defects and are not appropriate for diffuse lesions.

Osteotomy

- This is a reasonable option for the younger (less than approximately 50 to 60 years old), active patient with single-compartment

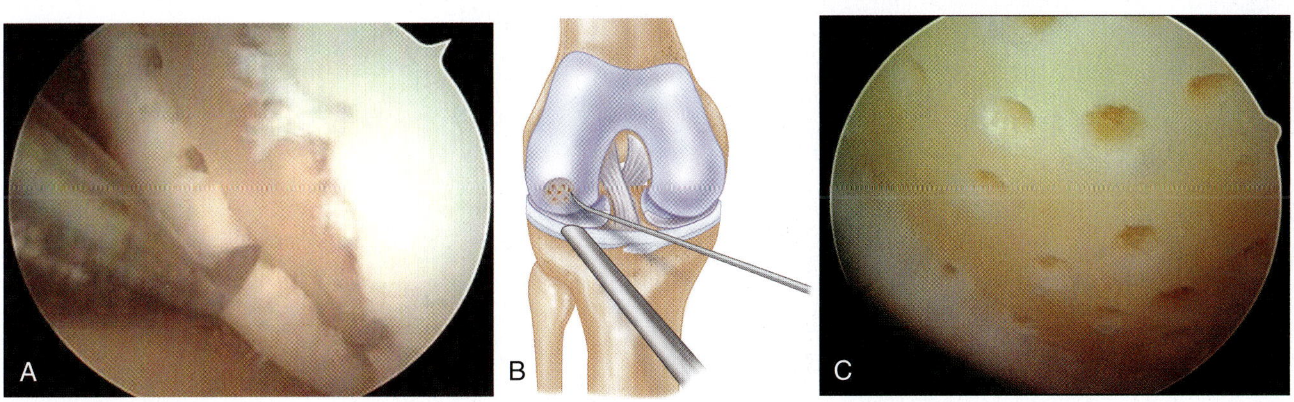

Figure 6–28 Operative technique for microfracture. **A,** A sharp awl is used to penetrate the subchondral plate. **B,** This step is repeated throughout the lesion. **C,** Completed microfracture. *(From Miller MD, Sekiya JK [eds]: Core Knowledge in Orthopaedics: Sports Medicine. Philadelphia, Mosby/Elsevier, 2006, p 175.)*

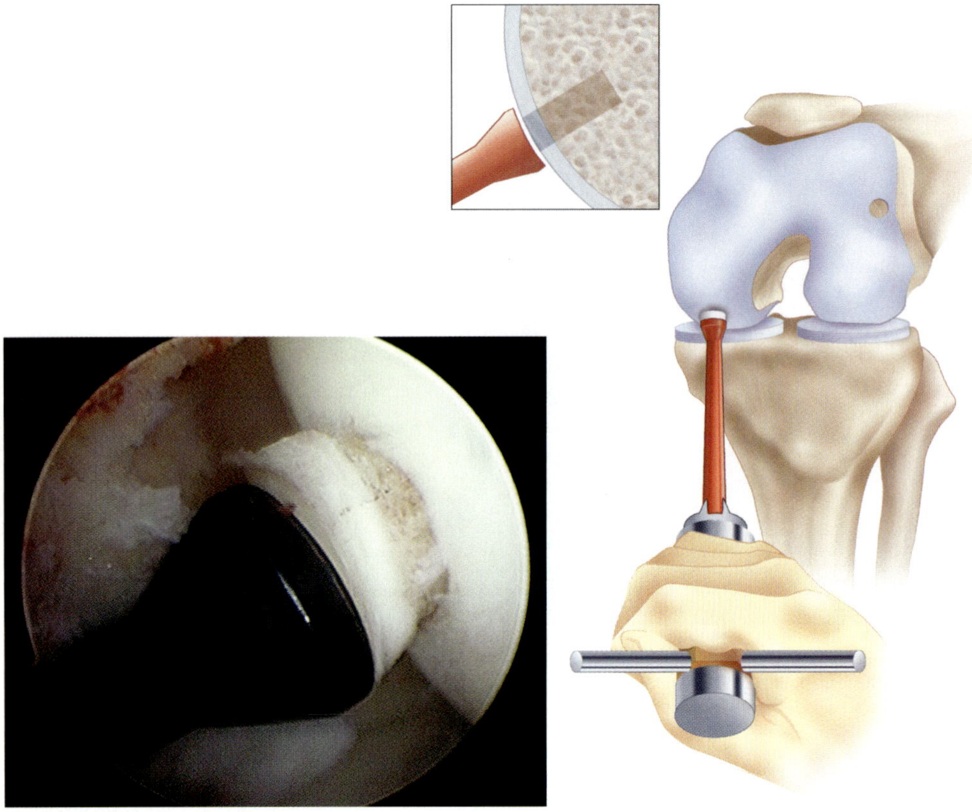

Figure 6–29 Operative technique for OATS. *(From Miller MD, Cole BJ, Cosgarea AJ, Sekiya JK [eds]: Operative Techniques: Sports Knee Surgery. Philadelphia, Saunders Elsevier, 2008, p 187.)*

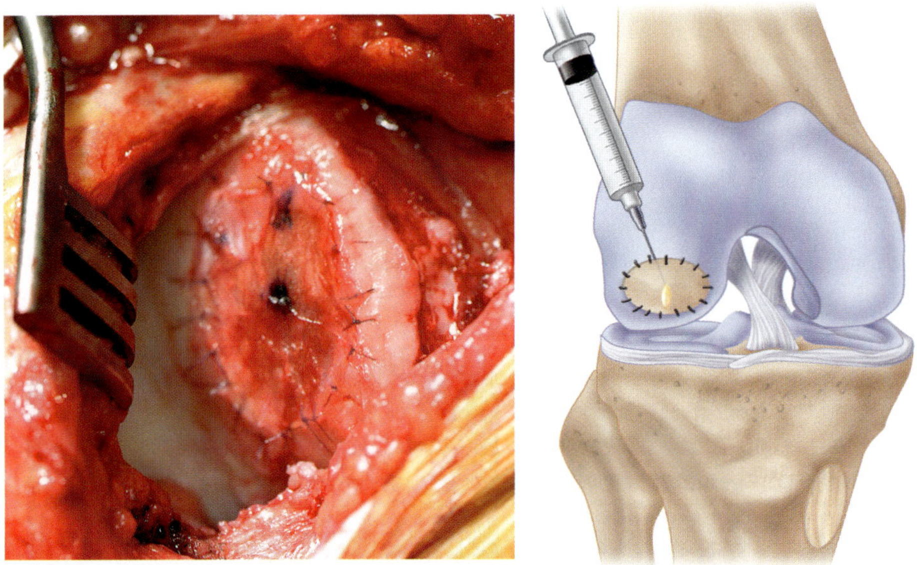

Figure 6–30 Operative technique for ACI. *(From Miller MD, Cole BJ, Cosgarea AJ, Sekiya JK [eds]: Operative Techniques: Sports Knee Surgery. Philadelphia, Saunders Elsevier, 2008, p 201.)*

involvement and a mechanical axis that falls into the affected compartment. There are several technical points that should be emphasized:

- Indications:
  - Osteotomies are best done in relatively younger, active patients with isolated involvement of either the medial (more common) or lateral compartment.
  - Contraindications include lateral tibial subluxation of more than 1 cm, flexion contracture of more than 10 degrees, knee flexion less than 90 degrees, and significant deformities (>20 degrees of varus/valgus).

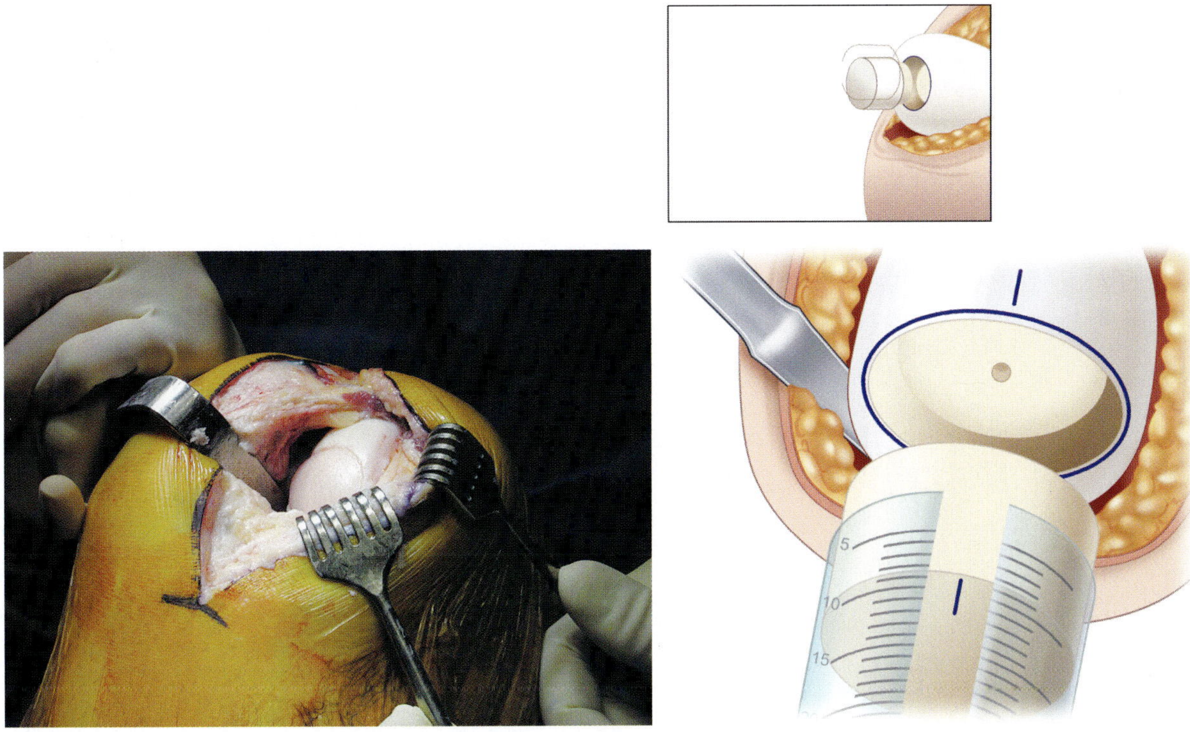

Figure 6–31 Operative technique for allograft transfer. *(From Miller MD, Cole BJ, Cosgarea AJ, Sekiya JK [eds]: Operative Techniques: Sports Knee Surgery. Philadelphia, Saunders Elsevier, 2008, p 216.)*

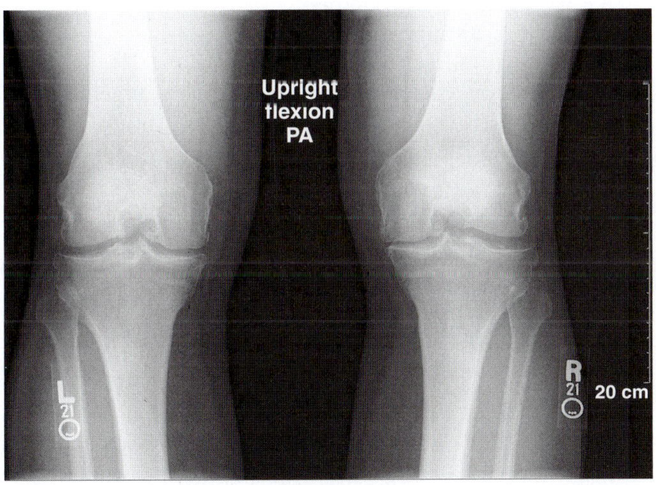

Figure 6–32 Flexion weight-bearing radiographs showing osteoarthritis of the knee. *(From Miller MD, Chhabra AB, Hurwitz SR, et al [eds]. Orthopaedic Surgical Approaches. Philadelphia, Saunders Elsevier, 2008, p 607.)*

- Planning for desired correction:
  - The goal is to place the weight-bearing axis 62% across the knee, into the unaffected compartment (Fig. 6–34).
- Technique:
  - For varus deformities (most common), either lateral closing or medial opening osteotomies of the proximal tibial are

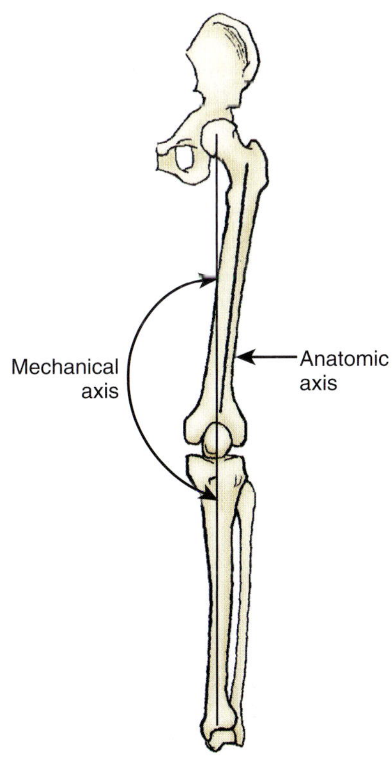

Figure 6–33 Hip-to-ankle radiograph for evaluating mechanical and anatomic axes of the lower extremity. *(From Insall WN [ed]: Insall & Scott's Surgery of the Knee, Vol 2, 4th ed. Philadelphia, Churchill Livingstone/Elsevier, 2006, p 1304.)*

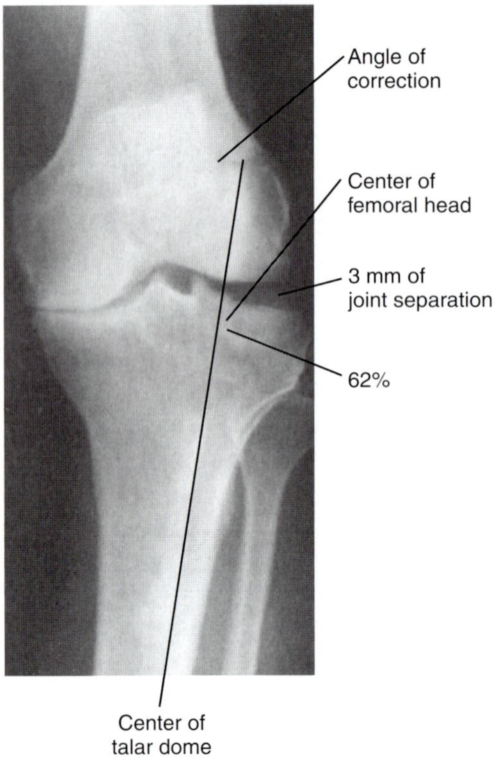

Figure 6–34 Osteotomy planning demonstrating placement of the weight-bearing axis placed at 62% across the knee. *(From Insall WN [ed]: Insall & Scott's Surgery of the Knee, Vol 2, 4th ed. Philadelphia, Churchill Livingstone/Elsevier, 2006, p 1305.)*

favored. Valgus deformities are usually addressed with medial femoral closing or lateral femoral opening osteotomies.
  - Fixation has transitioned from step-cut staples to plates. Special plates that incorporate a wedge for opening osteotomies are available.
  - Attention must be given to sagittal alignment as well as coronal alignment.
  - Complications of osteotomies include undercorrection (most common), overcorrection, and patella baja.

Osteonecrosis

- Atraumatic osteonecrosis: Similar to idiopathic osteonecrosis of the hip and shoulder. Can be related to steroid or alcohol use and sickle cell anemia. Treatment includes decompression and joint replacement.
- Spontaneous osteonecrosis of the knee (SONK): This is probably best considered an insufficiency fracture.
  - Is common after arthroscopy in elderly women.
  - Is a self-limited condition that is best treated with protected weight-bearing until it resolves.

Osteochondral Lesions Questions

1. A 40-year-old golfer has medial knee pain and minimal joint space narrowing on radiographs. He undergoes arthroscopy and a 1.5×1.5-cm focal chondral defect is identified. You elect to proceed with a marrow stimulation procedure. You later counsel the patient that he should expect:
A. Complete long-lasting relief of symptoms.
B. Improvement, but not complete or permanent resolution of symptoms.
C. Results equal to those of an osteochondral autograft.
D. Healing with normal articular cartilage.
E. That he will need a knee replacement within a couple of years.

2. When planning a tibial osteotomy for a varus knee, you would like to transfer the weight-bearing axis to a location:
A. Directly in the center of the tibial plateau.
B. 52% of the distance across the tibial plateau.
C. 57% of the distance across the tibial plateau.
D. 62% of the distance across the tibial plateau.
E. 67% of the distance across the tibial plateau.

3. A 60-year-old woman complains of aching and catching of her knee. Physical examination notes medial joint line tenderness. Plain radiographs, including a flexion weight-bearing PA view, demonstrate moderate to severe medial compartment narrowing. Anti-inflammatory medications and injections have not relieved the patient's symptoms. Treatment now should consist of:
A. Arthroscopic débridement.
B. Marrow stimulation procedure.
C. Osteochondral autograft.
D. ACI on discussion of knee replacement surgery options.
E. Continued nonoperative care.

Synovial Lesions

- Pigmented villonodular synovitis (PVNS) can be nodular or diffuse.
  - Consists of hemosiderin-laden cells, giant cells, and foam cells.
  - Nodular: Localized mass that is easily removed arthroscopically, with a low recurrence rate.
  - Diffuse: Requires a complete synovectomy with multiple portals and has a high recurrence rate (Fig. 6–35).
- Synovial chondromatosis: Proliferative disease of the synovium.
  - Seen most commonly in middle-aged men.
  - Mechanical symptoms are common.
  - Involves cartilaginous metaplasia with multiple loose bodies that must be completely removed.

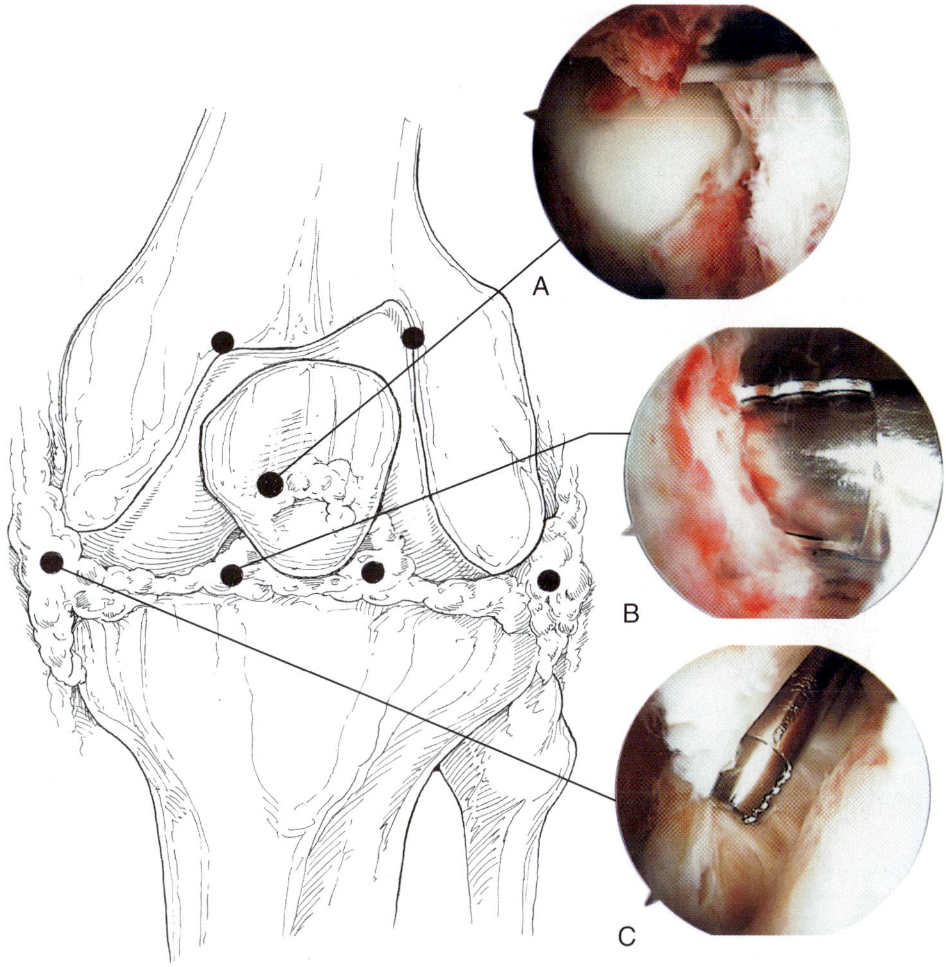

Figure 6–35 Synovectomy for diffuse pigmented villonodular synovitis using multiple portals. *(From Miller MD, Howard RF, Plancher KD: Surgical Atlas of Sports Medicine. Philadelphia, Saunders Elsevier, 2003, p 41.)*

- Other synovial processes also require complete synovectomy.
- Plicae:
  - Are synovial folds that are symptomatic only when they abrade articular cartilage (typically the medial femoral condyle).
  - Respond to arthroscopic excision, but the diagnosis of knee plicae as a source for knee pain is likely made more often than really exists.

Synovial Lesions Questions

1. Diffuse pigmented villonodular synovitis (PVNS):
  A. Has a low recurrence rate following arthroscopic synovectomy.
  B. Should best be treated with an open synovectomy.
  C. Is best treated with low-dose radiation therapy.
  D. Has a high recurrence rate following both arthroscopic and open synovectomy procedures.
  E. Has a much lower recurrence rate than nodular PVNS.

2. A rheumatologist has referred a patient with rheumatoid arthritis for a total synovectomy. He asks whether you are planning an open or arthroscopic procedure. You respond that:
  A. An open procedure is best in order to do a complete synovectomy.
  B. An arthroscopic procedure is best because of a lower postoperative recurrence rate.
  C. An arthroscopic procedure will have results similar to those of an open procedure as long as a complete synovectomy is done through multiple portals.
  D. An open or arthroscopic synovectomy is not indicated.
  E. Results of an arthroscopic procedure through standard portals are similar to those of open synovectomy.

3. Synovial plicae should be resected:
  A. Whenever they are identified arthroscopically.
  B. When direct evidence of chondral abrasion is seen.
  C. Never; they are not symptomatic.
  D. When they occur laterally.
  E. When they occur in the suprapatellar area.

Patellofemoral Disorders

Traumatic Injuries

- Quadriceps tendon rupture typically occurs in patients older than 40 years.
  - Is usually a result of indirect trauma.
  - The defect is noted when a patient is unable to do straight-leg raise.
  - Repair is performed with sutures through the patella and tied over the inferior patella.
- Patellar tendon rupture typically occurs in patients younger than 40 years.
  - Is also commonly a result of indirect trauma.
  - Consists of a defect and patella alta.
  - Patient is unable to do straight-leg raise.
  - Repair is performed with sutures through the patella and tied over the superior patella.
- Patellar fracture can be fixed with a variety of techniques (Fig. 6–36).

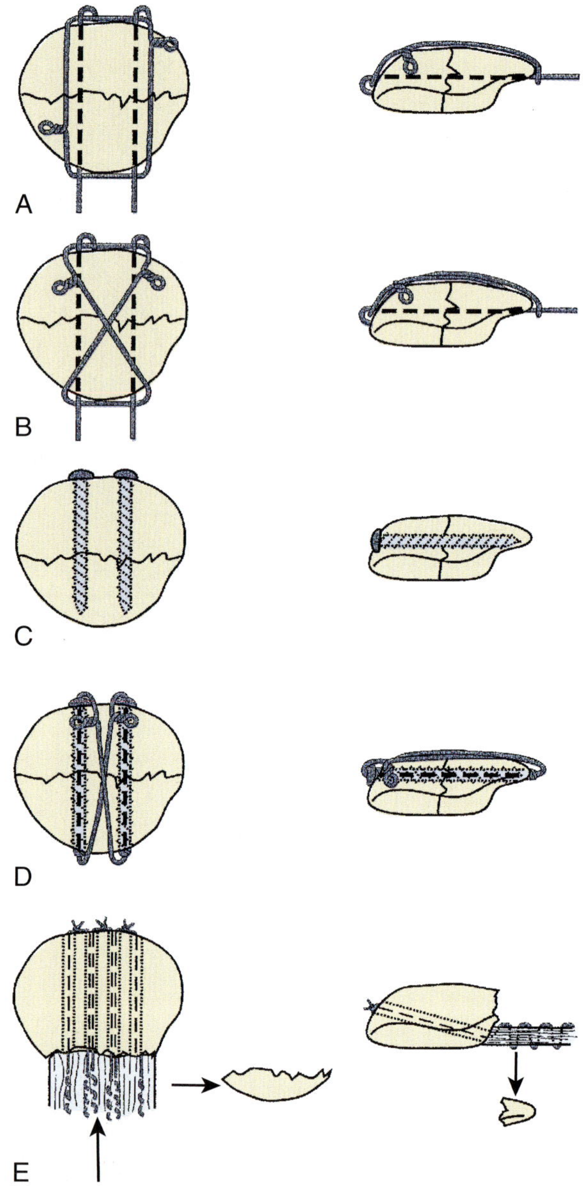

Figure 6–36 Techniques of patellar fracture fixation. **A**, Modified tension band with circular wire. **B**, Modified tension wire with figure-of-eight technique. **C**, Lag screw fixation. **D**, Combined cannulated lag screw and tension band wiring. **E**, Partial patellectomy. *(From Brinker MR: Review of Orthopaedic Trauma. Philadelphia, WB Saunders, 2001, p 103.)*

Overuse Injuries

- Patellar tendinosis (jumper's knee):
  - Degenerative fibrosis at the inferior border of the patella.
  - Symptoms and findings are worse in extension.
  - Treatment includes an orthosis (strap), modalities such as ultrasound, e-slim, and iontophoresis, and sometimes surgical excision.
- Quadriceps tendinosis:
  - Less common.
  - Occurs at the superior border of the patella.
- Prepatellar bursitis:
- Responds to symptomatic treatment (knee pads, etc.).
- Aspiration should be performed in wrestlers (to rule out infection from mats).
- Iliotibial band friction syndrome:
  - Occurs commonly in runners, especially with hill running.
  - Ober test result may be positive (Fig. 6–37).
  - Rehabilitation is typically effective. Modalities or injection helpful. Surgical excision rarely required.
- Pes anserinus bursitis:
  - Localized medial pain and swelling 5 to 7 cm below the joint line.
  - Symptomatic treatment and injections are usually curative.

Patellar Arthrosis

- Chondromalacia is measured according to the Outerbridge classification (Fig. 6–38).
- Treatment is difficult. Salvage procedures include patellar débridement, elevation (Maquet or modified Fulkerson), patellofemoral arthroplasty, and patellectomy.

Patellar Instability

- Lateral patellar compression syndrome:
  - Tight lateral retinaculum and excessive lateral tilt.
  - Quadriceps (VMO) strengthening helpful.
  - Lateral release may be indicated in refractory cases (but only with objective evidence of lateral tilting).

❑ Patella Subluxation or Dislocation
- May occur as a traumatic event and is almost always lateral.

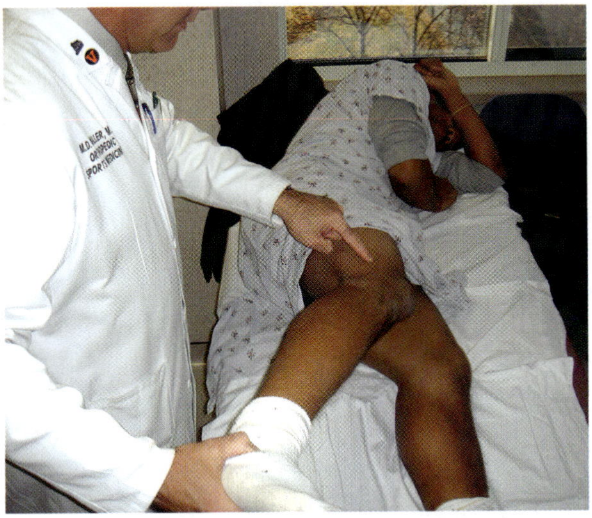

Figure 6–37 Ober test. Note that the leg is placed in hip abduction and extension with slight knee flexion. Pain occurs in a localized area with knee adduction. *(From Miller MD, Chhabra AB, Hurwitz SR, et al [eds]: Orthopaedic Surgical Approaches. Philadelphia, Saunders Elsevier, 2008, p 715.)*

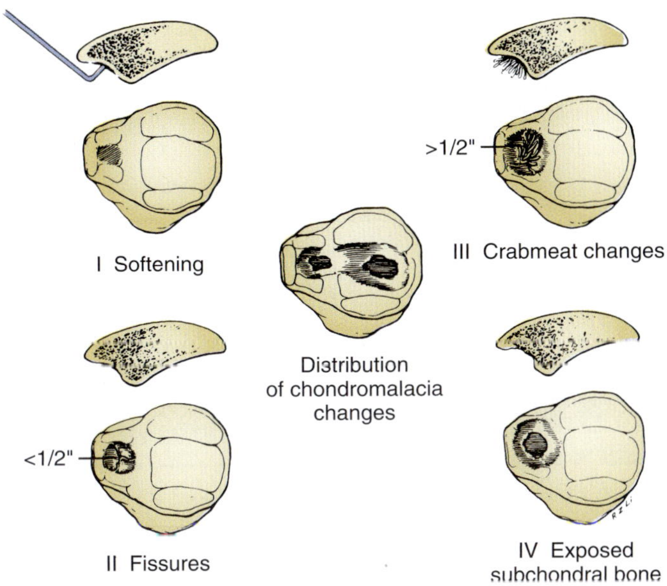

Figure 6–38 Outerbridge classification of chondromalacia. *(From Miller MD: Review of Orthopaedics, 5th ed. Philadelphia, Saunders Elsevier, 2008, p 265.)*

- May be associated with a flat trochlea and patella alta.
- Often injures the medial patellofemoral ligament, the key restraint to lateral displacement of the patella.
- Physical findings include lateral displacement (apprehension test) and abnormal Q angle (normal <10 degrees in men and 15 degrees in women).
- Often associated with chondral injury and/or loose bodies (medial facet of patella and lateral edge of lateral femoral condyle).
- Treatment is controversial but may include MPFL repair or reconstruction and/or distal realignment procedures (in patients with abnormal Q angle) in refractory cases.
  - Nonoperative management is preferred for first-time subluxations and/or dislocations unless loose bodies are present.
  - The most popular distal procedure is anteromedialization of the tibial tubercle, as popularized by Fulkerson (Fig. 6–39). This procedure unloads the distal and lateral patella and transfers the load proximally and medially (and therefore is contraindicated in patients with proximomedial patellar arthrosis).

Abnormalities of Patellar Height

- Patella alta: High-riding patella; associated with patellar instability.
- Patella baja: Low-riding patella; associated with arthrofibrosis.

Patellofemoral Disorders Questions

1. Which of the following structures contributes the most to patellar stability during lateral translation at 20 degrees of knee flexion?
   A. Lateral retinaculum.
   B. Medial patellofemoral ligament.
   C. Medial patellotibial ligament.
   D. Patellar tendon.
   E. Quadriceps tendon.

2. A 15 year-old basketball player says that her kneecap “slid out” while playing. She has a Q angle of 20 degrees, generalized ligamentous laxity, and 10 degrees of knee hyperextension bilaterally. What is the appropriate initial management for this patient?
   A. Open medial plication.
   B. Medial patellofemoral ligament reconstruction.
   C. Arthroscopic medial plication.
   D. Tibial tubercle osteotomy.
   E. Rehabilitation.

3. An 18-year-old rugby player complains of chronic anterior right knee pain. He has a history of recurrent patellar dislocations for which extended nonoperative management has failed. Physical examination demonstrates apprehension and patellar femoral crepitus. Which of the following procedures for this problem has the highest rate of recurrence?
   A. Arthroscopic lateral release combined with proximal and distal realignment procedures.
   B. Arthroscopic lateral release and patellar chondroplasty.
   C. Arthroscopic lateral release and proximal patellar realignment.
   D. Arthroscopic lateral release and distal patellar realignment.
   E. Open lateral release and distal patellar realignment.

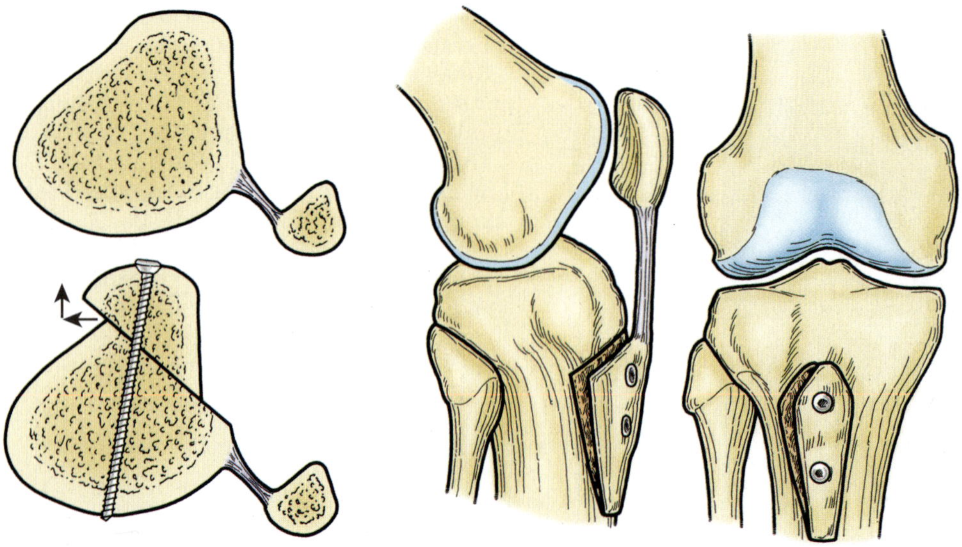

Figure 6–39 Fulkerson osteotomy. *(From Insall WN [ed]: Insall & Scott's Surgery of the Knee, Vol 2, 4th ed. Philadelphia, Churchill Livingstone/Elsevier, 2006, p 924.)*

Pediatric Sports Knee Disorders

Physeal Injuries

- Most often are Salter-Harris II fractures of the distal femoral physis.
- Stress radiographs are essential in evaluating adolescent knee injuries with varus/valgus instability.
- Knee physeal injuries often have a worse prognosis than other physeal injuries.

Ligamentous Injuries

❑ Avulsion Fractures
- Classification is shown in Figure 6–40.
- Treatment:
  - For irreducible and displaced fractures, open reduction and internal fixation (ORIF) with suture and/or screw(s) is appropriate.
  - Care must be taken to avoid injury to the physis (Fig. 6–41).

❑ Midsubstance Injuries
- Midsubstance injuries of the knee are occurring with increasing frequency, likely because of greater emphasis on competitive sports at an early age.
- Treatment may include ACL reconstruction that avoids eccentric tunnels (over-the-top position on the femur) to avoid the risk of physeal injury.

Traction Apophysitis (Fig. 6–42)

- Proximal apophysitis is known as Sinding-Larsen-Johansson disease.
- Distal (more common) apophysitis is also called Osgood-Schlatter disease.
- Treatment consists of activity modification. Late excision of ossicle(s) may occasionally be required.

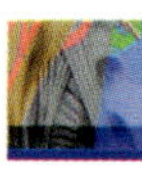

Pediatric Sports Knee Disorders

1. A 13-year-old quarterback is tackled and feels a pop in his knee. Plain radiograph findings and Lachman test results are normal. The patient has tenderness over the distal femoral physis. The next step in managing this patient should be:
   A. MRI.
   B. Arthroscopic examination.

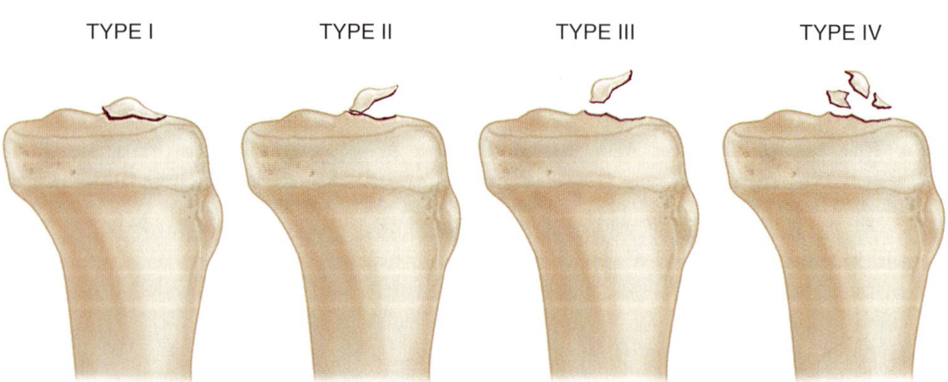

Figure 6–40 Classification of pediatric anterior crucial ligament tibial eminence avulsions. *(From Miller MD, Cole BJ, Cosgarea AJ, Sekiya JK [eds]: Operative Techniques: Sports Knee Surgery. Philadelphia, Saunders Elsevier, 2008, p 317.)*

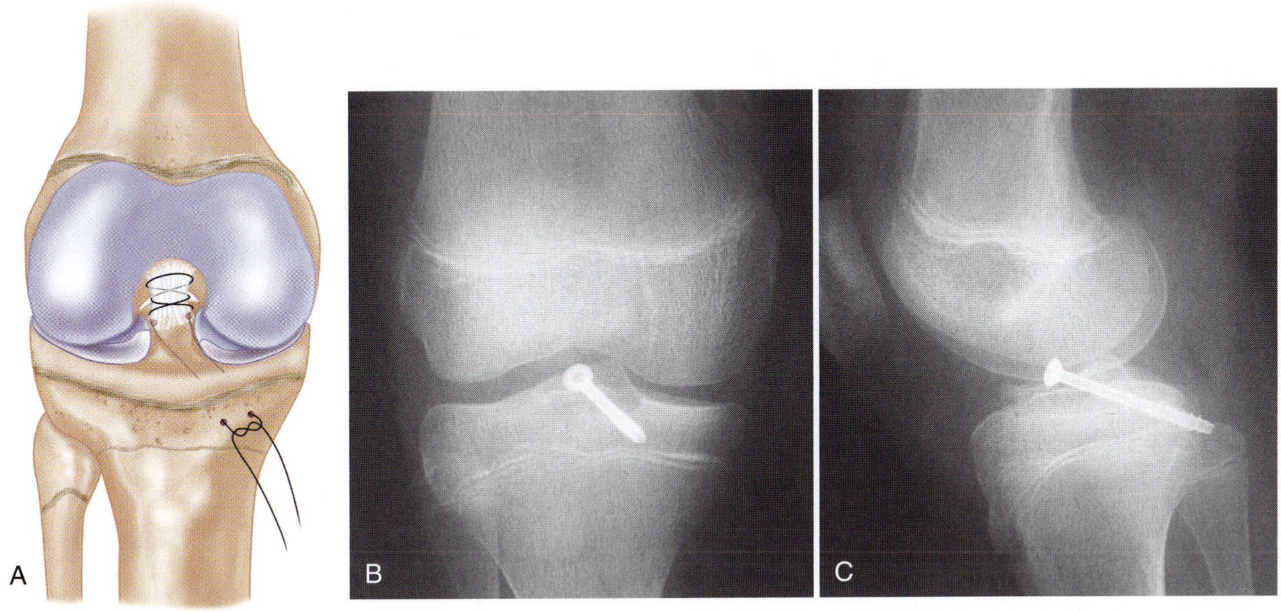

Figure 6–41 Open reduction with internal fixation of avulsion with screw avoiding the physis. **A,** Fixation of eminence with suture passed through drill holes. **B,** AP view of screw fixation A. **C,** Lateral view of screw fixation. *(From Miller MD, Cole BJ, Cosgarea AJ, Sekiya JK [eds]: Operative Techniques: Sports Knee Surgery. Philadelphia, Saunders Elsevier, 2008, p 320.)*

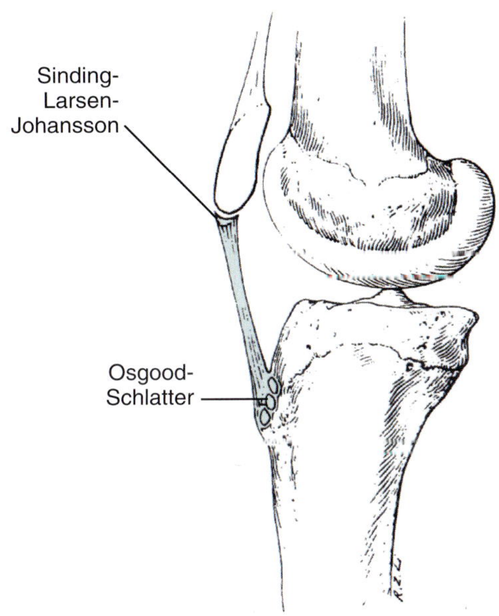

Figure 6–42 Traction apophysitis at the knee. *(From Miller MD: Review of Orthopaedics, 5th ed. Philadelphia, Saunders Elsevier, 2008, p 265.)*

C. AP and frog-leg lateral radiographs of the knee.
D. Varus and valgus stress radiographs of the knee.
E. Physical examination of the knee with the patient under anesthesia.

2. An 11-year-old gymnast injures her knee during a dismount from the high bars. Examination demonstrates a bony prominence in the notch and a positive Lachman test result. Extension of the knee does not reduce this prominence. The next step in treatment should be:

A. Percutaneous reduction of the prominence under fluoroscopy.
B. ACL reconstruction using a hamstring autograft.
C. Arthroscopic débridement.
D. Arthroscopic removal of loose bodies.
E. Arthroscopic or open reduction and fixation with a physis-sparing technique.

3. A 15-year-old boy complains of occasional pain at his tibial tubercle. He is on the school cross-country team and runs more than 25 miles a week. Initial treatment should consist of:

A. Excision of a bony prominence.
B. Tibial tubercle osteotomy.
C. Activity modification.
D. Arthroscopy.
E. Patellar tendon débridement.

■

Resources

Baer, G.S., Sekiya, J.K., 2008. Knee arthroscopy—the basics. In: Miller, M.D., Cole, B.J., Cosgarea, A.J., Sekiya, J.K. (Eds.), Sports Knee Surgery. Elsevier, Philadelphia, pp. 23–39.

Baumfeld, J.A., Hart, J.A., Miller, M.D., 2008. Sports medicine. In: Miller, M.D. (Ed.), Review of Orthopaedics, fifth ed. Elsevier Saunders, Philadelphia, pp. 245–305.

Cooper, D.E., Arnoaky, S.P., Warren, R.F., 1990. Arthroscopic meniscal repair. Clin. Sports Med. 9 (3), 589–608.

Diduch, D.R., Shen, F.R., Ong, B.C., et al., 2004. Knee: Diagnostic arthroscopy. In: Miller, M.D., Cole, B.J. (Eds.), Textbook of Arthroscopy. Elsevier, Philadelphia.

Ishibashi, Y., Yamamoto, Y., 2004. The history of arthroscopy. In: Miller, M.D., Cole, B.J. (Eds.), Textbook of Arthroscopy. Elsevier, Philadelphia.

Jackson, R.W., 1996. History of arthroscopy. In: McGinty, J.B., Jackson, R.W. (Eds.), Operative arthroscopy, second ed. Lippincott, Philadelphia.

Miller, M.D., 2008. Knee and lower leg. In: Miller, M.D., Chhabra, A.B., Hurwitz, S. (Eds.), Orthopaedic Surgical Approaches. Elsevier, Philadelphia, pp. 423–490.

Miller, M.D., Sekiya, J.K., 2006. Core Knowledge in Orthopaedics: Sports Medicine. Elsevier, Philadelphia.

Miller, M.D., Howard, R.F., Plancher, K.D., 2003. Surgical Atlas of Sports Medicine. Elsevier, Philadelphia.

Miller, M.D., Cole, B.J., Cosgarea, A.J., Sekiya, J.K., 2008. Sports Knee Surgery. Elsevier, Philadelphia.

Ong, B.C., Shen, F.H., Musahl, V., et al., 2004. Knee: Patient positioning, portal placement, and normal arthroscopy anatomy. In: Miller, M.D., Cole, B.J. (Eds.), Textbook of Arthroscopy. Elsevier, Philadelphia.

CHAPTER 7

Hip, Pelvis, and Thigh

Brian D. Busconi and Robert M. Masella

- Traditionally, the hip has received relatively minor attention among sports injuries. This situation is likely due to three reasons:
  - First, hip injuries are, perhaps, less common than injuries in other areas.
  - Second, investigative skills for the hip, including clinical assessment and imaging techniques, have been less sophisticated.
  - Third, fewer methods, both conservative and surgical, have been available to treat the hip.

Relevant Anatomy

Bones

- The hip comes closest to being a true ball-and-socket joint (Fig. 7–1). Its constrained bony architecture gives it greater stability, but less mobility, than the shoulder.
- The horseshoe or lunate articular surface of the acetabulum surrounds the acetabular fossa.
- The inferior portion of the fossa contains the acetabular attachment of the ligamentum teres.
- Above this attachment is a small fat pad encased in synovium that collectively forms the pulvinar.
- The articular surface of the acetabulum is encompassed by the fibrocartilaginous labrum, which is contiguous with the transverse acetabular ligament bridging the fossa inferiorly.
- The labrum in the hip is of lesser importance to joint stability. Nonetheless, it is likely important in the normal distribution of weight-bearing forces across the joint surface and may well have a role in facilitating normal joint lubrication.
- The abduction angle of the acetabulum relative to the horizontal plane averages 35 degrees with 20 degrees of forward flexion (Fig. 7–2).
- The femoral head forms two thirds of a sphere. Medially is a bare spot, the fovea capitis, which is the femoral attachment site of the ligamentum teres. The neck shaft angle averages 125–130 degrees and the femoral neck is anteverted 14 degrees relative to the bicondylar axis at the knee (see Fig. 7–2).

Ligaments

- The hip capsule is composed of the stout iliofemoral ligament anteriorly, the ischiofemoral ligament posteriorly, and the relatively weak pubofemoral ligament inferiorly (Figs. 7–3 and 7–4).
- The spiraling nature of the ligamentous configuration makes the capsule taut in extension with internal rotation and relaxed when the hip is slightly flexed and externally rotated.

Muscles

- The intricacies of dynamic muscle function across the hip joint are quite complex. The superficial layer consists of the tensor fascia lata, sartorius, and gluteus maximus (Fig. 7–5):
  - The fascia lata covers the entire hip region and splits to encase both the deep and superficial surfaces of the tensor fascia lata and gluteus maximus.
  - Distally, the tensor fascia lata and gluteus maximus become the iliotibial band.
  - The gluteus maximus also has a separate insertion to the proximal femur.
  - This fibromuscular sheath was termed the "pelvic deltoid" by Henry, reflecting how it covers the hip much as the deltoid muscle covers the shoulder. The gluteus maximus

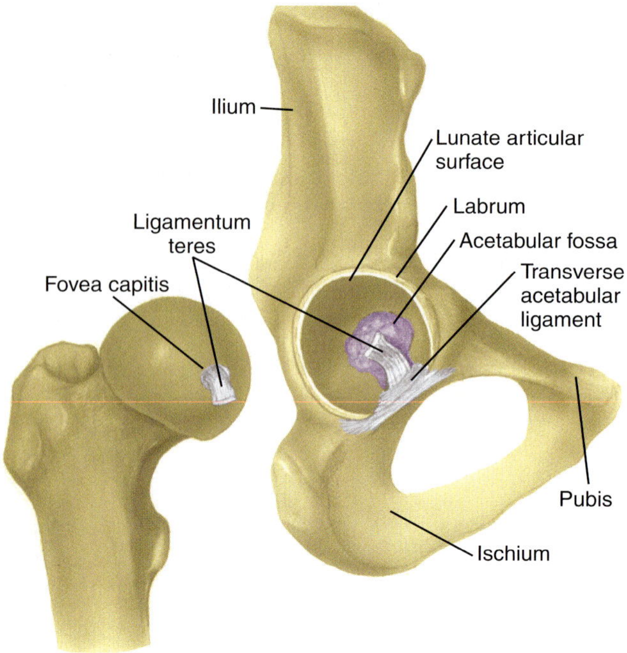

Figure 7–1 Formed from portions of the ilium, ischium, and pubis, the lunate (crescent-shaped) articular surface of the acetabulum surrounds the fossa containing the acetabular attachment of the ligamentum teres and fat, both encased in synovium. The labrum effectively deepens the socket and is contiguous with the transverse acetabular ligament inferiorly. The articular surface of the femoral head forms approximately two thirds of a sphere. Medially, the ligamentum teres attaches at the fovea capitis. The diameter of the femoral neck is only 65% of the diameter of the femoral head, an arrangement that allows for freer range of motion without marginal impingement. *(From Byrd JWT: Gross anatomy. In Byrd JWT [ed]: Operative Hip Arthroscopy. New York, Thieme, 1998, pp 69-82.)*

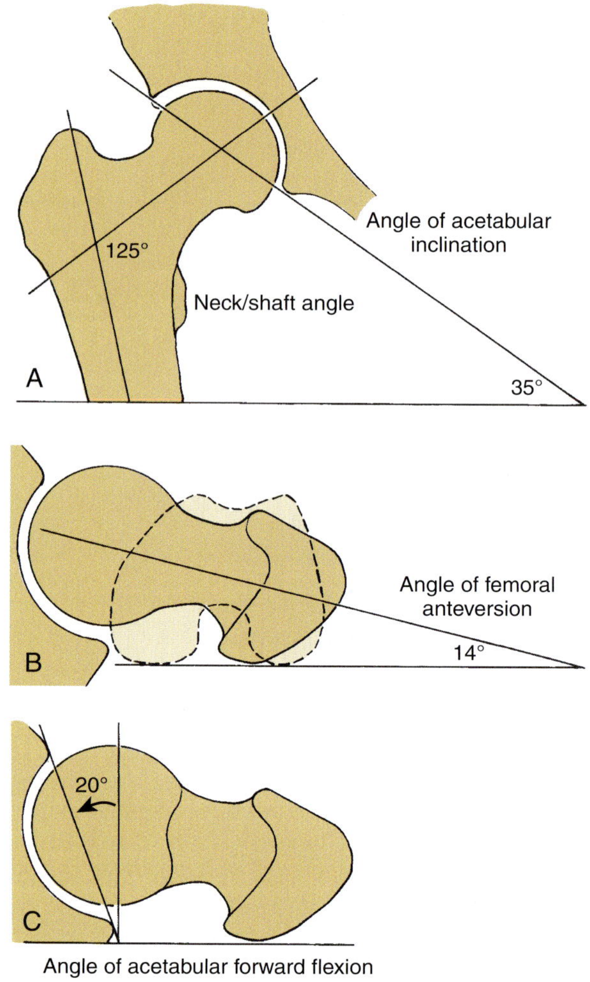

Figure 7–2 A, Acetabular orientation averages 35 degrees of abduction from the horizontal plane. The neck shaft angle formed between the axis of the femoral neck and femoral shaft averages 125 to 130 degrees. B, Femoral anteversion, determined by the angle created between the bicondylar axis of the knee and the axis of the femoral neck in the transverse plane, averages 14 degrees. C, The acetabulum is also oriented with 20 degrees of forward flexion relative to the sagittal plane. *(From Byrd JWT: Gross anatomy. In Byrd JWT [ed]: Operative Hip Arthroscopy. New York, Thieme, 1998, pp 69-82.)*

is the largest muscle in the body, whereas the sartorius is the longest.
  - The gluteus medius is transitional between the superficial and deep layers, with its origin superficial on the iliac crest covered by the fascia lata and its insertion deep on the greater trochanter.
- The deep layer includes posterior, lateral, anterior, and medial groups (Figs. 7–6 and 7–7).
  - Posteriorly are the piriformis, obturator internus, superior and inferior gemelli, obturator externus, and quadratus femoris.
  - Laterally is the gluteus minimus.
  - Anteriorly, the origin of the rectus femoris covers the capsule, and anterior to this is the iliopsoas tendon.
  - Medially are the adductor longus, adductor magnus, adductor brevis, pectineus, and gracilis.

Neurovascular Anatomy

- The lower extremity receives its innervation from the lumbosacral plexus, which forms the sciatic, femoral, and obturator nerves as well as various smaller branches:
  - The hip receives innervation from L2 to S1 of the plexus, but principally from L3 (Fig. 7–8).
  - This arrangement explains the presence of medial thigh pain often accompanying hip pathology, because symptoms may be referred to the L3 dermatome (Fig. 7–9).
- The femoral neurovascular structures (nerve, artery, and vein) exit the pelvis under the midportion of the inguinal ligament (Fig. 7–10). At the level of the hip joint, these structures lie on the anterior surface of the iliopsoas muscle, which separates them from the hip.
  - The lateral femoral cutaneous nerve, providing sensation to the lateral thigh, exits the pelvis under the inguinal ligament, close to the anterior superior iliac spine.
  - Posteriorly, 10 neurovascular structures exit the sciatic notch, including the sciatic nerve, the superior and inferior gluteal nerves, and the arteries (Fig. 7–11).

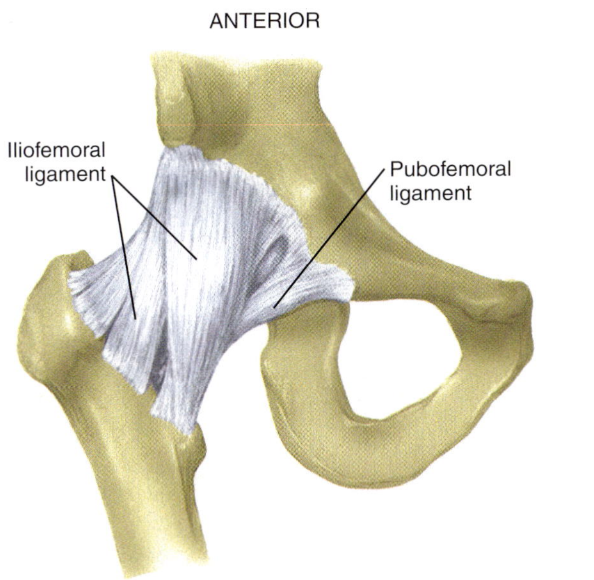

Figure 7–3 The iliofemoral ligament (ligament of Bigelow) has the shape of an inverted Y as it spirals from its attachment on the iliac portion of the superior acetabulum to its femoral attachment on the anterior neck. It is quite powerful and becomes taut in extension. The relatively weak pubofemoral ligament reinforces the inferior and anterior capsule where it blends with the medial edge of the iliofemoral ligament. *(From Byrd JWT: Gross anatomy. In Byrd JWT [ed]: Operative Hip Arthroscopy. New York, Thieme, 1998, pp 69-82.)*

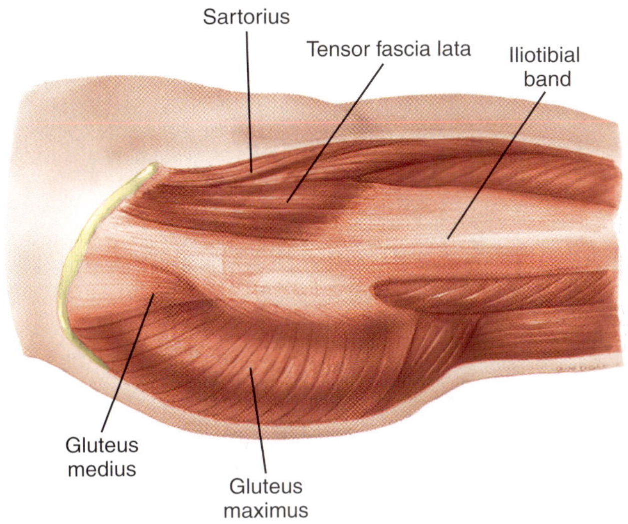

Figure 7–5 Superficial muscle layer of the hip. *(From Byrd JWT: Gross anatomy. In Byrd JWT [ed]: Operative Hip Arthroscopy. New York, Thieme, 1998, pp 69-82.)*

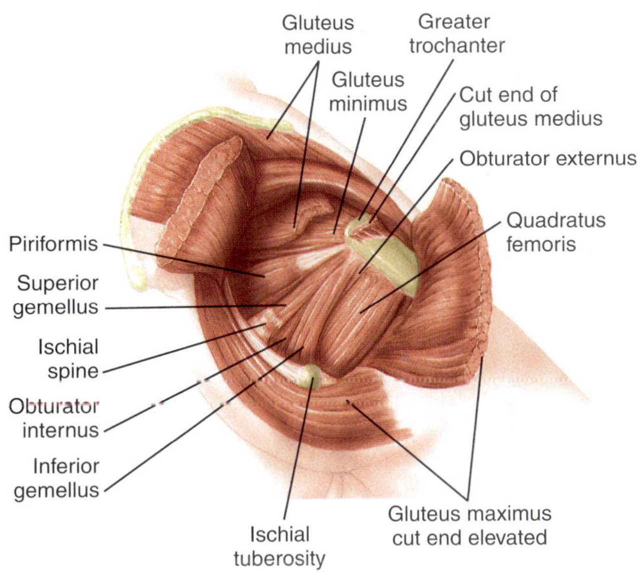

Figure 7–6 Deep structures (posterior view). *(From Byrd JWT: Gross anatomy. In Byrd JWT [ed]: Operative Hip Arthroscopy. New York, Thieme, 1998, pp 69-82.)*

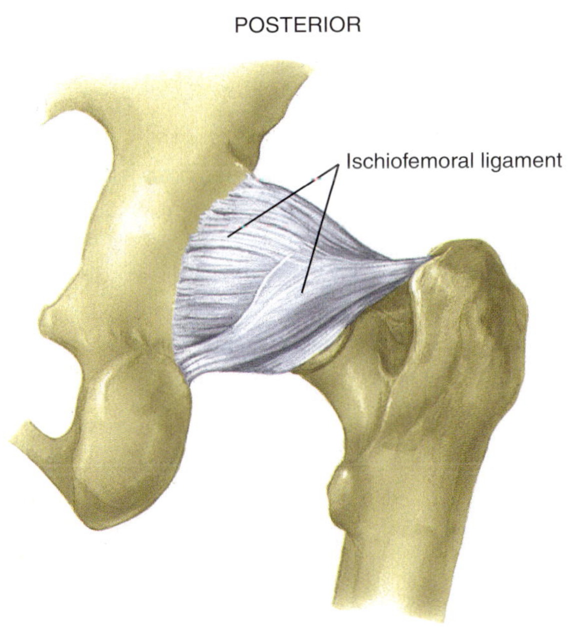

Figure 7–4 The ischiofemoral ligament reinforces the posterior capsule, spiraling from its attachment on the ischial portion of the posterior acetabulum to the superolateral aspect of the femoral neck. *(From Byrd JWT: Gross anatomy. In Byrd JWT [ed]: Operative Hip Arthroscopy. New York, Thieme, 1998, pp 69-82.)*

- The hip has an intricate vascular anastomosis (Fig. 7–12):
  - Ascending branch of the first perforating artery.
  - Descending branch of the inferior gluteal artery.
  - Transverse branches of the medial and lateral circumflex femoral arteries.
  - Terminal branches of the medullary artery from the shaft of the femur.
  - The artery of the ligamentum teres, which arises from a posterior division of the obturator artery.
  - Retinacular arteries, superior-anterior/posterior-inferior.

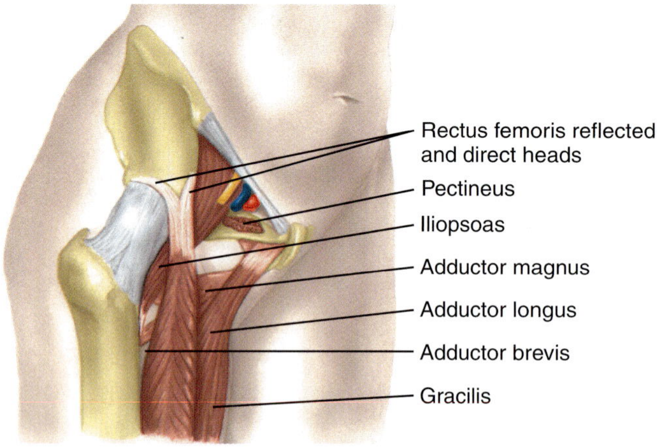

Figure 7–7 Deep structures (anterior view). *(From Byrd JWT: Gross anatomy. In Byrd JWT [ed]: Operative Hip Arthroscopy. New York, Thieme, 1998, pp 69-82.)*

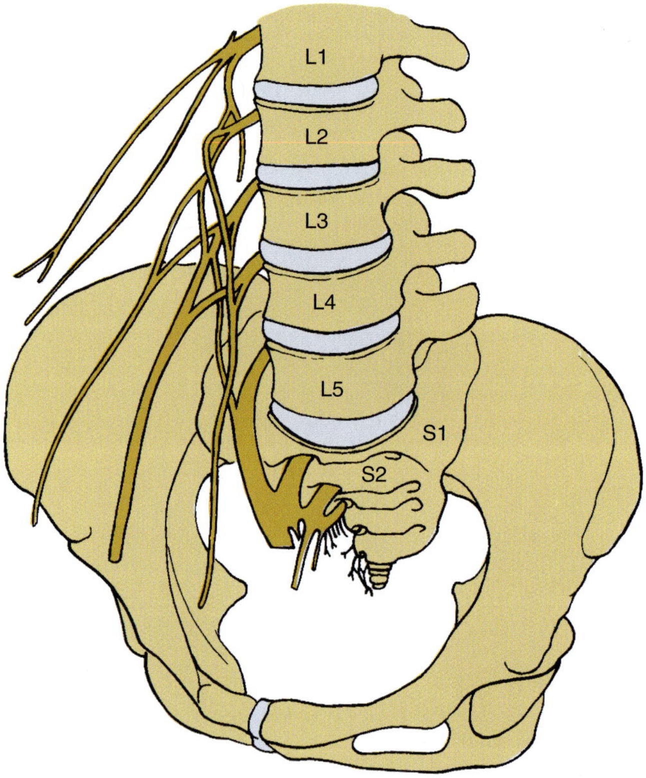

Figure 7–8 The hip joint receives innervation from branches of L2 to S1 of the lumbosacral plexus, but predominantly from the L3 nerve root. *(From Byrd JWT: Investigation of the symptomatic hip: Physical examination. In Byrd JWT [ed]: Operative Hip Arthroscopy. New York, Thieme, 1998, pp 25-41.)*

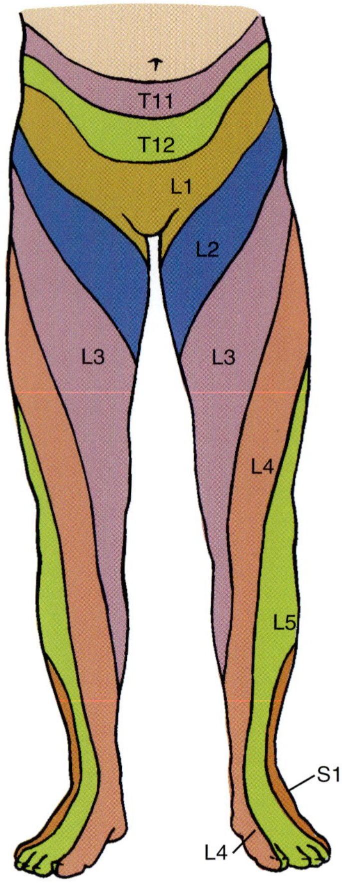

Figure 7–9 The L3 dermatome crosses the anterior thigh and extends distally along the medial thigh to the level of the knee. *(From Byrd JWT: Investigation of the symptomatic hip: Physical examination. In Byrd JWT [ed]: Operative Hip Arthroscopy. New York, Thieme, 1998, pp 25-41.)*

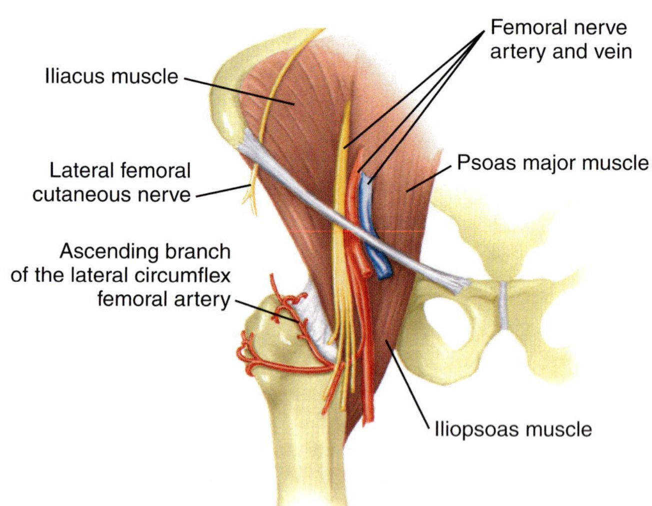

Figure 7–10 Neurovascular structures (anterior view). *(From Byrd JWT: Gross anatomy. In Byrd JWT [ed]: Operative Hip Arthroscopy. New York, Thieme, 1998, pp 69-82.)*

Anatomy Questions

1. Which of the following muscles functions as an internal rotator of the hip?
   A. The iliopsoas.
   B. The sartorius.
   C. The gluteus medius.
   D. The obturator internus.
   E. The gluteus maximus.

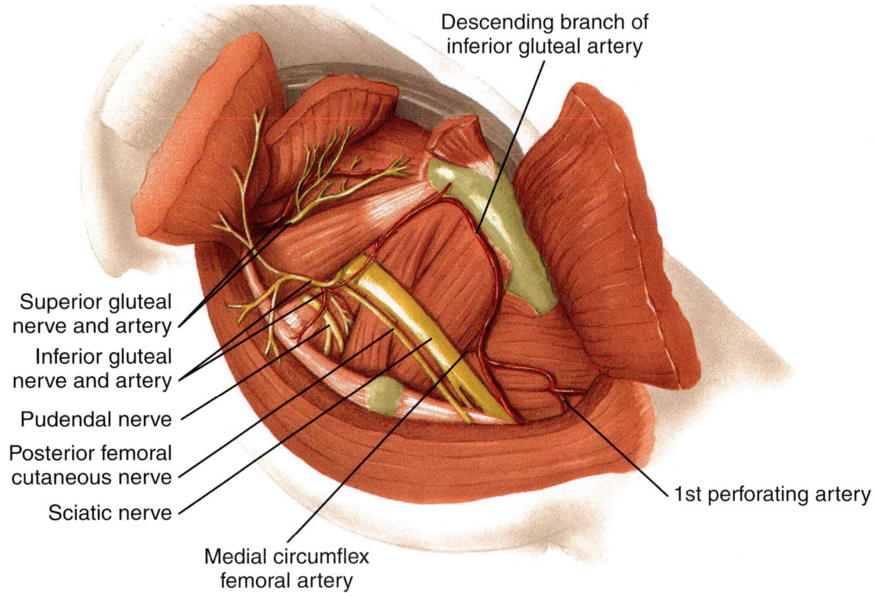

Figure 7–11 Neurovascular structures (posterior view). *(From Byrd JWT: Gross anatomy. In Byrd JWT [ed]: Operative Hip Arthroscopy. New York, Thieme, 1998, pp 69-82.)*

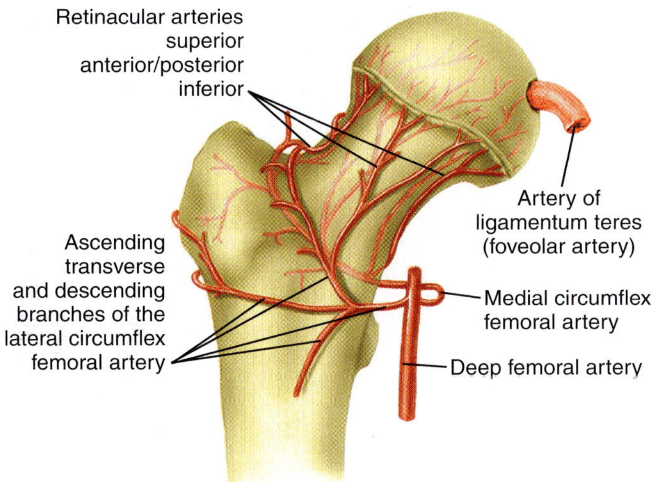

Figure 7–12 The femoral head receives arterial blood flow from an anastomosis of three sets of arteries: (1) the retinacular vessels, primarily from the medial circumflex femoral artery and, to a lesser extent, the lateral circumflex femoral artery; (2) terminal branches of the medullary artery from the shaft of the femur; and (3) the artery of the ligamentum teres from the posterior division of the obturator artery. *(From Byrd JWT: Gross anatomy. In Byrd JWT [ed]: Operative Hip Arthroscopy. New York, Thieme, 1998, pp 69-82.)*

2. All of the following structures exit the greater sciatic notch distally to the piriformis except:
A. The inferior gluteal nerve.
B. The obturator nerve.
C. The posterior femoral cutaneous nerve.
D. The sciatic nerve.
E. The pudendal nerve.

3. Which two nerves enter the pelvis through the lesser sciatic foramen?
A. The nerve to the obturator externus and the pudendal nerve.
B. The nerve to the obturator externus and the genitofemoral nerve.
C. The pudendal nerve and the genitofemoral nerve.
D. The nerve to the obturator internus and the genitofemoral nerve.
E. The nerve to the obturator internus and the pudendal nerve.

4. What separates the greater and lesser sciatic foramina?
A. Sacrotuberous ligament.
B. Ischiofemoral ligament.
C. Inguinal ligament.
D. Sacrospinous ligament.

5. What nerve is associated with hip pain referred to the knee?
A. Lateral femoral cutaneous nerve.
B. Sciatic nerve.
C. Anterior branch of the obturator nerve.
D. Femoral nerve.

Bursitis

- There are at least 13 consistent bursae around the hip region, and numerous others that are variably present.
- Bursitis can be a significant source of pain.
- Bursitis may be difficult to differentiate from other types of soft tissue inflammation and may coexist with tendinitis, tendinosis, and other friction syndromes.
- Inflammation of the larger bursae is usually the most clearly recognized (Fig. 7–13).

Trochanteric Bursitis

- This condition is characterized by lateral pain and tenderness to palpation of the bursa overlying the greater trochanter.
- Commonly seen in association with friction of the overlying iliotibial band, which is

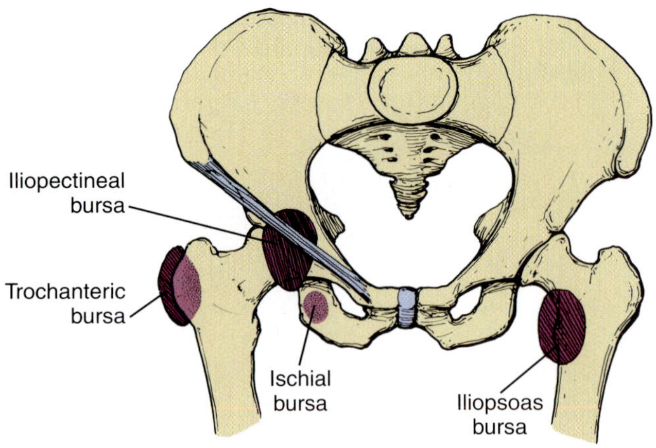

Figure 7–13 Location of the major pelvic bursae. *(From Fross ML, Nasser S, Finerman GAM: Hip and pelvis. In DeLee JC, Drez D Jr [eds]: Orthopaedic Sports Medicine. Philadelphia, WB Saunders, 1994, pp 1063-1085.)*

characteristically seen in runners and may be associated with training on banked surfaces.
- More commonly encountered in girls and women, in whom a wide pelvis and prominent trochanter are implicated.
- Magnetic resonance imaging (MRI) may show increased fluid within the bursal region.
- Treatment includes nonsteroidal anti-inflammatory drugs (NSAIDs), modification of the offending activities, and stretching to reduce the tension of the overlying abductor mechanism. Judicious use of corticosteroid injection of the bursa is appropriate for recalcitrant cases.
- Rarely, bursectomy may be indicated.

Ischial Bursitis

- This condition may be caused by direct trauma or prolonged sitting. It can be difficult to differentiate from disorders of hamstring origin.
- Conservative treatment is the standard, and judicious injection may be appropriate.

Iliopsoas Bursitis

- Usually coexists with mechanical irritation of the iliopsoas tendon.
- MRI may show excessive fluid within this bursa.
- Bursography and concomitant injection of anesthetic and corticosteroid are diagnostic and may be therapeutic in cases unresponsive to conventional conservative treatment.
- Surgery is usually directed at the offending iliopsoas tendon.

Iliopectineal Bursitis

- Also causes anterior hip pain. It accompanies irritation to the iliopsoas tendon as it exits the pelvis.
- Treatment is conservative, whereas surgery is directed at the offending iliopsoas tendon.

Contusions

- The most common injury in this region.
- The degree of injury is variable, and most cases resolve with minimal intervention.
- The key to treatment is proper recognition, because in some circumstances contusions can have lasting consequences if neglected or mismanaged.

Iliac Crest Contusion (Hip Pointer)

- Occurs from a direct blow incurred from a fall or collision. Occasionally, periostitis or exostosis may develop.
- In adolescents, radiographs should be carefully inspected to rule out avulsion of the iliac apophysis.
- The common principles of treatment are to reduce swelling and pain and then gently implement range-of-motion (ROM) exercises, followed by strengthening. Occasional judicious use of local corticosteroid injection has sometimes been advocated.
- The hallmark of return to sports is full pain-free function. Additional padding over the affected area may also be helpful to prevent recurrence.

Quadriceps Contusion

- Common in contact and collision sports, quadriceps contusion results from a direct blow to the thigh with resultant hemorrhage and muscle fiber disruption.
- Myositis ossificans may also develop as a consequence of this injury.
- Treatment:
  - Acute treatment consists of the usual modalities to reduce swelling, including cold, compression, elevation, and rest.
  - Resting the extremity with the knee in flexion maintains tension on the quadriceps muscle, possibly helping reduce pooling and lessening the likelihood of contracture and scar. Also, during the acute phase, it is important to monitor for compartment syndrome of the thigh; although this complication is uncommon, numerous cases have been reported.
  - Crutches should be used as necessary until the athlete can achieve painless, normal gait.
  - Once the acute phase has passed, formal quadriceps rehabilitation begins. Gentle ROM exercises are emphasized, but aggressive passive stretching should be avoided because it could potentiate the development of myositis ossificans.
  - As painless range of motion is achieved, gentle strengthening is begun, and functional progression continues as dictated by the patient's response to treatment.
  - If myositis ossificans develops, treatment is still conservative. Occasionally, surgical

excision of the lesion may be considered, but it should be delayed many months, until the lesion is fully matured, to minimize the likelihood of recurrence.

Groin Contusions

- Direct contusion to the groin can occur.
- Potential serious consequences that must be assessed include traumatic phlebitis, thrombosis, and femoral neuropathy.

Bursitis and Contusions Question

1. Your high school running back takes a direct blow to his anterior thigh from another player's helmet. You evaluate him on the sideline trainer's table. He has soft tissue swelling over the anterior thigh, pain with restricted knee extension, and no extensor lag. The initial evaluation reveals no evidence of fracture or compartment syndrome. Because of the severe quadriceps contusion, he is unable to continue to play. What should be included in initial management?
   A. No weight-bearing, with 30 degrees of knee flexion.
   B. Immobilization of the knee in 120 degrees of flexion.
   C. Placement of the leg into a knee immobilizer at 0 degrees of flexion.
   D. Alternating electrical muscle stimulation with moist heat.
   E. Institution of immediate continuous passive motion of the knee and hip.

■

Myositis Ossificans

- Occurs in areas of deep soft tissue injury with hematoma or around a joint or the insertion or origin of a tendon.
- Manifests as a painful mass associated with a loss of motion.
- Radiographic findings often lag behind clinical diagnosis.
- Treatment starts with avoidance of increased bleeding and maintenance of the ROM. Rehabilitation with active stretching and strengthening may be given, but massage and manipulation should be avoided.
- If surgery is needed, it should be delayed for 9 to 12 months to allow the lesion to mature. Bone scan can help delineate immature vs. mature with regards to hot vs. cold respectively.

Muscle Strains

- Muscle strains usually occur at the myotendinous junction (Fig. 7–14). An exception to this generality is a previously contused muscle; with incomplete healing, the injury may occur at the site of previous muscle contusion.
- The hip region most clearly illustrates the difference between one- and two-joint muscles:
  - One-joint muscles such as the gluteals are located close to bone and are important for maintaining posture. They tend to have slower speed of contraction but greater strength, and are less susceptible to injury.
  - In contrast, two-joint muscles such as the hamstrings are important for control and the regulation of joint motion. They often contract eccentrically, have higher percentages of type II (fast-twitch) muscle fibers, and are more susceptible to injury.
- Most commonly, strains develop from a violent eccentric force while the muscle is attempting to contract.
- Treatment focuses on reducing pain and swelling with compression, ice, elevation, and rest while maintaining normal muscle length. After subsidence of the acute symptoms,

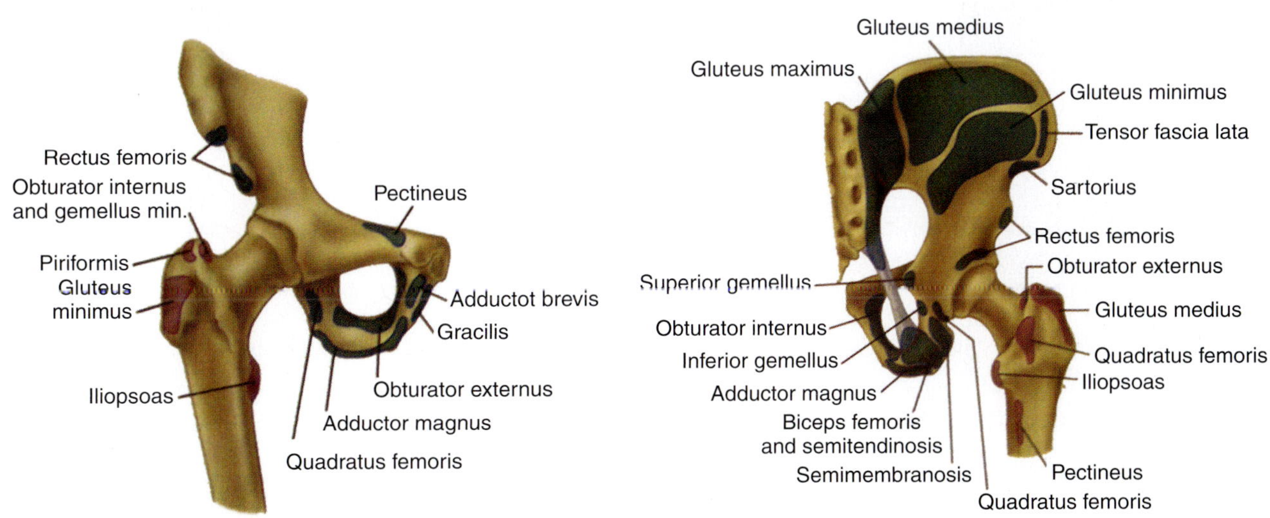

Figure 7–14 Muscle insertions and attachments around the pelvis. *(From DeLee: DeLee and Drez's Orthopaedic Sports Medicine, 3rd ed. Philadelphia, WB Saunders, 2009.)*

gentle flexibility followed by conditioning is implemented. Strengthening begins with isometric exercises and then progresses to isotonic and isokinetic methods as symptoms allow.

- Return to sport is dictated mostly by the athlete's functional performance. General guidelines include full pain-free range of motion and 90% of strength.
- In general, re-injuries tend to be more severe, and recovery from them longer. Therefore, good judgment is necessary in determining when the athlete should return to play.
- MRI may help define the location, size, and, to some extent, severity of injury. It does not forecast the length of recovery, but may provide useful adjunct information.

Adductor Strain

- Adductor injuries are especially common in soccer and ice hockey.
- The adductor longus is the most frequently injured (Fig. 7–15).
- Location of the injury can be determined by careful palpation and the presence of pain with resisted adduction.
- A distinct entity characterized by injury of the tendinous origin of the adductor musculature can occur as a consequence of either acute trauma or repetitive microtrauma. Referred to as "athletic pubalgia," this entity is discussed further in the syndromes section.

External Oblique Strain

- The injury mechanism for external oblique strain is usually a forceful contracture of the muscle while the trunk is forced to the contralateral side.
- It manifests as difficulty straightening the trunk and symptoms of local tenderness and possibly a palpable defect.
- The injury often results in partial tearing of the external oblique fibers from the iliac crest.
- Treatment involves rest, taping may help, and surgical repair to restore anatomy is rarely required.

Hamstring Strain

- The hamstrings are one of the most frequently injured muscle groups.
- Because these muscles are hip extensors and knee flexors, a common mechanism of injury occurs during sprinting, with hip flexion and knee extension.
- Because of the variable locations of the musculotendinous junction in this group, strain can occur anywhere along the posterior thigh (Fig. 7–16).

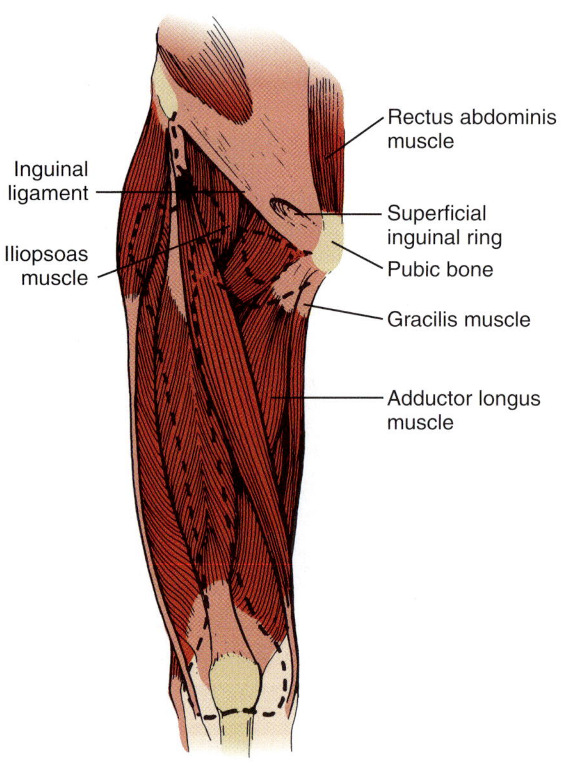

Figure 7–15 Anterior view of the hamstring muscles illustrates the geographic location of the anterior and medial thigh musculature. *(From Brunet ME, Hontas RB: The thigh. In DeLee JC, Drez D Jr [eds]: Orthopaedic Sports Medicine. Philadelphia, WB Saunders, 1994, pp 1086-1112.)*

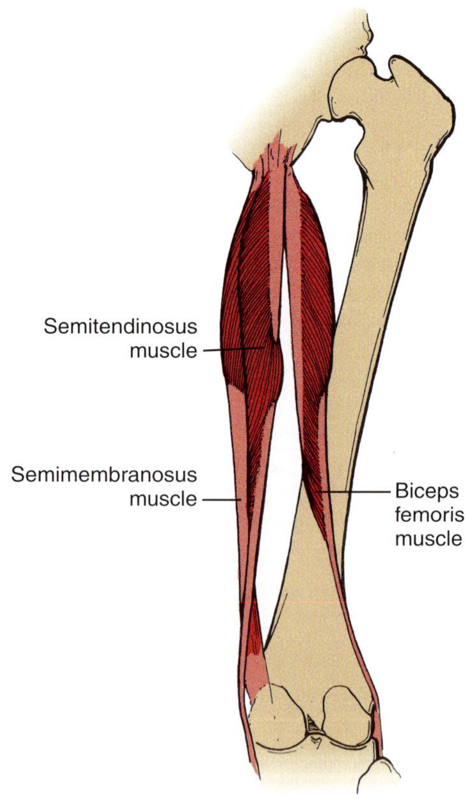

Figure 7–16 Posterior view of the hamstring muscles illustrates the various musculotendinous junctions and overlap of the tendons of origin with the tendons of insertion. *(From Brunet ME, Hontas RB: The thigh. In DeLee JC, Drez D Jr [eds]: Orthopaedic Sports Medicine. Philadelphia, WB Saunders, 1994, pp 1086-1112.)*

- Complete avulsion of the tendinous origin of the hamstrings from the ischium can also occur. This is most commonly reported as a water-skiing injury.
- For patients with chronic symptoms and dysfunction, surgical repair of the tendinous origin may result in significant improvement. Perhaps this possibility might also suggest that acute repair of select cases may provide a better functional outcome. Apart from the relative ease of surgical repair in the acute setting where anatomy is not distorted, early surgery would allow for early functional rehabilitation and also avoid the potential neurologic symptoms of gluteal sciatica (Chakravarthy et al, 2005).

Iliopsoas Strain

- Injury to the iliopsoas can occur but is probably not common.
- Careful assessment is necessary to differentiate the numerous structures anterior to the hip.
- Iliopsoas strain can usually be distinguished from strain of the origin of the rectus femoris. Iliopsoas strain elicits pain with resisted hip flexion but no pain with resisted knee extension.

Rectus Femoris Strain

- As a two-joint muscle, the rectus femoris is the most injury-prone of the quadriceps group (Fig. 7–15).
- Accompanying pain is usually elicited with either resisted hip flexion or knee extension.
- In general, acute injuries tend to occur distally in the thigh, and chronic injuries to occur near the origin at the hip.
- Avulsion of the anterior inferior iliac spine may also occur, especially in adolescence; it is discussed in the fractures section.

Syndromes

Snapping Iliopsoas Tendon

- Snapping of the iliopsoas tendon is caused as it transiently lodges against the anterior femoral head and capsule or pectineal eminence during its glide across the front of the hip and pelvic brim.
- The onset of symptoms may accompany trauma or, more frequently, overuse repetitive microtrauma associated with certain disciplines, such as ballet.
- The characteristic "clunk" occurs as the hip comes from a flexed, abducted, externally rotated position toward extension with internal rotation (Fig. 7–17). The clunk is often quite prominent and can be heard from across the room.
- Bursography is useful in the diagnosis, and injection of the bursa may be therapeutic.
- Treatment begins with recognition of the entity. Most cases can be managed conservatively with emphasis on a stretching program, anti-inflammatory medications, and modification of offending activities.
- Surgery has been successfully reported for recalcitrant cases. Partial lengthening can be performed by relaxation incisions placed at the myotendinous junction. Arthroscopic release of the tendinous insertion from the lesser trochanter has also been described. There may be variable loss of hip flexor strength associated with complete release.

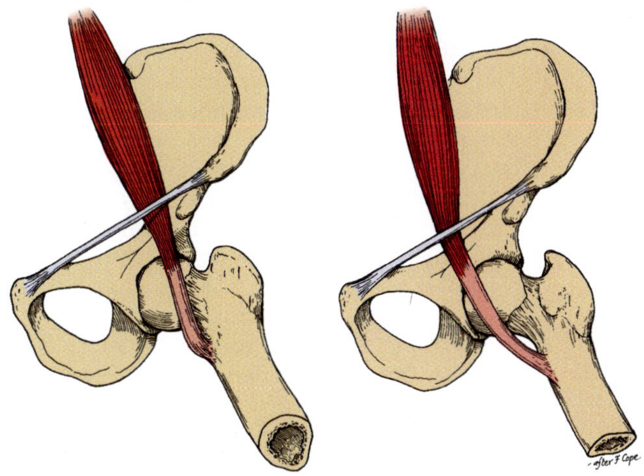

Figure 7–17 *Left,* With flexion of the hip, the iliopsoas tendon shifts laterally in relation to the center of the femoral head. *Right,* With extension of the hip, the iliopsoas tendon shifts medially in relation to the center of the femoral head. *(From Allen WC, Cope R: Coxa saltans: The snapping hip revisited. J Am Acad Orthop Surg 1995;3:303-308.)*

Snapping Iliotibial Band

- Snapping across the prominence of the greater trochanter is created by the tensor fascia lata at its site of convergence with the gluteus maximus, forming the iliotibial band.
- This condition is visually quite prominent, because it is usually best actively demonstrated by the patient while standing. The patient may feel as if the hip is subluxating; subluxation may be suggested by the visual appearance, but it is rarely the case.
- Like snapping of the iliopsoas tendon, this condition may be the result of acute trauma or, more frequently, repetitive microtrauma.
- If necessary, radiography can be used to confirm that the hip remains concentrically reduced.
- Treatment focuses on conservative measures, including stretching, conditioning, modalities to reduce inflammation, and modification of the offending activities.
- If these measures fail, selective corticosteroid injection deep to the tendon, within the trochanteric bursa, may be appropriate.
- Success has been described with a variety of surgical procedures for recalcitrant cases. The common principle is relaxation of the tendinous portion directly overlying the greater trochanter.

Piriformis Syndrome

- A relatively uncommon condition, piriformis syndrome is probably overdiagnosed and overlooked in equal proportions. The principal feature is compression of the sciatic nerve by the piriformis muscle, which may be a consequence of trauma from a direct blow to the piriformis or an anomalous relationship of the piriformis muscle with the sciatic nerve (Fig. 7–18). Typically, the result is sciatica-type symptoms that may culminate in an unrewarding workup of the lumbar spine.
- The term "piriformis syndrome" is often inaccurately used to describe many causes of poorly defined posterior hip pain. Many other posterior soft tissue structures can be injured or painful in the absence of involvement of the piriformis. The diagnosis of piriformis syndrome should be questioned in the absence of accompanying radicular pain.
- The piriformis functions most clearly as an external rotator when the hip is in extension. With flexion, it may serve more to internally rotate the hip. Palpation for posterior tenderness is performed, and symptoms may be provoked with either resisted external rotation or passive internal rotation of the extended hip.
- The most characteristic physical finding is the elicitation of symptoms by direct palpation of the piriformis muscle against the anterior sacrum on either rectal or vaginal examination.
- Neurodiagnostic studies may be helpful when they reveal selective preservation of normal signals from muscles innervated by the sciatic nerve above the piriformis (i.e., superior gluteal nerve to the gluteal maximus).

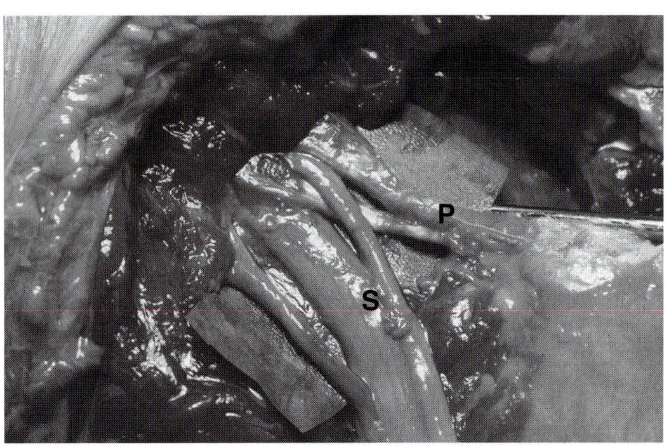

Figure 7–18 Anatomic specimen demonstrates the anomalous relationship of the sciatic nerve and piriformis, often implicated in piriformis syndrome. Three trunks converge to form the sciatic nerve after exiting the sciatic notch distal to the piriformis. The superior trunk passes through two separate muscle bellies of the piriformis. P, piriformis muscle; S, sciatic nerve. *(From Byrd JWT, Pappas JN, Pedley MJ: Hip arthroscopy: An anatomic study of portal placement and relationship to the extra-articular structures. Arthroscopy 1995;11:418-423.)*

- Treatment is conservative, but surgical release of the piriformis tendon and decompression of the sciatic nerve have been reported, with good results in properly selected cases.
- If surgery is performed, it is important to be aware of the numerous anomalous variations that exist between the piriformis and sciatic nerve, including interdigitation of the two, which require careful exploration both to ensure adequate decompression and to avoid iatrogenic injury.

Athletic Pubalgia (Sports Hernia)

- Sports hernia results from either acute microtrauma or repetitive microtrauma to the region constituting the insertion of the rectus abdominis and the origin of the hip abductors at the pubis. It is increasingly diagnosed in ice hockey and soccer players as well as athletes in other elite-level sports in which the typical mechanism of injury is common.
- The diagnosis is usually based on a high index of suspicion when pain localized to this area remains unresponsive to conservative treatment.
- Investigative studies are usually unrevealing, although MRI is becoming more sensitive at detecting signal changes within the substance of the tendon.
- For recalcitrant cases, surgical exploration with repair of the pelvic floor, including the rectus abdominis and release of the adductor longus, has met with success in high-performance athletes. The results in lower-demand individuals have been less predictable.

Syndromes Questions

1. Which of the following best describes athletic pubalgia?
   A. A syndrome of lower abdominal and adductor pain.
   B. Painful symptoms emanating from the symphysis pubis.
   C. Painful symptoms associated with dysfunction of the iliopsoas tendon.
   D. Stress fracture of the pubic ramus.
   E. Entrapment of the pudendal nerve.
2. A 16-year-old lacrosse player complains of audible popping and pain in her hip when she runs. Physical examination demonstrates mild pain with resisted hip flexion. A click can be elicited with hip adduction with the knee in extension. The location of the pathology is most likely to be:
   A. Intra-articular.
   B. Between the IT band and the greater trochanter.
   C. Between the iliopsoas muscle and the anterior hip capsule.
   D. Near the adductor longus origin.
   E. Between the rectus femoris and anterior hip capsule.

3. For the past 2 weeks, a 19-year-old ballet dancer has experienced a "clicking" sensation about the hip with extension. Ultrasonography confirms a diagnosis of internal snapping hip syndrome. What should the recommended treatment be?
   A. Crutches and no weight-bearing for 4 weeks.
   B. Rest, stretching, and analgesics.
   C. Z-plasty lengthening of the iliopsoas tendon.
   D. Intra-articular corticosteroid injection.
   E. Arthroscopic hip capsulotomy.
4. A 25-year-old professional hockey player is referred to your office by the team trainer after 6 weeks of physical therapy failed to improve his symptoms. Radiographic and MRI findings in the pelvis were normal. The patient complains of diffuse groin and lower abdominal pain that increases with heavy weight training. Examination reveals bilateral adductor tightness but no pubic or adductor tenderness. What is the best next step in management of this patient?
   A. Bone scan.
   B. Referral to a general surgeon.
   C. Decreased weight training.
   D. Administer a corticosteroid injection.
   E. CT scan of the pelvis.
5. What injury mechanism is postulated to result in athletic pubalgia?
   A. Traumatic flexion, abduction, external rotation.
   B. Repetitive flexion, internal rotation.
   C. Repetitive extension, abduction.
   D. Traumatic extension, external rotation.
6. What groin adductor muscle is most commonly strained?
   A. Adductor longus.
   B. Adductor magnus.
   C. Gracilis.
   D. Adductor brevis.
7. What quadriceps tendon is most commonly injured?
   A. Vastus medialis.
   B. Vastus lateralis.
   C. Rectus femoris.
   D. Vastus intermedius.
8. What type of muscle contraction force is the leading cause of most muscle strains?
   A. Isometric.
   B. Isokinetic.
   C. Eccentric.
   D. Isotonic.

Hernias

Inguinal Hernia

- Symptoms of inguinal hernia include tenderness, a sense of fullness, or a bulge localized to the area of the inguinal canal. There may be an accompanying mass. Small defects may be palpated or tenderness elicited laterally at the level of the internal ring.
- Herniography has been reported as a useful investigative method. Painful occult hernias are characterized as "sports hernia," especially when there is involvement of the wall of the inguinal canal without a detectable herniation.

Femoral Hernia

- A femoral hernia extends underneath the inguinal ligament, occupying the space medial to the femoral vein within the femoral triangle.
- Examination reveals tenderness localized to this area, and careful inspection for an accompanying mass helps substantiate the diagnosis.
- A high index of suspicion is necessary to avoid overlooking this entity. When it is suspected on clinical grounds, a general surgical consultation is recommended.

Osteitis Pubis

- This disorder of the symphysis pubis occurs as a consequence of repetitive trauma. It may occur with any intense activity but is seen with greatest frequency in soccer and hockey players, and runners.
- Physical findings are characterized by tenderness localized to the region of the symphysis, but there may be accompanying tenderness or spasm within the adductor musculature.
- With chronic osteitis pubis, radiographs show irregularities around the symphysis, including both cystic formation and sclerosis.
- Radionuclide scanning demonstrates increased activity, and MRI may show surrounding edema.
- Treatment includes rest, anti-inflammatory medication, and local modalities such as ultrasound, electric stimulation and deep tissue massage/release.
  - Occasional judicious use of local corticosteroid injection has been advocated for recalcitrant conditions.
  - Resolution can be expected in most cases, but the period of morbidity may be several months.

Fractures

Acute or Traumatic Fractures

- Acute or traumatic fractures of the hip require more force in athletes than similar fractures in the elderly. The higher energy translates into increased soft tissue damage and an increased risk of avascular necrosis (AVN). Anatomic rigid fixation is essential with acute fractures in the proximal femur.

- Pediatric hip fractures are rare. Slipped capital femoral epiphysis (SCFE) is the most common hip disorder in adolescents. A poorly diagnosed condition, SCFE should be suspected in a skeletally immature patient with hip or knee pain or a limp.
  - Anteroposterior (AP) and frogleg lateral radiographs are diagnostic.
  - SCFE is classified according to the ability to bear weight, with stable cases allowing weight-bearing.
  - Although unstable cases are associated with higher incidence of AVN, all cases of SCFE must be stabilized with in situ pinning.

Stress Fractures

- As with most stress fractures, radiographs of stress fracture in the hip may initially be unrevealing but with time show evidence of remodeling in response to the stress lesion. Radionuclide scanning and MRI are equally sensitive at detecting stress fractures, but MRI is more specific.
- Femoral neck stress fractures are, in general, of most concern because of the risk of propagating a displaced fracture. Stress fractures of this region may initiate from the medial or lateral side, and the treatment strategies differ.
  - Medial neck stress fractures are on the compressive surface of the bone and inherently more stable.
    - Conservative treatment is an appropriate option. It is imperative that the athlete's activity be kept below the threshold of symptoms, a requirement that may necessitate protected weight-bearing with crutches for a time.
    - Surgical fixation is generally reserved for cases in which symptoms do not respond promptly to conservative measures.
    - Healing typically requires 3 to 6 months of activity modification. Although radiographic findings may initially be normal, radiography usually is a useful method of monitoring the healing and remodeling process. Radionuclide scanning is a relatively inexpensive method of assessing resolution of the lesion.
  - Lateral neck stress fracture involves the tensile surface and represents a fracture at risk. Early surgical intervention is recommended because of the high risk of displacement.
- Stress fractures of the femoral shaft can usually be managed conservatively but still require some caution because of the potential for displacement. As with other fractures in this area, whether the lesion involves the compressive or tensile cortex partially influences the extent of necessary precautions.
- Stress fractures of the pelvis can occur, including the sacrum and pubis. The diagnosis can be easily made through clinical suspicion and imaging studies. Caution is sometimes needed so as not to misinterpret these fractures as neoplastic lesions.

Avulsion Fractures

- Avulsion fractures are most commonly seen in adolescent boys. These apophyseal avulsion injuries occur because the physis is the weakest site in such patients, having not yet closed, while muscle power has markedly increased in conjunction with the appearance of androgens.
- As with musculotendinous strains, the injury is usually the result of a sudden ballistic maneuver with accompanying eccentric loading of the tendinous insertion site to bone.
- The diagnosis is usually evident from the clinical assessment and radiographic findings. The amount of initial displacement rarely widens over time, although follow-up radiographs may be prudent.
- Sites of involvement, in order of decreasing frequency, are the anterior superior iliac spine, ischium, lesser trochanter, anterior inferior iliac spine, iliac crest, and greater trochanter.
- Treatment of these injuries is nonoperative, with an excellent prognosis for return to unrestricted activities. Crutches are often necessary to development of a painless gait. Gentle ROM and conditioning exercises are implemented as symptoms allow. Return to unrestricted sports can be anticipated within 6 to 10 weeks, depending on location and severity of the injury and the age of the athlete.
- Surgery has occasionally been postulated for severely displaced avulsion fractures, especially those involving the ischium, but there is no evidence of a better outcome than with conservative management.

Apophysitis

- Apophysitis may occur anywhere within the hip girdle, but the most common site of involvement is the iliac crest. It generally represents an overuse phenomenon, although the onset of symptoms may be acute or may be associated with a period of intense activity.
- The diagnosis may be purely clinical, because apophysitis is often characterized by pain and tenderness to palpation along the iliac crest in a skeletally immature athlete.
- With chronic involvement, radiographs may demonstrate slight asymmetric physeal widening on the side of involvement.
- Treatment is symptomatic, principally involving modification of the offending activities while the discomfort subsides.

Fracture Questions

1. A 32-year-old marathon runner complains of 5 weeks of increasing pain in the left groin during training. Radiographic findings are negative. MRI demonstrates linear increased signal in the medial 50% of the left femoral neck, with no disruption of the vascular supply to the femoral head and no displacement of the trabeculae. What is the best management of this condition?
   A. No weight-bearing for 6 weeks.
   B. Limitation of all running, full weight-bearing, and physical therapy.
   C. Strict bed rest for 6 weeks.
   D. Immediate gadolinium-enhanced MRI.
   E. Immediate in situ fixation followed by no weight-bearing for 6 weeks.
2. A 13-year-old football player presents with left hip pain and pain with passive internal rotation. Radiographs reveal an unstable, acute slipped capital femoral epiphysis. The patient's mother expresses concern that her son will gain more weight in the postoperative period because of activity limitations. Review of systems reveals that the patient has had increased fatigue, loss of interest in school, and patchy hair loss. What is the most likely underlying medical disorder?
   A. Hyperthyroidism.
   B. Hypothyroidism.
   C. Depression.
   D. Hyperparathyroidism.
   E. Adrenal adenoma.
3. A 39-year-old man presents with severe left buttock and posterior hip pain that began 2 days ago, after a fall during water skiing. He says he has no numbness in the left leg but that it feels weak when ascending and descending stairs. Examination reveals point tenderness over the ischial region and ecchymoses of the proximal posterior thigh. What is the next most appropriate step in management of this patient?
   A. Plain radiographs of the hip and pelvis.
   B. Rest, NSAIDs, rehabilitation, and gradual return to sports.
   C. MRI of the lumbosacral spine.
   D. Aspiration and an appropriate course of antibiotics.
   E. Nerve conduction studies.
4. Which of the following physical examination findings differentiates an apophyseal avulsion fracture from an acute episode of apophysitis?
   A. Passive stretch reproduces pain.
   B. Swelling and tenderness.
   C. Weakness.
   D. Bruising and ecchymosis.
5. A serious complication associated with an avulsion of the greater trochanter is:
   A. Sciatic nerve palsy.
   B. Weakness of adduction.
   C. Femoral nerve palsy.
   D. Osteonecrosis of the femoral head.
6. Pelvic avulsion injuries matching. Column A is "Boney Landmarks" and Column B is "Muscle Unit":

A. ASIS.	1. Gluteus.
B. AIIS.	2. Sartorius.
C. Lesser trochanter.	3. Hamstring.
D. Greater trochanter.	4. Iliopsoas.
E. Ischial tuberosity.	5. Rectus femoris.

Dislocation

- Nascent hip dislocations require a violent force. The majority are posterior, with only 8% to 15% being anterior.
- The patient with posterior hip dislocation usually presents with the affected lower extremity flexed, adducted, and internally rotated.
- The patient with anterior dislocation presents with the affected lower extremity flexed, abducted, and externally rotated. The violent force necessary to cause this position should alert the diagnostician to look for associated pelvic, acetabular, femoral, and patellar fractures as well as ligamentous knee injuries and sciatic nerve injuries.
- Treatment consists of urgent reduction, which usually requires general anesthesia or induction of total paralysis.
- Post-reduction hip ROM should be checked carefully for stability.
- A computed tomography (CT) scan is helpful to identify fracture fragments that may not be seen with adequate post-reduction radiographs.
- AVN may occur up to 2 to 5 years after a posterior hip dislocation. Usually the patient is followed up with serial radiographs for up to 2 years after dislocation.

Avascular Necrosis

- Osteonecrosis of the femoral head may be causally related to trauma, especially dislocation or subluxation of the hip.
- AVN may be idiopathic, but a search should be made for other causative factors (e.g., alcohol abuse, catabolic steroid use, decompression sickness).
- Radiographic findings will vary from normal to signs of advanced collapse, depending on the stage of the disease. MRI is the study of choice for both diagnosis and accurate staging.
- It is suggested that clinical trochanteric bursitis, especially when refractory to local corticosteroid treatment, may be the initial sign of AVN in the hip.

- Treatment starts with activity modification. Medications such as bisphosphonates and anticoagulation agents (Enoxaparin) have been utilized to prevent the progression of both the femoral head collapse and the arthrosis.
- Surgical treatments include core decompression, free vascularized fibular grafting, and resurfacing arthroplasty as well as hemiarthroplasty and total arthroplasty.

Nerve Entrapment

- Nerve entrapment around the hip can be a source of significant disability.
- Essentially, any nerve arising from the lumbosacral plexus may be involved (Figs. 7–19 and 7–20).
- Often no motor dysfunction is present, and the areas of sensory innervation overlap (Table 7–1). Thus, the symptoms may be confusing and the diagnosis elusive.
- Treatment is sometimes controversial, but an understanding of these entities is important for an accurate assessment.

Sciatic Nerve

- Entrapment of the sciatic nerve may potentially occur anywhere along its course from the abdomen to the knee.
- One recognized site is at the level of the ischial tuberosity from the fibrous edge of the biceps femoris origin.
- Another entity is compression of the sciatic nerve by the piriformis muscle, referred to as "piriformis syndrome" (discussed previously).

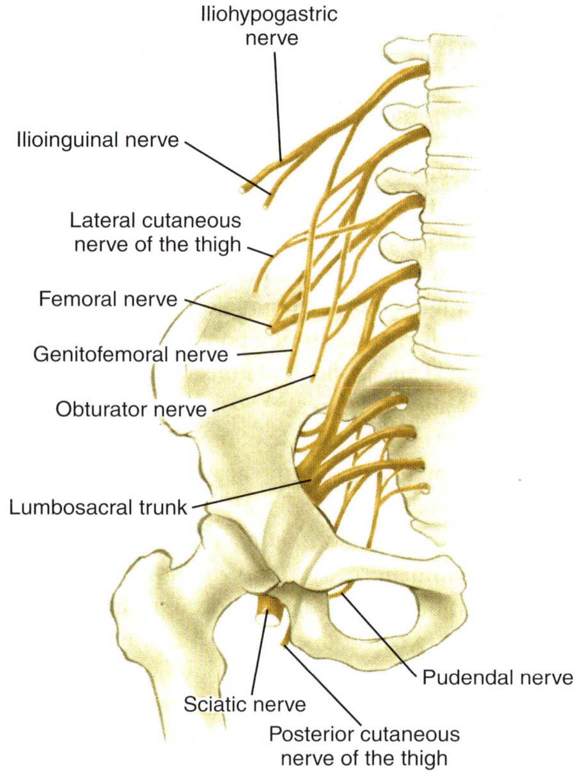

Figure 7–19 Diagrammatic anatomy of the lumbosacral plexus. *(From McCrory P, Bell S: Nerve entrapment syndromes as a cause of pain in the hip, groin and buttock. Sports Med 1999;27:261-274.)*

Obturator Nerve

- Entrapment of the obturator nerve in athletes has been reported as resulting from fascial band compression of the nerve as it exits the obturator canal.
- Surgical release has been reported to be successful in properly selected cases.

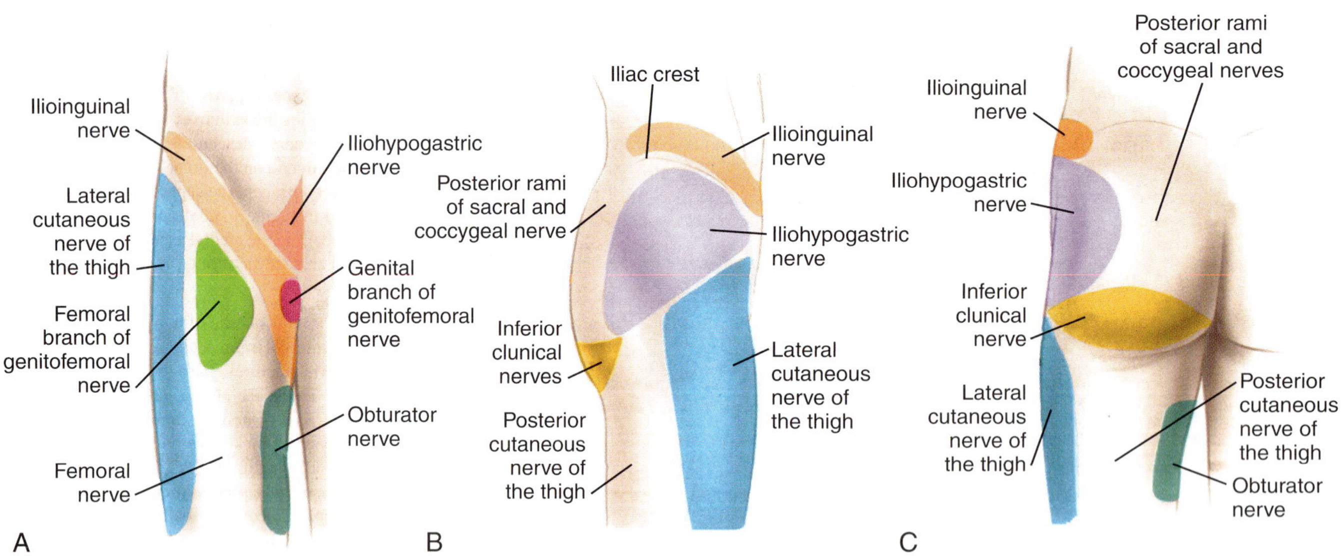

Figure 7–20 Cutaneous sensory innervation of the hip, groin, and buttock. **A**, Anterior view; **B**, lateral view; **C**, posterior view. *(From McCrory P, Bell S: Nerve entrapment syndromes as a cause of pain in the hip, groin and buttock. Sports Med 1999;27:261-274.)*

Table 7–1 Motor and Sensory Distribution of the Lumbosacral Plexus

Nerve	Motor Innervation	Cutaneous Sensory Distribution
Iliohypogastric nerve	Abdominal wall muscles	Upper buttock Suprapubic
Ilioinguinal nerve	Internal oblique, transversalis	Inguinal ligament Upper medial thigh Lateral scrotal skin or mons/labia
Genitofemoral nerve	—	Anterior thigh Lateral scrotal skin or mons/labia
Obturator nerve	Adductor longus, adductor brevis, gracilis, pectineus, adductor magnus, obturator externus	Distal medial thigh, knee joint (hip joint)
Femoral nerve	Quadriceps muscle	Anterior thigh
Lateral cutaneous nerve of the thigh	—	Anterolateral thigh
Sciatic nerve	Hamstring muscles	—
Pudendal nerve	External anal sphincter, perineal muscles, external urethral sphincter	Perineal skin, scrotal or labial skin, perianal skin
Superior and inferior gluteal nerves	Gluteus medius, gluteus minimus, gluteus maximus, tensor fasciae latae	—
Posterior cutaneous nerve of the thigh	—	Lower buttock, posterior thigh, perineum

From McCrory P, Bell S: Nerve entrapment syndromes as a cause of pain in the hip, groin and buttock. Sports Med 1999;27:261-274.

Pudendal Nerve

- Compression of the pudendal nerve has been reported in cyclists, with resulting neuropraxia characterized by sensory loss to the perineum and impotence in severe cases. The condition is usually transient, although recovery may be incomplete.
- This condition has also been reported as a complication of hip arthroscopy and other fracture management necessitating distraction on a fracture table.

Ilioinguinal Nerve

- Ilioinguinal nerve entrapment is most often caused by hypertrophied abdominal muscles (bodybuilders or pregnancy), but it can also be iatrogenic, from iliac crest bone graft harvesting.
- It manifests as pain in the inguinal region that radiates to the genitals. There is usually tenderness to palpation approximately 2 to 3 cm medial and inferior to the anterior superior iliac spine (ASIS). Symptoms can be reproduced with hip extension.
- Treatment is conservative, with rest, ice, and anti-inflammatory medication. Surgical release is beneficial but rarely necessary.

Lateral Femoral Cutaneous Nerve Entrapment (Meralgia Paresthetica)

- Meralgia paresthetica is the most easily recognized of the nerve conditions around the hip. The lateral femoral cutaneous nerve is susceptible to compression as it exits underneath the ASIS and becomes superficial. It can occur from tight belts or pads or long periods of hip flexion.
- Manifests as anterolateral thigh numbness/paresthesias with no motor symptoms and the detection of tinel sign 1 cm medial and inferior to the ASIS.
- Relief from the offending activity may be helpful. Surgical release is rarely necessary.

Dislocation, Avascular Necrosis, and Nerve Entrapment Questions

1. A 27-year-old power lifter complains of dysesthesias at the anterolateral aspect of his left thigh. The remainder of peripheral neurologic findings in the hip are unremarkable. Which of the following would be the most appropriate initial clinical step?
A. Lumbar myelography.
B. Lumbar MRI.
C. Digital rectal examination.
D. Electromyography.
E. Adjustment of the fit of his weight belt.

2. What is the most common direction of traumatic hip dislocation?
A. Anterior.
B. Posterior.
C. Inferior.
D. Medial.

3. What is the principal complication following a hip dislocation with stable reduction without fracture?
A. Post-traumatic osteoarthritis.
B. AVN.
C. Gait abnormality.
D. Hip pain.

4. What is the most common etiology of ilioinguinal nerve entrapment?
   A. Fascial band.
   B. Hip arthroscopy.
   C. Abdominal muscle hypertrophy.
   D. Long periods of hip flexion.
5. All of the following are commonly believed to be risk factors for avascular necrosis of the femoral head except:
   A. Caisson disease.
   B. Sickle cell anemia.
   C. Gaucher disease.
   D. Intra-articular glucocorticoid injection.
   E. Pancreatitis.
6. A 28-year-old man is involved in a head-on motor vehicle accident. A pelvic CT scan obtained in the emergency room reveals a posterior dislocation of the femoral head with no associated fracture. The least common complication of this injury is:
   A. Avascular necrosis of the femoral head.
   B. Recurrent dislocation.
   C. Sciatic nerve palsy.
   D. Post-traumatic arthritis.
   E. Irreducibility.
7. What injuries result from an acute posterior subluxation event of the hip?

Arthroscopy

- Arthroscopy of the hip is well-established, with numerous reports highlighting its efficacy. The constrained ball-and-socket architecture of the joint, the dense surrounding soft tissue envelope, and thick capsule with limited compliance each provide a unique challenge but can be overcome by following basic principles and giving attention to the details of carrying out this technique.
- For obvious forms of pathology, such as symptomatic loose bodies, arthroscopy offers an excellent alternative to the traditional open techniques necessary in the past. Perhaps more importantly, arthroscopy now offers a method of treatment for many elusive forms of intra-articular pathology that previously went untreated and largely unrecognized, forcing the patient to simply resign himself/herself to living within the constraints of the symptoms.

Indications

- There are numerous indications for hip arthroscopy (Table 7–2).
- The largest potential group of candidates is patients with degenerative disease of the hip, most typically osteoarthritis. However, arthroscopic débridement is rarely indicated because the results can be unpredictable with regard to appreciable symptomatic improvement. Even with careful patient selection, the results of débridement are not as successful in the hip as those reported in the knee.

Table 7–2 Indications for Hip Arthroscopy

Loose bodies
Labral tears
Degenerative disease
Chondral injuries
Avascular necrosis
Synovial disease
Ruptured ligamentum teres
Impinging osteophytes
Instability
Joint sepsis
Status post–total hip arthroplasty
Unresolved hip pain
Association with open procedures

- Loose bodies represent the clearest indication for arthroscopy. The diagnosis is frequently evident with various investigative techniques, and the importance of loose body removal to slow the occurrence of secondary damage due to third-body wear has been well documented by Epstein (1973).
- Three common sources of hip pain associated with acute trauma in young active individuals are damage to the acetabular labrum, acute fragmentation of the articular surface, and rupture of the ligamentum teres.
- In general, when assessing acute hip pain, the surgeon must always be wary of underlying degenerative disease or some other predisposition, such as acetabular dysplasia, that may have made the individual more vulnerable to injury. This may be a harbinger of a less successful response to surgery or of greater potential for long-term problems. In general, patients with a specific traumatic event and those with mechanical symptoms such as a sharp stabbing pain, catching, or locking are more likely to have a good response to arthroscopy.

Contraindications

- Contraindications specific to the hip joint are uncommon. Restricted ROM of the hip suggests there is insufficient capsular mobility to achieve distraction necessary for introducing the instruments into the joint.
- Ankylosis would be the most absolute contraindication.
- Severely osteoporotic bone or stress risers might prevent sufficient distraction for performing the procedure.
- Wound problems or severely altered soft tissue anatomy, whether from previous trauma or surgery, might also be a consideration.

Setup

- Arthroscopy of the hip can be effectively performed in either the supine or lateral decubitus position. Positioning is principally influenced by the surgeon's preference.

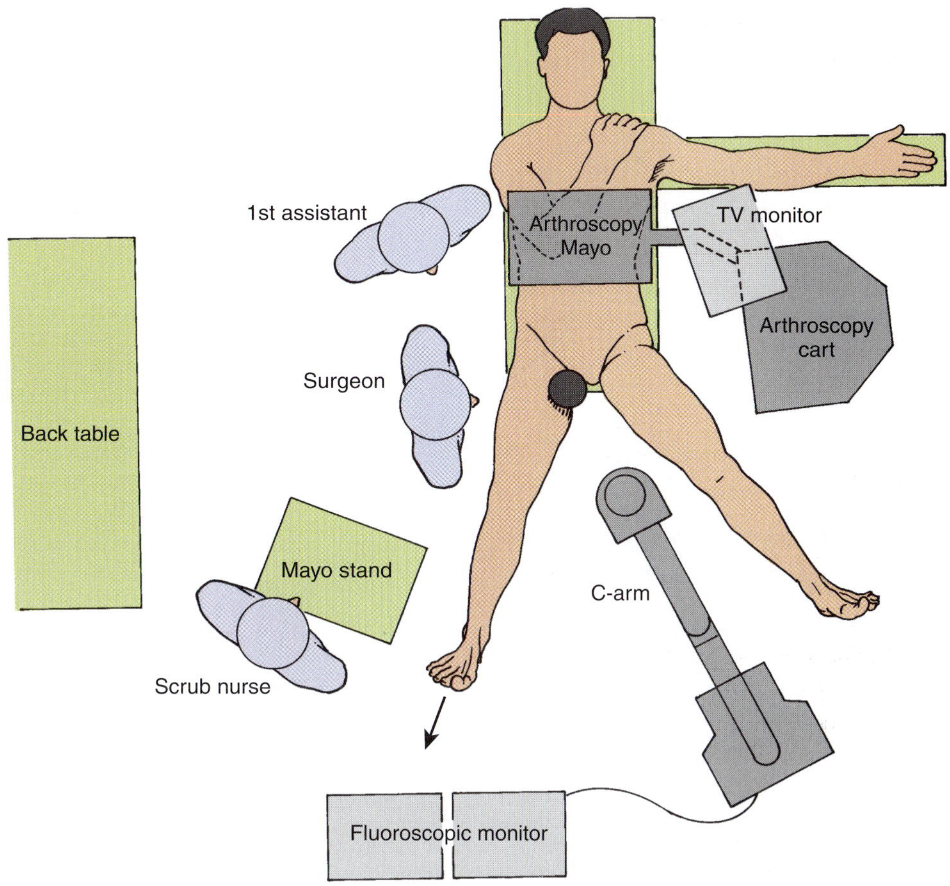

Figure 7–21 Schematic of the operating room layout showing the position of the surgeon, assistant, scrub nurse, arthroscopy cart, monitor and Mayo, scrub nurse's Mayo, C-arm, and back table. *(From Byrd JWT: The supine position. In Byrd JWT [ed]: Operative Hip Arthroscopy. New York, Thieme, 1998, pp 123-138.)*

- Minor advantages of the supine approach include use of a standard fracture table and simplicity of patient positioning and setup (Fig. 7–21).
- Regardless of whether the patient is place supine or lateral, careful positioning of the torso and lower extremities is critical to carrying out a successful and safe procedure.

- The perineal post is lateralized against the medial thigh of the operative hip (Figs. 7–22 and 7–23). This arrangement helps open up the hip joint with distraction and reduces direct pressure on the perineum, lessening the risk of pudendal neuropraxia.
- Typically, about 50 lb of force is necessary to adequately distract the joint.
  - In general, use the minimal force necessary to achieve adequate distraction, and keep traction time as brief as possible to minimize the risk of traction neuropraxia of the sciatic or femoral nerve.
  - Two hours is usually recognized as a reasonable limit for traction. Also of note, there have been a few reports describing arthroscopy without distraction.

Equipment

- Use of the C-arm of the fluoroscope is important for precise placement of the instrumentation within the joint.
- Extra-length arthroscopy instruments are also available to accommodate the dense surrounding soft tissue of the hip. Standard-length instruments may be adequate for thin patients, although caution should be exercised

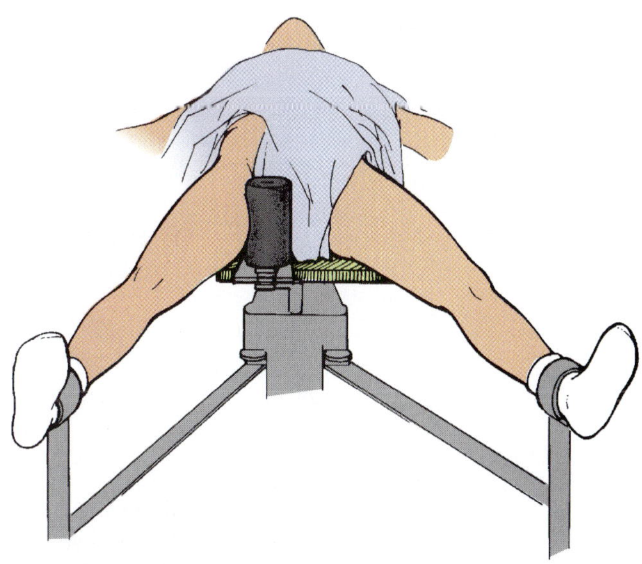

Figure 7–22 Supine position for hip arthroscopy requires a perineal post lateralized to the operative side. The operative hip is placed in extension, approximately 25 degrees of abduction, and neutral rotation. *(From Byrd JWT: Hip Arthroscopy: Principles and Application. Andover, MA, Smith & Nephew Endoscopy, 1996.)*

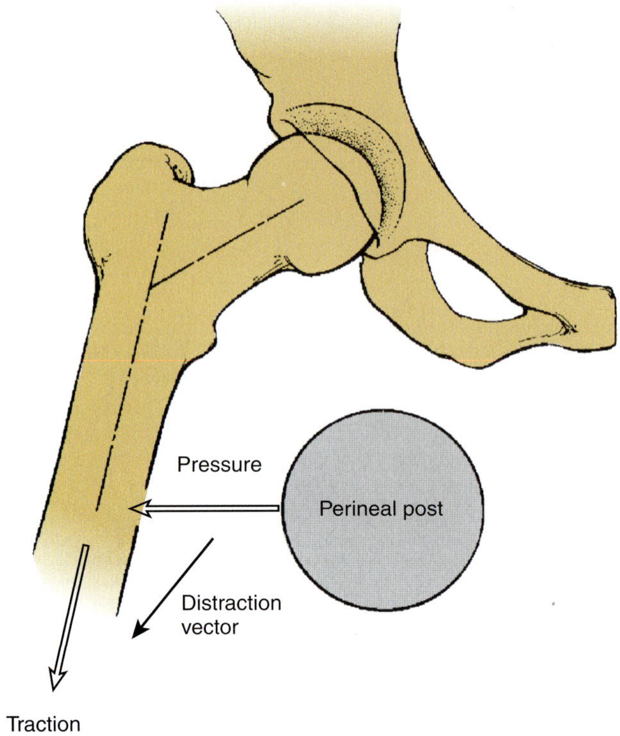

Figure 7–23 The optimal vector for distraction is oblique relative to the axis of the body and more closely coincides with the axis of the femoral neck than the femoral shaft. This oblique vector is partially created by hip abduction and partially accentuated by the small transverse component achieved by lateralizing the perineal post. *(From Byrd JWT: Hip Arthroscopy: Principles and Application. Andover, MA, Smith & Nephew Endoscopy, 1996.)*

in patients in whom the instrumentation may be marginal for accessing the joint, especially once a modest degree of soft tissue fluid extravasation has occurred.

Portals

- Three standard portals are utilized for hip arthroscopy (Figs. 7–24 and 7-25).
- Two of these (anterolateral and posterolateral) are placed laterally over the superior margin of the greater trochanter at its anterior and posterior borders.
- The anterior portal is placed at the site of intersection of a sagittal line drawn distally from the anterior superior iliac spine and a transverse line across the tip of the greater trochanter.
- With careful orientation to the landmarks in relation to the joint, these portals are a safe distance from the surrounding major neurovascular structures (Figs. 7–26 and 7–27; Table 7–3).

Complications

- With careful attention to the details of performing hip arthroscopy, complications are rare. In a review of almost 1500 cases from several centers, an overall complication rate of 1.3% was identified (Table 7–4).
- Direct injury to the major neurovascular structures is avoided by careful orientation during portal placement.

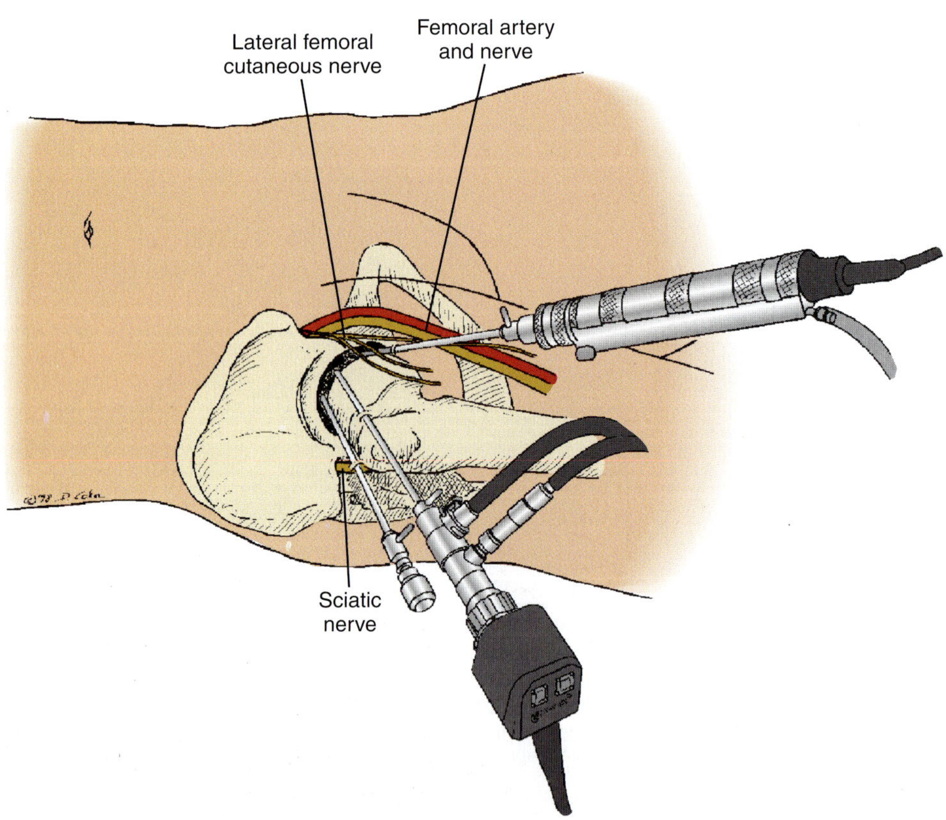

Figure 7–24 The site of the anterior portal coincides with the intersection of a sagittal line drawn distally from the anterior superior iliac spine and a transverse line across the superior margin of the greater trochanter. The direction of this portal courses approximately 45 degrees cephalad and 30 degrees toward the midline. The anterolateral and posterolateral portals are positioned directly over the superior aspect of the trochanter at its anterior and posterior borders.

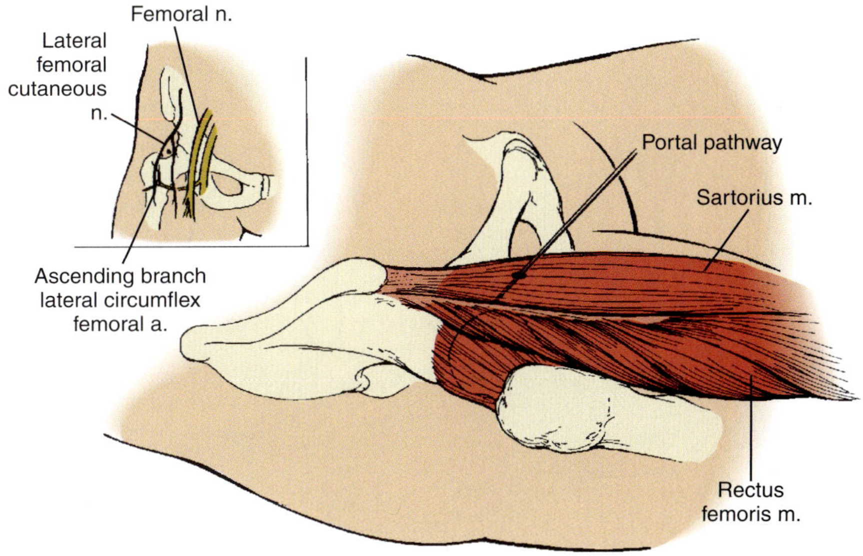

Figure 7–25 The relationship of the major neurovascular structures to the three standard portals. The femoral artery and nerve lie well medial to the anterior portal. The sciatic nerve lies posterior to the posterolateral portal. The lateral femoral cutaneous nerve lies close to the anterior portal. Injury to this structure is avoided by utilizing proper technique in portal placement. The anterolateral portal is established first because it lies most centrally in the safe zone for arthroscopy. a., artery; m., muscle; n., nerve.

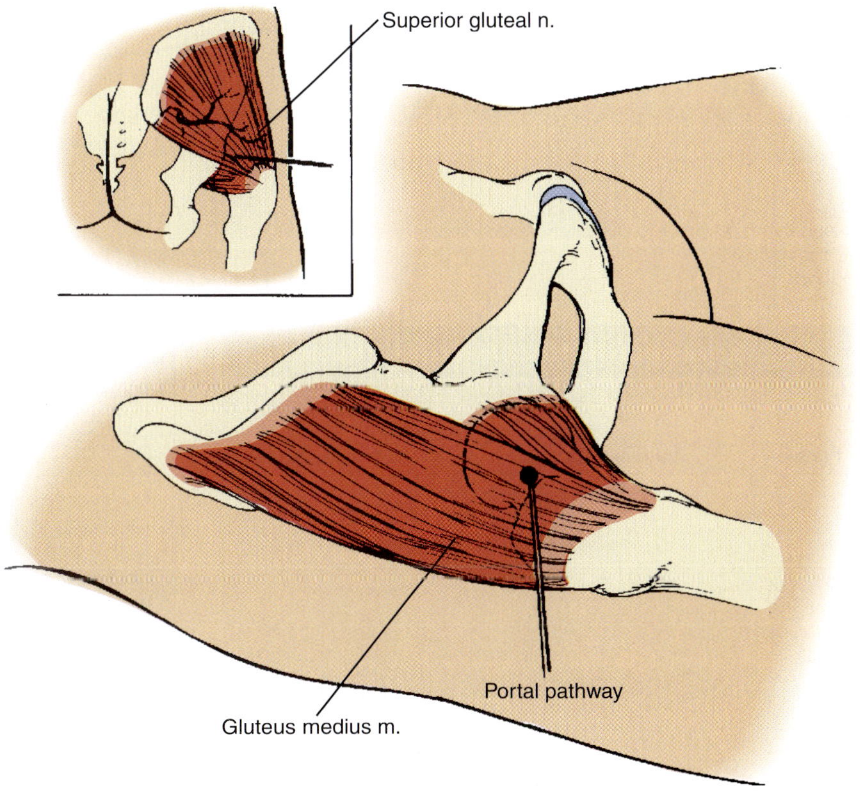

Figure 7–26 Anterior portal pathway: Relationship to the lateral femoral cutaneous nerve, femoral nerve, and lateral circumflex femoral artery. m., muscle; n., nerve. *(From Byrd JWT: Hip Arthroscopy: Principles and Application. Andover, MA, Smith & Nephew Endoscopy, 1996.)*

- The risk of traction and compression injuries is minimized by careful attention to patient positioning, the amount of traction force being utilized, and the length of time that traction is applied.
- Disturbance of one of the small branches of the lateral femoral cutaneous nerve is a unique concern with the anterior position. This complication is uncommon and results in only a small patchy area of reduced sensation, not the painful symptoms attributed to meralgia paresthetica.
- It is likely that the most common complication, which goes largely unreported, is iatrogenic intra-articular damage. Even with careful attention to the details of the procedure, this possibility cannot be minimized, emphasizing the importance of meticulous technique in performing this procedure.

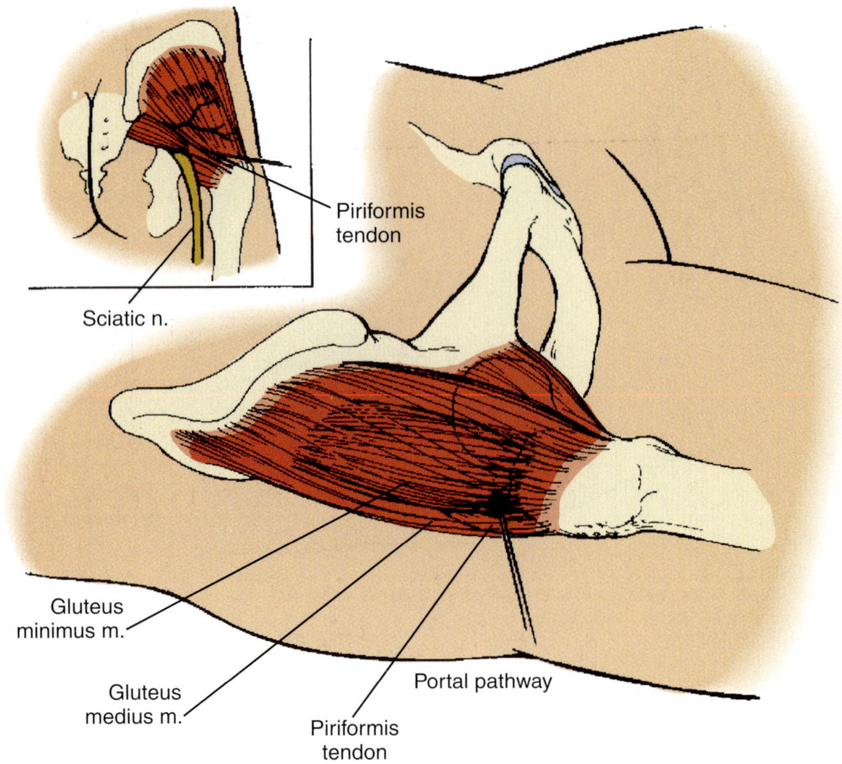

Figure 7–27 Relationship of the anterolateral portal pathway to the superior gluteal nerve. m., muscle; n., nerve. *(From Byrd JWT: Hip Arthroscopy: Principles and Application. Andover, MA, Smith & Nephew Endoscopy, 1996.)*

Table 7–3 Distance from Portal to Anatomic Structures*

Portals	Anatomic Structure	Distance (cm) Average	Range
	Anterior superior iliac spine	6.3	6.0-7.0
	Lateral femoral cutaneous nerve†	0.3	0.2-1.0
Anterior	Femoral nerve‡		
	Level of sartorius	4.3	3.8-5.0
	Level of rectus femoris	3.8	2.7-5.0
	Level of capsule	3.7	2.9-5.0
	Lateral circumflex femoral artery		
	Ascending branch	3.7	1.0-6.0
	Terminal branch§	0.3	0.2-0.4
Anterolateral	Superior gluteal nerve	4.4	3.2-5.5
Posterolateral	Sciatic nerve	2.9	2.0-4.3

*Based on an anatomic dissection of portal placements in eight fresh cadaver specimens.
†The nerve had divided into three or more branches, and measurement was made to the closest branch.
‡Measurement was made at superficial surfaces of sartorius, rectus femoris, and capsule.
§Small terminal branch of ascending branch of lateral circumflex femoral artery was identified in three specimens.
From Byrd JWT, Pappas JN, Pedley MJ: Hip arthroscopy: An anatomic study of portal placement and relationship to the extra-articular structures. Arthroscopy 1995;11:418-423.

Table 7–4 Complications Associated with 1491 Arthroscopic Hip Procedures*

Transient pudendal nerve neurapraxia (5)
Permanent pudendal nerve neurapraxia (1)
Transient sciatic nerve neurapraxia (4)
Intra-abdominal fluid extravasation (3)
Partial lateral femoral cutaneous nerve neurapraxia (2)
Laceration of the lateral femoral cutaneous nerve (1)
Scrotal skin necrosis (1)
Femoral nerve palsy (1)
Instrument breakage (1)
Heterotopic ossification (1)

*Numbers in parentheses represent the actual number of complications in 1491 hip procedures.

Loose Bodies

- Symptomatic loose bodies may occur as a result of trauma or disease such as synovial chondromatosis (Fig. 7–28). Most sizable loose bodies can be diagnosed with various imaging techniques, but some form of arthrography combined with either CT or MRI is often needed.
- Arthroscopic removal of loose bodies represents an excellent alternative to traditional open methods. The importance of loose body removal to slow the secondary damage incurred by third-body wear has been well documented by Epstein (1973).

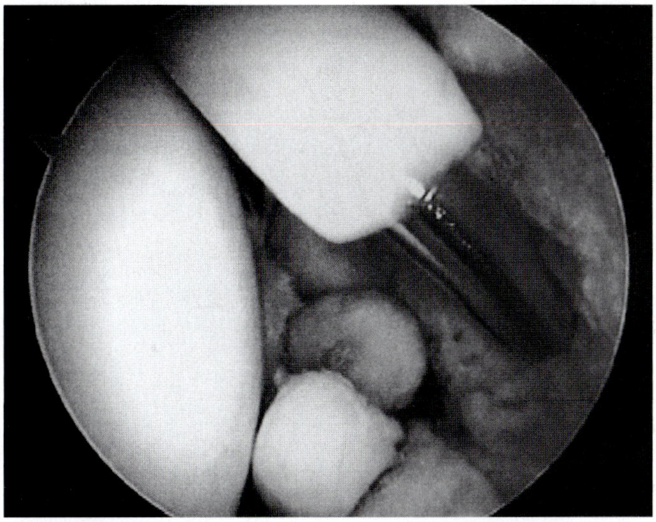

Figure 7–28 Arthroscopic view of a patient with synovial chondromatosis reveals numerous intra-articular loose bodies.

Labral Tears

- Labral tears represent a significant source of mechanical hip pain (Fig. 7–29). Tears may be degenerative or traumatic. Even in the presence of a clear history of trauma, some predisposition to tearing must be suspected, because of either the morphology of the labrum or underlying degeneration.
- There is a particularly high incidence of labral anomalies and tearing in the presence of acetabular dysplasia.
- High-resolution MRI and gadolinium-enhanced MRI are steadily improving the recognition of this entity.
- Arthroscopic débridement of labral tears can have very gratifying results. However, the response is sometimes modulated by accompanying degenerative disease or uncertain circumstances.

Chondral Injuries

- Chondral injuries exist on a spectrum ranging from acute isolated fragments to diffuse degenerative disease (Fig. 7–30).
- Current MRI technology occasionally reveals articular surface defects but in general is poor at discerning the extent of articular involvement.
- Fragments from acute trauma are increasingly recognized as a cause of recalcitrant mechanical hip pain and respond well to excision.
- The long-term prognosis of these lesions is still of concern. Microfracture of the subchondral bone may be effective for focal lesions.

Ruptured Ligamentum Teres

- Rupture uniformly accompanies dislocation of the hip. However, rupture can also occur as a consequence of a twisting injury or subluxation episode in the absence of dislocation (Fig. 7–31). The ruptured portion can catch within the joint and be a significant source of mechanical hip pain.
- MRI may suggest involvement of the ligamentum teres but is rarely conclusive.
- Arthroscopic débridement of the ruptured portion can result in pronounced symptomatic improvement. The vessel of the ligamentum teres may contribute to vascularity of the femoral head. However, it is unlikely that débridement of the ruptured portion would have an adverse effect on the head's viability.

Femoroacetabular Impingement

- The history of an athlete with femoroacetabular impingement (FAI) usually involves a groin ache or pain that is worse with flexion activities, with accompanying stiffness or tightness.
- Physical examination often demonstrates limited hip flexion; limitations of passive ROM are greater with internal rotation than with external rotation. The anterior impingement test result is positive with demonstration of pain upon passive hip flexion, adduction, and internal rotation.

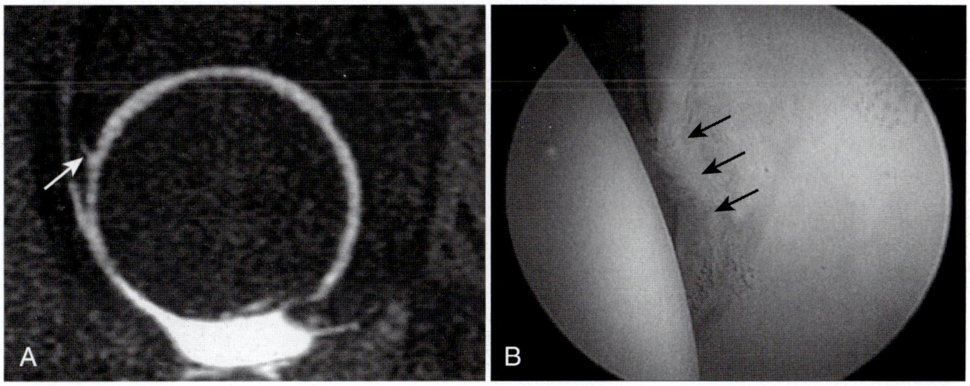

Figure 7–29 A 27-year-old woman with pain and catching of the left hip. **A**, Sagittal magnetic resonance image with gadolinium arthrography reveals a tear of the anterior labrum (*arrow*). **B**, Arthroscopic view illustrates the tear of the anterior labrum at the articular labral junction (*arrows*).

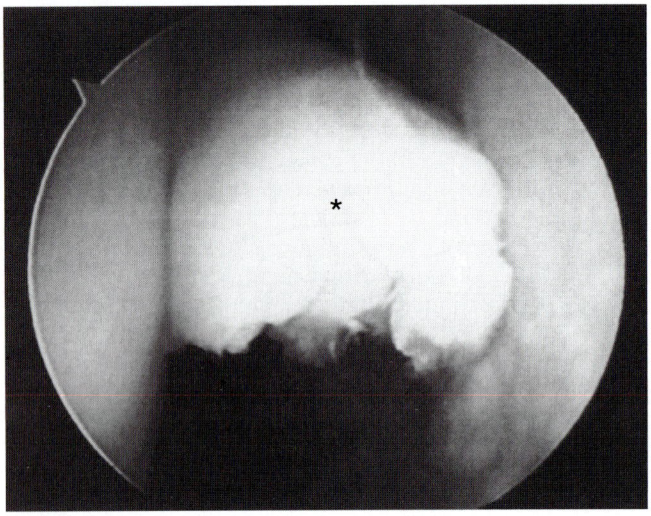

Figure 7–30 Arthroscopic view of a 20-year-old college basketball player with persistent mechanical hip pain following an acute injury. A grade IV unstable articular fragment (*) is identified.

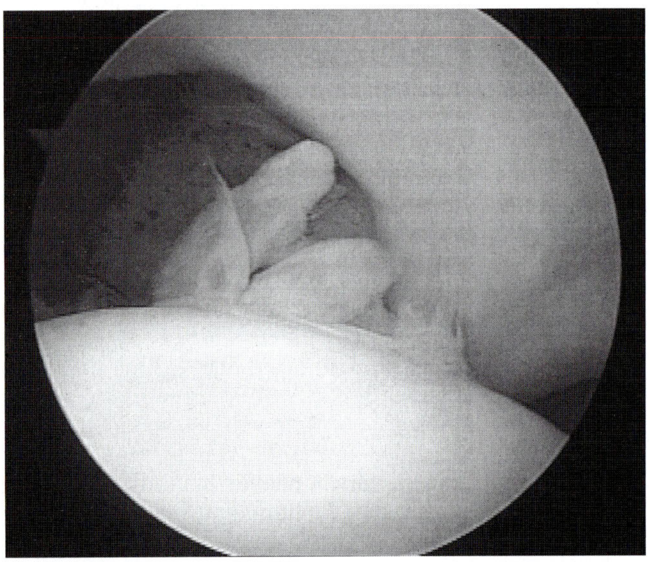

Figure 7–31 A 19-year-old woman sustained a dashboard injury to her right hip. There was no history of dislocation. Arthroscopy reveals a complete rupture of the ligamentum teres. *(From Byrd JWT: Indications and contraindications. In Byrd JWT [ed]: Operative Hip Arthroscopy. New York, Thieme, 1998, pp 7-24.)*

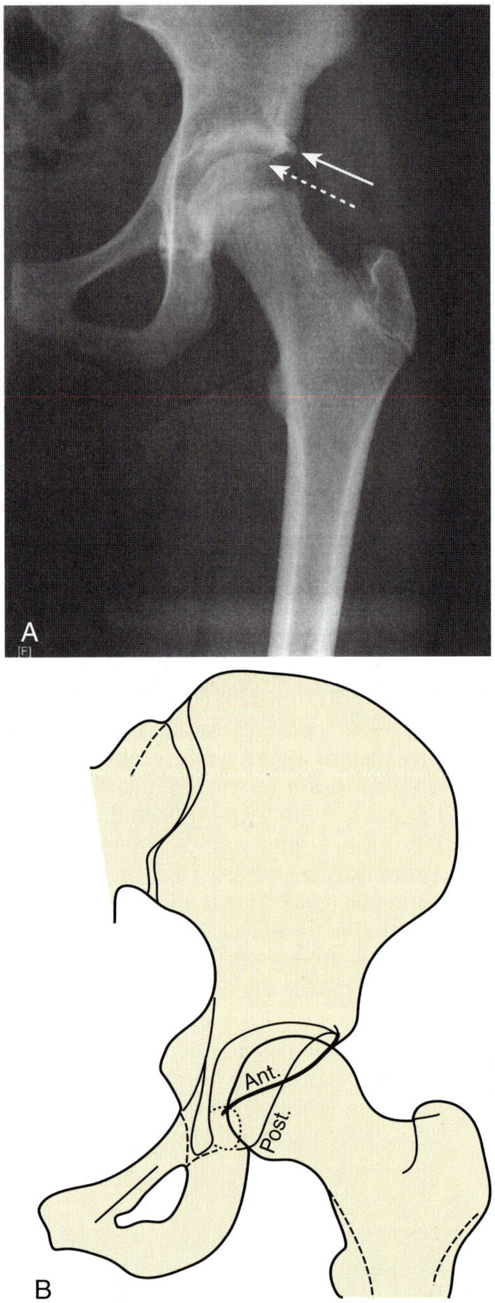

Figure 7–32 A, Anteroposterior radiograph of the hip with pincer impingement (*solid arrow*) showing the crossover sign (*dotted arrow*). The other signs of pincer impingement present are ossification of the labrum and coxa profunda. B, The crossover sign described by Reynolds and colleagues was that the anterior wall of the acetabulum (Ant.) is more lateral to the posterior wall (Post.) on an anteroposterior hip radiograph. This is an indication of global or local acetabular retroversion. *(From Sink EL, Gralla J, Ryba A, Dayton M: Clinical presentation of femoracetabular impingement in adolescents. J Pediatr Orthop 2008; 28(8):806-11.)*

- Imaging
  - Imaging modalities usually start with AP and lateral radiographs of the symptomatic hip to check for femoroacetabular joint space and asymmetry. Notable radiographic features include the acetabular cross-over sign, demonstrated on the AP view, which shows the anterior acetabular wall crossing over the posterior wall superiorly (Fig. 7–32). The posterior wall sign, also demonstrated on the AP view, consists of the femoral head appearing lateral or medial to the posterior wall.
  - MRI and MR angiography (MRA) are useful for diagnosing labral lesions as well as loose bodies, chondral damage, and foveal abnormalities.
  - CT can show asphericity and offset balance of the femoroacetabular articulation as well as herniation pits.

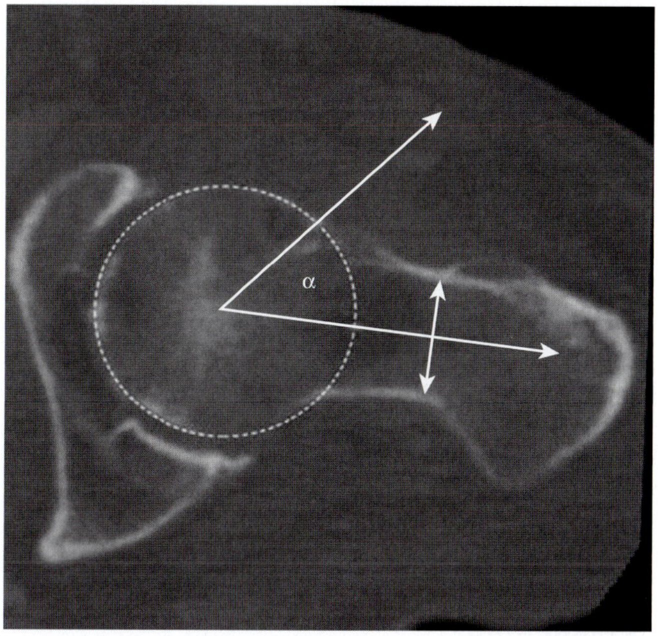

Figure 7–33 Measurement of the angle a on a paraxial reformation computed tomography scan in a patient with herniation pits (HP). The α angle was used to measure the degree of femoral head sphericity. It is defined as follows: a *dotted circle* is drawn overlying the femoral head. Two lines are drawn, one from the center of the femoral head through the center of the femoral neck (*two-headed arrow*) and a second line from the center of the femoral head to the place where the head-and-neck bone becomes outside the circle. The angle of these two lines is the α angle. *(From Panzer S, Augat P, Esch U: CT assessment of herniation pits: Prevalence, characteristics, and potential association with morphological predictors of femoracetabular impingement. Eur Radiol 2008;18:1869-1875.)*

- Oblique coronal scanning can be utilized to measure the α angle—the angle between a line along the neck shaft axis and a line bisecting from the center of the head to the point of femoral head asphericity (Fig. 7–33).
- An α angle greater than 55 degrees is significant for cam-type FAI (see later). Three-dimensional reconstructions also help in diagnosis.

❑ Types
- Cam type: The pathoanatomy is femur-based and involves asphericity of the femoral head or insufficient offset at the head-neck junction. It results in continuous loading of the anterior acetabular cartilage and labrum, with the greatest stress at the acetabular rim (Fig. 7–34).
- Pincer type: The pathoanatomy is acetabulum-based, with a deep or retroverted socket. It produces high stress and causes extensive direct damage by the femoral neck to the overhanging anterior and anterolateral labrum. There is a large zone of labral crush injury and indirect damage to the adjacent cartilage (see Fig. 7–34).

❑ Treatment
- For recalcitrant cases, surgical goals aim at resecting impinging tissue, débriding damaged cartilage and labral tissue, and, possibly, repairing the labrum.
- Open surgery involves surgical dislocation and arthrotomy with possible osteotomies.
  - Advantages include easy access to all structures and the ability to intraoperatively test and accurately measure dynamic ROM.
  - Disadvantages are that the surgical procedure is highly invasive and carries a risk of AVN from 0% to 18%.
- Arthroscopic management is less invasive and offers the ability to repair labral tears. The disadvantages are that hip arthroscopy is technically challenging and that it is difficult to perform dynamic assessment secondary to the applied traction.
- Postoperative management usually includes protected weight-bearing for 4 to 6 weeks. This restriction is secondary to the higher risk for femoral neck fractures. Patients can return to high-impact activities at 12 weeks.

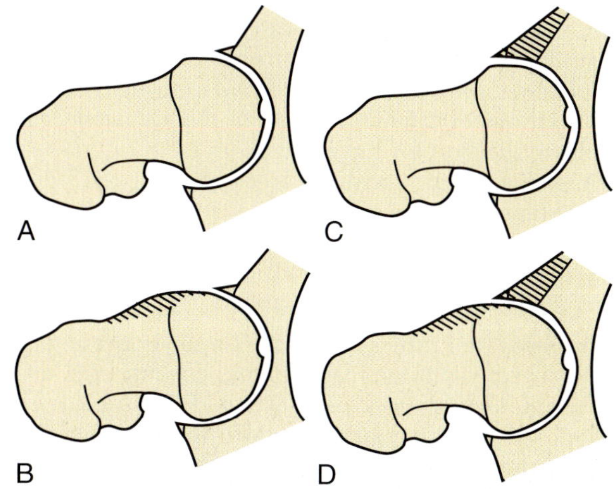

Figure 7–34 Femoroacetabular disease patterns. The reduced clearance during joint motion leads to repetitive abutment between the proximal part of the femur and the anterior acetabular rim. **A,** The normal clearance of the hip. **B,** Reduced femoral head and neck offset (cam impingement). **C,** Excessive overcoverage of the femoral head by the acetabulum (pincer impingement). **D,** A combination of reduced head and neck offset and excessive anterior overcoverage (combined impingement). *(From Clohisy JC, Beaulé PE, O'Malley A, et al: AOA Symposium: Hip Disease in the Young Adult: Current concepts of etiology and surgical treatment. J Bone Joint Surg Am 2008;90A:2267-2281.)*

Arthroscopy Questions

1. A 45-year-old executive is concerned that he has scrotal numbness after hip arthroscopy for removal of loose bodies. What is the most likely cause of this complication?

A. Pudendal nerve injury.
B. Direct inguinal hernia.
C. Adductor compartment syndrome.
D. Analgesic-induced prostatitis.
E. Acute lumbar disc herniation.

2. A 55-year-old triathlete has catching and popping in his left hip that is keeping him from running comfortably. Examination reveals painful ROM with mechanical sensations of catching. Which of the following is the best indication for hip arthroscopy?
   A. Management of osteonecrosis.
   B. Management of intra-articular loose bodies.
   C. Treatment of moderate osteoarthritis.
   D. Treatment of osteochondritis dissecans.
   E. Treatment of crystalline arthropathy.
3. A 24-year-old professional squash player presents with persistent right inguinal pain and clicking after an episode of lunging for a backhand shot. A plain radiograph is unremarkable. MRI reveals a labral tear. A 3-month course of rest, stretching, and NSAIDs has failed to help the problem. Which is the most appropriate treatment plan?
   A. Hip arthroscopy and débridement.
   B. Arthrotomy and repair.
   C. Right inguinal herniorrhaphy.
   D. Electromyography.
   E. CT-guided needle biopsy.
4. During decompression of the peripheral compartment for arthroscopic treatment of hip FAI, what artery is most likely to be injured?
   A. Artery of ligamentum teres.
   B. Ascending branch of the lateral circumflex femoral artery.
   C. Retinacular arteries, superior-anterior/posterior-inferior.
   D. Terminal branches of the medullary artery from the shaft of the femur.
5. What two structures are at risk with use of the anterior arthroscopic portal?
   A. Lateral femoral cutaneous nerve and femoral vessels.
   B. Superior gluteal nerve and lateral femoral cutaneous nerve.
   C. Lateral femoral circumflex artery and superior gluteal nerve.
   D. Sciatic nerve and superior gluteal nerve.
6. What two structures are at risk with use of the anterolateral arthroscopic portal?
   A. Lateral femoral cutaneous nerve and femoral vessels.
   B. Superior gluteal nerve and lateral femoral cutaneous nerve.
   C. Lateral femoral circumflex artery and superior gluteal nerve.
   D. Sciatic nerve and superior gluteal nerve.
7. What two structures are at risk with use of the posterolateral arthroscopic portal?
   A. Lateral femoral cutaneous nerve and femoral vessels.
   B. Superior gluteal nerve and lateral femoral cutaneous nerve.
   C. Lateral femoral circumflex artery and superior gluteal nerve.
   D. Sciatic nerve and superior gluteal nerve.
8. In FAI, what is the usual location of the corresponding labral injury?
   A. Anteroinferior.
   B. Anterosuperior.
   C. Posteroinferior.
   D. Posterosuperior.
9. *True or false:* Noncontrast MRI has been shown to be 94% effective in identifying the acetabular labrum and articular cartilage.
10. What is the typical position of the hip to exacerbate FAI?
11. *True or false:* The abnormalities with cam-type femoroacetabular impingement are restricted to the osseous protuberance of the femoral neck.

References and Resources

INTRODUCTION

Agur, A.M.R., 1999. Grant's Atlas of Anatomy, tenth ed. Williams & Wilkins, Baltimore.

Byrd, J.W.T., 1998. Gross Anatomy. In: Byrd, J.W.T. (Ed.), Operative Hip Arthroscopy. Thieme, New York, pp. 69–82.

Henry, A.K., 1973. Extensile Exposure, second ed. Churchill Livingstone, New York.

Hoppenfeld, S., deBoer, P. (Eds.), 1994. Surgical Exposures in Orthopaedics: The Anatomic Approach, second ed. JB Lippincott, Philadelphia.

BURSITIS

Gross, M.L., Nasser, S., Finerman, G.A.M., 1994. Hip and Pelvis. In: DeLee, J.C., Drez Jr., D. (Eds.), Orthopaedic Sports Medicine. WB Saunders, Philadelphia, pp. 1063–1085.

CONTUSIONS

Crisco, J.J., Jokl, P., Heinen, G.T., et al., 1994. A muscle contusion injury model, biomechanics, physiology, and histology. Am. J. Sports Med. 22, 702–710.

Jackson, D.R., Feagin, J.A., 1973. Quadriceps contusions in young athletes. J. Bone Joint Surg. Am. 55, 95–105.

Rooser, B., Bengston, S., Hagglund, G., 1991. Acute compartment syndrome from anterior thigh muscle contusion: A report of eight cases. J. Orthop. Trauma 5, 57–59.

Ryan, J.B., Wheeler, J.H., Hopkinson, W.J., et al., 1991. Quadriceps contusions: West Point Update. Am. J. Sports Med. 19, 229–304.

Winternitz, W.A., Metheny, J.A., Wear, L.C., 1992. Acute compartment syndrome of the thigh in sports-related injuries not associated with femoral fractures. Am. J. Sports Med. 20, 476–478.

MUSCLE STRAINS

Akermark, C., Johansson, C., 1992. Tenotomy of the adductor longus tendon in the treatment of chronic groin pain in athletes. Am. J. Sports Med. 20, 640–643.

Best, T.M., 1995. Muscle-tendon injuries in young athletes. Clin. Sports Med. 14, 669–686.

Brunet, M.E., Hontas, R.B., 1994. The thigh. In: DeLee, J.C., Drez Jr., D. (Eds.), Orthopaedic Sports Medicine. WB Saunders, Philadelphia, pp. 1086–1112.

Chakravarthy, J., Ramisetty, N., Pimpalnerkar, A., et al., 2005. Surgical repair of complete proximal hamstring tendon ruptures in water skiers and bull riders: a report of four cases and review of the literature. Br. J. Sports Med. 39, 569–572.

Gross, R.H., 1994. Acute musculotendinous injuries. In: Stanitski, C.L., DeLee, J.C., Drez Jr., D. (Eds.), Pediatric and Adult Sports Medicine. WB Saunders, Philadelphia, pp. 131–143.

Hughes, C., Hasselman, C.T., Best, T.M., et al., 1995. Incomplete, intrasubstance strain injuries of the rectus femoris muscle. Am. J. Sports Med. 23, 500–506.

Merrifield, H., Cowan, R.F.J., 1973. Groin strain injuries in ice hockey. J. Sports Med. 1, 41–42.

Noonan, T.J., Garrett Jr., W.E., 1992. Injuries at the myotendinous junction. Clin. Sports Med. 11, 783–806.

Renstrom, P.A., 1992. Tendon and muscle injuries in the groin area. Clin. Sports Med. 11, 815–832.

Sallay, P.I., Friedman, R.L., Coogan, P.G., Garrett, W.E., 1996. Hamstring muscle injuries among water skiers: Functional outcome and prevention. Am. J. Sports Med. 24, 130–136.

SYNDROMES

Allen, W.C., Cope, R., 1995. Coxa saltans: The snapping hip revisited. J. Am. Acad. Orthop. Surg. 3, 303–308.

Benson, E.R., Schutzer, S.F., 1999. Posttraumatic piriformis syndrome: Diagnosis and results of operative treatment. J. Bone Joint Surg. Am. 81, 941–949.

Brignall, C.G., Stainsby, G.D., 1991. The snapping hip: Treatment by Z-plasty. J. Bone Joint Surg. Br. 73, 253–254.

Jacobson, T., Allen, W.C., 1980. Surgical correction of the snapping iliopsoas tendon. Am. J. Sports Med. 18, 470–474.

Meyers, W.C., Foley, D.P., Garrett, W.E., et al., 2000. Management of severe lower abdominal or inguinal pain in high performance athletes. Am. J. Sports Med. 18, 2–8.

Pariziale, J.R., Hudgins, T.H., Fishman, L.M., 1997. The piriformis syndrome. Am. J. Orthop. 26, 316–318.

Taylor, D.C., Meyers, W.C., Moylan, J.A., et al., 1991. Abdominal musculature abnormalities as a cause of groin pain in athletes. Inguinal hernias and pubalgia. Am. J. Sports Med. 19, 239–242.

Zoltan, D.J., Clancy Jr., W.G., Keene, J.S., 1986. A new operative approach to snapping hip and refractory trochanteric bursitis in athletes. Am. J. Sports Med. 14, 201–204.

HERNIAS

Gilmore, J., 1998. Groin pain in the soccer athlete: Fact, fiction, and treatment. Clin. Sports Med. 17, 787–793.

Jenkins, D.B., 1998. The abdomen and pelvis. In: Jenkins, D.B. (Ed.), Hollinshead's Functional Anatomy of the Limbs and Back, seventh ed. WB Saunders, Philadelphia, pp. 389–402.

Lacroix, V.J., 2000. A complete approach to groin pain. Phys. Sports Med. 28, 66–86.

FRACTURES

Boden, B.P., Speer, K.P., 1997. Femoral stress fractures. Clin. Sports Med. 16, 307–317.

Canale, S.T., Beaty, J.H., 1996. Pelvic and hip fractures. In: Rockwood Jr., C.A., Wilkins, K.E., Beaty, J.H. (Eds.), Fractures in Children, fourth ed. Lippincott-Raven, Philadelphia, pp. 1109–1193.

Cooper, D.E., Warren, R.F., Barnes, R., 1991. Traumatic subluxation of the hip resulting in aseptic necrosis and chondrolysis in a professional football player. Am. J. Sports Med. 19, 232–234.

DeLee, J.C., 1996. Fractures and dislocations of the hip. In: Rockwood, C.A., Green, D.P., Bucholz, R.W., Heckman, J.D. (Eds.), Rockwood and Green's Fractures in Adults, fourth ed. Lippincott-Raven, Philadelphia, pp. 1659–1825.

Fullerton Jr., L.R., Snowdy, H.A., 1988. Femoral neck stress fractures. Am. J. Sports Med. 16, 365–377.

Holt, M.A., Keene, J.S., Graf, B.K., Helwig, D.C., 1995. Treatment of osteitis pubis in athletes: Results of corticosteroid injections. Am. J. Sports Med. 23, 601–606.

Johnson, A.W., Weiss Jr., C.B., Wheeler, D.L., 1994. Stress fractures of the femoral shaft in athletes—more common than expected: A new clinical test. Am. J. Sports Med. 22, 248–256.

Mont, M.A., Hungerford, D.S., 1995. Non-traumatic avascular necrosis of the femoral head. J. Bone Joint Surg. Am. 7, 459–474.

Paletta Jr., G.A., Andrish, J.T., 1995. Injuries about the hip and pelvis in the young athlete. Clin. Sports Med. 14, 591–628.

Tornetta, P., Mostafavi, H.R., 1997. Hip dislocation. J. Am. Acad. Orthop. Surg. 5, 27–36.

NERVE ENTRAPMENT

Bradshaw, C., McCrory, P., Bell, S., et al., 1997. Obturator nerve entrapment: A cause of groin pain in athletes. Am. J. Sports Med. 25, 402–408.

Byrd, J.W.T., 1998. Complications associated with hip arthroscopy. In: Byrd, J.W.T. (Ed.), Operative Hip Arthroscopy. Thieme, New York, pp. 171–176.

Hofmann, A., Jones, R., Schoenvogel, R., 1982. Pudendal nerve neuropraxia as a result of traction on the fracture table. J. Bone Joint Surg. Am. 64, 136–138.

McCrory, P., Bell, S., 1999. Nerve entrapment syndromes as a cause of pain in the hip, groin and buttock. Sports Med. 27, 261–274.

Puranen, J., Orava, S., 1988. The hamstring syndrome: A new diagnosis of gluteal sciatic pain. Am. J. Sports Med. 16, 517–521.

Weiss, B.D., 1994. Clinical syndromes associated with bicycle seats. Clin. Sports Med. 13, 175–186.

ARTHROSCOPY

Byrd, J.W.T., 1996. Hip arthroscopy for post-traumatic loose fragments in the young active adult: Three case reports. Clin. Sports Med. 6, 129–134.

Byrd, J.W.T., 1996. Hip arthroscopy: Principles and application. Smith & Nephew Endoscopy, Andover, MA.

Byrd, J.W.T., 1996. Labral lesions: An elusive source of hip pain: Case reports and review of the literature. Arthroscopy 2, 603–612.

Byrd, J.W.T., 1997. Low velocity lateral impact injury to the hip: A source of occult hip pathology. J. South Orthop. Assoc. 6, 151.

Byrd, J.W.T. (Ed.), 1998. Operative Hip Arthroscopy. Thieme, New York.

Byrd, J.W.T., 2000. Avoiding the labrum in hip arthroscopy. Arthroscopy 16, 770–773.

Byrd, J.W.T., 2001. Arthroscopy of the hip and applications: Supine position. In: Chow, J.C. (Ed.), Advanced arthroscopy. Springer-Verlag, New York, pp. 293–321.

Byrd, J.W.T., Jones, K.S., 2000. Prospective analysis of hip arthroscopy. Arthroscopy 16, 578–587.

Byrd, J.W.T., Pappas, J.N., Pedley, M.J., 1995. Hip arthroscopy: An anatomic study of portal placement and relationship to the extra-articular structures. Arthroscopy 11, 418–423.

Clohisy, J.C., Beaulé, P.E., O'Malley, A., et al., 2008. AOA Symposium: Hip Disease in the Young Adult: Current concepts of etiology and surgical treatment. J. Bone Joint Surg. Am. 90, 2267–2281.

Czerny, C., Hofmann, S., Neuhold, A., et al., 1996. Lesions of the acetabular labrum: Accuracy of MR imaging and MR arthrography in detection and staging. Radiology 200, 225–230.

Danzig, L.A., Gershuni, D.H., Resnick, D., 1982. Diagnosis and treatment of diffuse pigmented villonodular synovitis of the hip. Clin. Orthop. 168, 42–77.

Dorr, L.D., 1991. Arthritis and athletics. Clin. Sports Med. 10, 343–357.

Epstein, H.C., 1961. Posterior fracture-dislocations of the hip: Comparison of open and closed methods of treatment of certain types. J. Bone Joint Surg. Am. 43, 1079–1098.

Epstein, H.C., 1973. Traumatic dislocations of the hip. Clin. Orthop. 92, 116–142.

Epstein, H.C., 1974. Posterior fracture-dislocations of the hip: Long-term follow up. J. Bone Joint Surg. Am. 56-A, 1103–1127.

Epstein, H.C., Wiss, D.A., Cozen, L., 1985. Posterior fracture dislocation of the hip with fractures of the femoral head. Clin. Orthop. 20, 9–17.

Farjo, L.A., Glick, J.M., Sampson, T.G., 1999. Hip arthroscopy for acetabular labrum tears. Arthroscopy 15, 132–137.

Ganz, R., Gill, T.J., Gautier, E., et al., 2001. Surgical dislocation of the adult hip: A technique with full access to the femoral head and acetabulum without the risk of avascular necrosis. J. Bone Joint Surg. Br. 83, 1119–1124.

Glick, J.M., Sampson, T.G., 1995. Hip arthroscopy by the lateral approach. In: McGinty, J., Caspari, R., Jackson, R., Poehling, G. (Eds.), Operative Arthroscopy, second ed. Raven Press, New York, pp. 1079–1090.

Gray, A.J.R., Villar, R.N., 1997. The ligamentum teres of the hip: An arthroscopic classification of it pathology. Arthroscopy 13, 575–578.

Klapper, R.C., Dorfman, H., Boyer, T., 1998. Hip arthroscopy without traction. In: Byrd, J.W.T. (Ed.), Operative Hip Arthroscopy. Thieme, New York, pp. 139–152.

Lavigne, M., Parvizi, J., Beck, M., et al., 2004. Anterior femoroacetabular impingement. Part I: Techniques of joint preserving surgery. Clin. Orthop. Relat. Res. 418, 61–66.

McCarthy, J.C., Bono, J.V., Wardell, S., 1997. Is there a treatment for synovial chondromatosis of the hip joint? Arthroscopy 13, 409–410.

O'Leary, J.A., Berend, K., Vail, T.P., 2001. The relationship between diagnosis and outcome in arthroscopy of the hip. Arthroscopy 17, 181–188.

Reynolds, D., Lucas, J., Klaue, K., 1999. Retroversion of the acetabulum: a cause of hip pain. J. Bone Joint Surg. Br. 81-B (2), 281–288.

Sampson, T.G., Farjo, L., 1998. Hip arthroscopy by the lateral approach. In: Byrd, J.W.T (Ed.), Operative Hip Arthroscopy. Thieme, New York, pp. 105–122.

Sampson, T.G., Glick, J.M., 1995. Indications and surgical treatment of hip pathology. In: McGinty, J., Caspari, R., Jackson, R., Poehling, G. (Eds.), Operative Arthroscopy, second ed. Raven Press, New York, pp. 1067–1078.

Sink, E.L., Gralla, J., Ryba, A., Dayton, M., 2008. Clinical presentation of femoracetabular impingement in adolescents. J. Pediatr. Orthop. 28, 806–811.

CHAPTER 8

Ankle and Foot

David A. Joos and Anish R. Kadakia

Anatomy and Biomechanics

Bones and Joints

- Distal Tibia (Fig. 8–1)
  - Plafond:
    - Concave inferior articular surface.
    - Posterior lip forms the "posterior malleolus."
  - Medial malleolus.
  - Incisura fibularis:
    - Articulation of the distal tibiofibular joint.
- Distal Fibula (Fig. 8–1)
  - Lateral malleolus.
- Talus (Fig. 8–2)
  - Head: Articulates with the navicular.
  - Neck.
  - Body/dome: Articulates with the ankle mortise.
    - Wedge-shaped and wider anteriorly.
  - Inferior talus:
    - Anterior, middle, and posterior calcaneal articulations.
  - No tendinous insertions.
- Calcaneus (Fig. 8–3)
  - Anterior, middle, and posterior facets:
    - Form subtalar articulation with talus.
  - Tuberosity:
    - Insertion of Achilles tendon.
- Other Tarsal Bones (Figs. 8-3 and 8-4)
  - Navicular.
  - Cuboid.
  - Medial, middle, and lateral cuneiform.
- Five Metatarsals (Fig. 8–4)
  - Numbered 1 through 5 with great toe metatarsal number 1.
- Toes (see Fig. 8–4)
  - Numbered 1 through 5 with great toe number 1.
  - Great toe has only proximal and distal phalanges.
  - Lesser toes have proximal, middle, and distal phalanges.
- Tibiotalar Joint
  - Ginglymus or hinge joint.
  - Responsible for most sagittal plane motion of the foot and ankle:
    - 23 to 48 degrees of plantarflexion.
    - 10 to 23 degrees of dorsiflexion.
  - The ankle mortise is formed by the tibial plafond, medial malleolus, and lateral malleolus.
    - The mortise articulates with the dome of the talus.
    - The mortise widens and the ankle becomes more stable in dorsiflexion because of the shape of the talar dome.
    - The mortise also contributes to inversion/eversion and rotation.
- Distal Tibiofibular Joint
  - Distal fibula: Convex medial surface.
  - Incisura fibularis: Concave surface of the distal lateral tibia.
  - The fibula rotates (≈2 degrees) within the incisura during ankle motion and ambulation.
  - The mortise widens 1 to 1.5 mm during motion from plantarflexion to dorsiflexion.
- Subtalar Joint
  - Talus articulation with the calcaneus through their three respective facets.
  - Responsible for inversion and eversion motions.
  - Makes small contribution to plantarflexion and dorsiflexion.

Ligaments and Tendons

- Medial Ankle: Deltoid Ligament Complex
  - Deep deltoid ligament:
    - From the apex of the medial malleolus to the medial talar body.
    - Functions primarily to resist lateral talar translation.

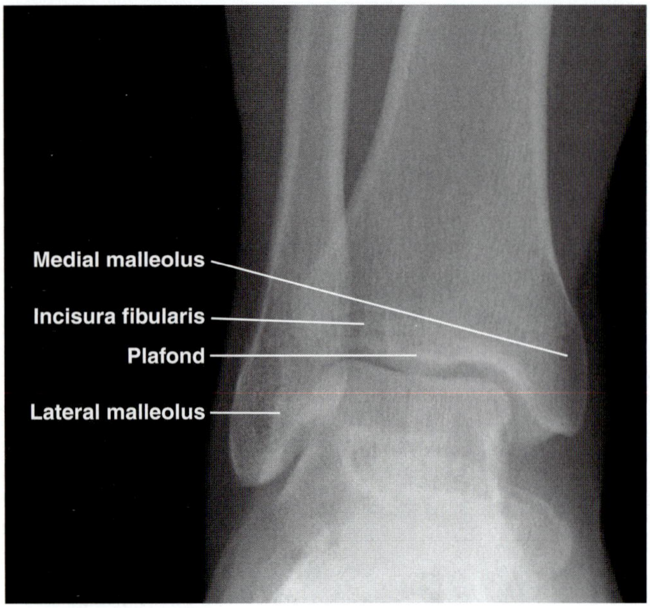

Figure 8–1 Anteroposterior standing radiograph of the ankle. *(From Miller M, Hart J, MacKnight J [eds]: Essential Orthopaedics. Philadelphia, Elsevier Saunders, 2008, p 724.)*

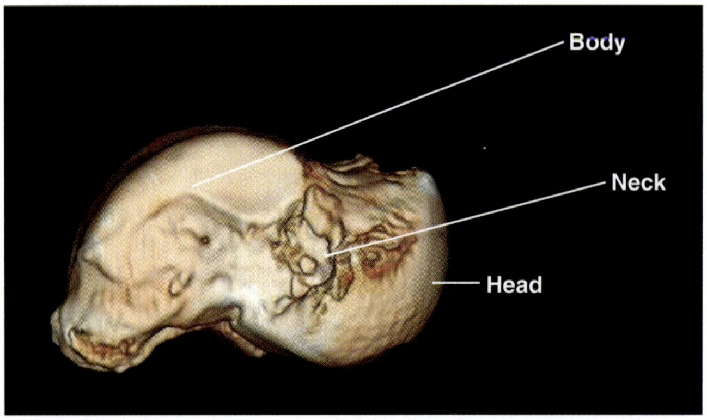

Figure 8–2 Three-dimensional reconstruction of the talus.

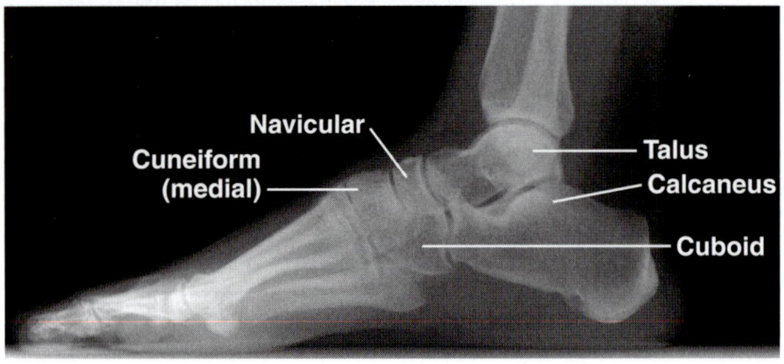

Figure 8–3 Lateral standing radiograph of the foot. *(From Miller M, Hart J, MacKnight J [eds]: Essential Orthopaedics. Philadelphia, Elsevier Saunders, 2008, p 724.)*

- Superficial deltoid ligament:
  - From the distal medial malleolus to the navicular, spring ligament, sustentaculum tali, and medial talus.
  - Functions primarily to resist valgus forces at the ankle.

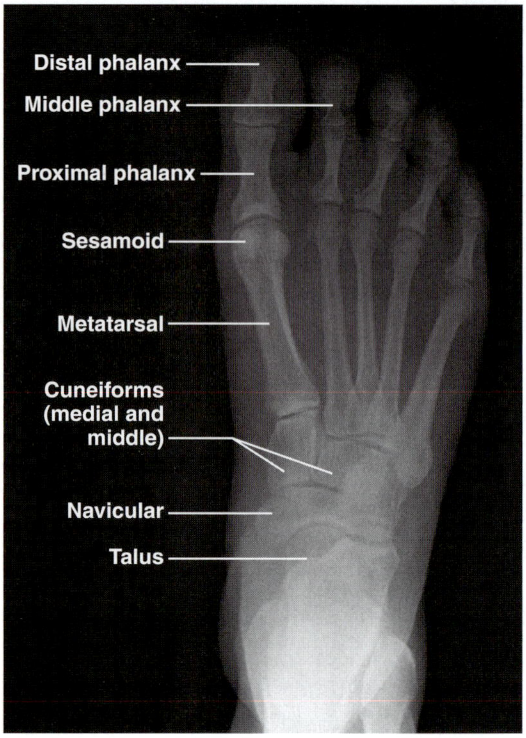

Figure 8–4 Anteroposterior standing radiograph of the foot. *(From Miller M, Hart J, MacKnight J [eds]: Essential Orthopaedics. Philadelphia, Elsevier Saunders, 2008, p 724.)*

- ❑ Lateral Ankle Ligaments
  - Anterior talofibular ligament (ATFL).
  - Calcaneofibular ligament (CFL).
  - Posterior talofibular ligament (PTFL).
- ❑ Syndesmosis Ligaments
  - Anterior inferior tibiofibular ligament (AITFL).
  - Posterior inferior tibiofibular ligament (PITFL).
  - Interosseous tibiofibular ligament.
  - Interosseous membrane.
- ❑ Achilles Tendon (Fig. 8–5)
  - Common tendon of triceps surae (gastrocnemius and soleus), inserting on calcaneal tuberosity.
  - Its primary action is plantarflexion.
  - Fibers rotate 90 degrees from proximal to distal:
    - Gastrocnemius fibers are posterior proximally and insert laterally on the calcaneus.
    - Soleus fibers are anterior proximally and insert medially on the calcaneus.
  - There is a watershed vascular area 2 to 6 cm proximal to the tendon's insertion on calcaneus.
- ❑ Flexor Tendons (Fig. 8–6)
  - Posterior tibialis: Foot inversion and plantarflexion.
  - Flexor hallucis longus: Great toe flexion.
  - Flexor digitorum longus: Lesser toe flexion.
  - Tendons pass posterior to the medial malleolus.

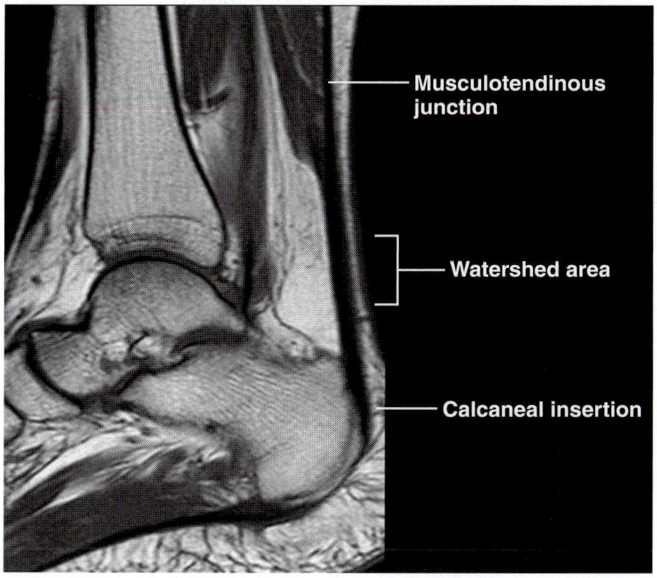

Figure 8–5 Sagittal T1-weighted magnetic resonance image of the ankle. Note the Achilles tendon and its musculotendinous junction, watershed area, and insertion on the calcaneus.

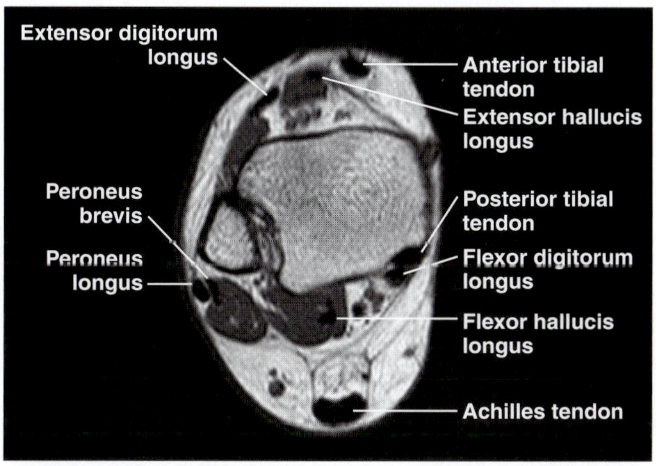

Figure 8–6 Axial T1-weighted magnetic resonance image of the distal leg. The tendons at this level are denoted.

- ❑ Extensor Tendons (see Fig. 8–6)
  - Anterior tibialis: Foot dorsiflexion.
  - Extensor hallucis longus: Great toe extension.
  - Extensor digitorum longus: Lesser toe extension.
  - Tendons pass over the anterior ankle beneath the extensor retinaculum.
- ❑ Peroneal Tendons (see Fig. 8–6)
  - Peroneus longus: Plantarflexion of the first ray.
  - Peroneus brevis: Foot eversion.
  - Tendons pass posterior to the lateral malleolus.

Nerves

- ❑ Tibial Nerve
  - Major division of the sciatic nerve.
  - Part of the posterior neurovascular bundle traveling posterior to the medial malleolus.
  - Divides into medial and lateral plantar branches.
  - Innervates plantar intrinsic foot musculature.
  - Provides plantar foot and toe sensation.
- ❑ Superficial Peroneal Nerve
  - Branch of the common peroneal nerve.
  - Travels subcutaneously from the lateral distal leg to the dorsal foot.
  - Provides dorsal foot sensation.
- ❑ Deep Peroneal Nerve
  - Branch of the common peroneal nerve.
  - Part of the anterior neurovascular bundle traveling directly anterior to the ankle.
  - Innervates dorsal intrinsic foot musculature.
  - Provides sensation to the first web space.
- ❑ Sural Nerve
  - Formed by branches of the tibial and common peroneal nerves.
  - Travels subcutaneously with the small saphenous vein from the posterior leg to the lateral foot.
  - Provides lateral foot sensation.
- ❑ Saphenous Nerve
  - Terminal branch of the femoral nerve.
  - Travels subcutaneously with the great saphenous vein over the anterior aspect of the medial malleolus.
  - Provides medial ankle and foot sensation.

Vessels

- ❑ Anterior Tibial Artery
  - Branch of the popliteal artery.
  - Travels with the deep peroneal nerve over the anterior ankle to the dorsum of the foot.
  - Forms an anastomotic connection with the plantar arch through a communicating artery between the first and second metatarsals.
- ❑ Posterior Tibial Artery
  - Branch of the popliteal artery.
  - Travels with the tibial nerve posterior to the medial malleolus.
  - Forms the plantar arch.

Anatomy and Biomechanics Questions

1. Dysfunction and weakness of the peroneus brevis will lead to loss of:
   A. Inversion.
   B. Eversion.
   C. Dorsiflexion.
   D. Plantarflexion.

2. The syndesmosis is composed of the articulation between the:
   A. Tibia and talus.
   B. Talus and calcaneus.
   C. Fibula and talus.
   D. Tibia and fibula.
3. The five superficial nerves of the foot and ankle are:
   A. Anterior tibial, deep peroneal, superficial peroneal, sural, lateral plantar.
   B. Posterior tibial, anterior tibial, sural, deep peroneal, saphenous.
   C. Tibial, superficial peroneal, deep peroneal, saphenous, sural.
   D. Tibial, lateral plantar, superficial peroneal, sural, deep peroneal.

History, Physical Examination, and Imaging

History

- Elicit history of trauma and mechanism for acute injuries.
- Pain is a common complaint:
  - Determine the location, character, timing, chronicity, and aggravating factors.
- Other complaints include deformity, instability, neurologic symptoms, popping, snapping, and swelling.
- Ask about previous symptoms, injuries, operations, therapies, and treatments.
- Associated medical conditions, including diabetes mellitus, inflammatory arthritis, and neurologic conditions, are also important.
- Obtain social history, especially of tobacco use, employment, activities, and pending litigation or worker's compensation claims.

General Physical Examination

- The lower extremities should be visible from the foot to knee.
  - Always evaluate both limbs for comparison.
- Begin with visual inspection of the patient in the standing position and evaluation of gait, if possible. Alter as necessary for acute injuries.
  - Inspection of shoe wear may also be helpful for chronic complaints.
  - Identify specific areas of swelling, ecchymosis, and other skin changes.
- Evaluate for hair loss, edema, venous stasis changes, ulcerations, and calluses.
- A seated inspection of the plantar skin surface should be included.
  - Plantar ecchymosis should raise the suspicion of a Lisfranc injury.
- Palpate each bone, joint, ligament, and tendon to localize tenderness.
- Evaluate active and passive range of motion of the ankle and subtalar joints. Note any associated pain with joint motion.
- Neurovascular examination should include evaluation of light touch for all nerves of the foot, with examination of dorsal pedis and posterior tibial pulses.
- A focused physical examination, including specialized and provocative tests to evaluate for specific pathology, may then be performed.

❑ Imaging
- Appropriate imaging should be obtained on the basis of the history and physical findings.
- Plain radiographs are the most common initial imaging:
  - When evaluating the ankle, always obtain anteroposterior (AP), lateral, and mortise views.
  - When evaluating the foot, always obtain AP, lateral, and oblique views.
  - Weight-bearing views should also be obtained, except in the evaluation of acute injuries.
- Computed tomography (CT) scan, magnetic resonance imaging (MRI), ultrasound, and nuclear medicine studies may then be obtained as indicated.

History, Physical Examination, and Imaging Questions

1. Increased dorsiflexion of the ankle can be a subtle sign of:
   A. Anterior tibial tendon rupture.
   B. Posterior tibial tendon rupture.
   C. Achilles tendon rupture.
   D. Flexor hallucis longus tendon rupture.
2. The presence of plantar ecchymosis in the setting of an acute injury most likely indicates:
   A. Talus fracture.
   B. Tarsometatarsal fracture-dislocation.
   C. Ankle fracture.
   D. Navicular fracture.
3. Inspection of the patient's shoe wear reveals increased wear of the lateral aspect of the heel. This can be a sign of:
   A. Cavovarus deformity.
   B. Pes planovalgus.
   C. Calcaneovalgus.
   D. Equinovarus.

Ankle Arthroscopy

Indications

- Diagnostic arthroscopy alone is often of limited benefit in ankle injuries because a diagnosis is usually established from findings of the history, physical examination, and radiography.

- Other indications for arthroscopy are:
  - Débridement of synovitis.
  - Osteochondral lesions.
  - Loose body.
  - Anterior ankle impingement.
  - Arthroscopic ankle arthrodesis.
- Arthroscopy may be performed with the use of general or spinal anesthesia.

Positioning

- The patient is positioned supine with a bolster under the ipsilateral pelvis to achieve neutral foot rotation.
- The hip on the operative side must be flexed with the use of a beanbag or thigh holder.
- A noninvasive ankle distractor should be applied.

Equipment

- A 2.7-mm, 30-degree arthroscope is suitable for almost all ankle arthroscopy needs.
- Probe.
- Small joint grasper and biter.
- Motorized shaver: 3.5-mm full-radius shaver.
- Motorized bur: 4-mm round bur, to facilitate anterior tibial osteophyte removal.
- Microfracture awls.

Portals

❏ Anteromedial Portal
- The first portal made.
- The incision is made at a soft spot at the level of the joint line, 0.5 cm medial to the tibialis anterior tendon.
  - Immediately inferior to the tibial plafond.
  - Variability in anatomy minimizes the utility of using the medial malleolus as a landmark.
- Incise the skin only; then bluntly dissect through the subcutaneous tissues to the joint capsule.
- Introduce the blunt trocar and cannula, then the arthroscope after removing the trocar.

❏ Anterolateral Portal
- Made after the arthroscope has been introduced into the anteromedial portal.
- Soft spot at level of joint line, just lateral to peroneus tertius tendon.
- A spinal needle may be used to access the joint under visualization through the arthroscope.
- The superficial peroneal nerve is at risk of damage.
  - Use careful bluntly dissection through the subcutaneous tissues.
  - The nerve can be palpated preoperatively in some patients and marked to avoid injury.
- This is most commonly used working portal, but the portals may be switched for easier access if necessary.

❏ Posterior Portal
- Posterior portals are not routinely used but may be necessary in certain situations:
  - Posterior osteochondral lesions.
  - Posterior impingement.
  - Loose body.

Diagnostic Arthroscopy

- Anterior tibia, osteophytes, synovitis, loose bodies, and scar tissue may be visualized in the anterior ankle.
- Tibiotalar articulation is evaluated with careful introduction of the arthroscope over the dome of the talus.
- Medial and lateral gutters are also visualized and inspected:
  - Evidence of chondral damage or syndesmotic injury may be present in the gutters.

Complications

- Complications of arthroscopy include neurologic injury, neuroma formation, chondral damage, infection, and complex regional pain syndrome.
- Reported rates range from 3.4% to 17%.
- Most commonly reported complication is nerve injury, with the superficial peroneal nerve being the most commonly injured.
  - Lower rates are reported when arthroscopy is performed without mechanical distraction.
- Damage to the deep peroneal nerve and anterior tibial artery has been reported with aggressive anterior débridement.
  - To avoid such damage, the shaver blades should never be directed toward the anterior ankle.

Arthroscopy Questions

1. Use of which portal places the superficial peroneal nerve at risk?
A. Anteromedial.
B. Anterolateral.
C. Posteromedial.
D. Posterolateral.

2. The posteromedial portal is not commonly used because of risk of damage to the:
A. Deep peroneal nerve.
B. Superficial peroneal nerve.
C. Tibial nerve.
D. Saphenous nerve.

3. Use of an anterocentral portal is contraindicated because of the risk of damage to the:
A. Saphenous nerve and vein.
B. Tibial nerve and posterior tibial artery.
C. Superficial peroneal nerve.
D. Deep peroneal nerve and anterior tibial artery.

Acute Sprains

- Ankle sprains are common sports-related injuries; 85% are lateral sprains.
- Undertreatment may lead to weakness, recurrence, pain, or instability.

Evaluation

- Evaluation begins with history and physical examination.
- After a general foot and ankle examination, a focused examination starts with palpation of the ankle musculoskeletal structures:
  - Medial and lateral malleoli.
  - Bones of the hindfoot and midfoot:
    - Lateral process of talus.
    - Anterior process of calcaneus.
    - Tarsometatarsal joints.
  - Base of the fifth metatarsal.
  - Deltoid ligament (distal to tip of medial malleolus).
  - ATFL (distal and anterior to tip of lateral malleolus).
  - CFL (distal to tip of lateral malleolus).
  - Achilles tendon.
  - Peroneal tendons (posterior to lateral malleolus).

Imaging

❑ Radiography
- Patients who present with an acute injury and pain should be assessed with weight-bearing radiographs of the ankle and/or foot.
- Use of the Ottawa ankle rules in clinical practice can lead to missed injuries, because this classification is not 100% sensitive.
- Given the low morbidity of a plain radiograph and the high morbidity of a missed fracture/dislocation, radiographs are recommended for all injuries.

❑ Magnetic Resonance Imaging
- Use of MRI is not required in the initial treatment of a standard lateral ankle sprain.
- Persistent pain, swelling, or mechanical complaints at 6 weeks may be related to an osteochondral injury, and an MRI is indicated at this time if there is clinical concern.

Acute Lateral Sprains

- *Acute lateral sprains* are a result of inversion and internal rotation of the hindfoot relative to the leg. The patient may give a history of "rolling" the ankle.
- The ligaments damaged are the ATFL, CFL, and PTFL:
  - The ATFL is weakest, and is involved in virtually all lateral injuries.
  - The CFL is involved in 50% to 75% of lateral injuries.
  - The PTFL is involved in less than 10% of lateral injuries.

❑ Classification
- Grade I: Partial ATFL injury. Mild swelling and little or no ecchymosis. Point tenderness over the ATFL. No limitation to range of motion. No laxity.
- Grade II: Complete ATFL tear with possible partial CFL injury. Localized swelling and ecchymosis. Diffuse lateral ligament tenderness. Less than 10-degree decrease in range of motion. Mild laxity may be present.
- Grade III: Complete ATFL and CFL tears, with possible PTFL and capsular injury. Diffuse swelling, ecchymosis, and tenderness laterally.
- It can be difficult to distinguish between grade II and grade III injuries in the acute setting.

❑ Management
- Nonsurgical management is the mainstay of treatment for acute lateral ankle injuries.
- Grade I or II injuries are managed with functional bracing (ankle stirrup orthosis or similar brace) and rest, ice, compression, elevation (RICE) therapy, followed by rehabilitation and return to activity.
- Grade III injuries are treated with a period of immobilization and RICE therapy, followed by functional bracing, and, finally, rehabilitation and return to activity.
  - Some controversy exists over the role of casting for immobilization. Many studies have shown no benefit of casting over a cast boot or other types of immobilization. There is conflicting data regarding return to work, return to sport, and pain.
  - Our preferred method of treatment is immobilization for 6 weeks in a removable cast boot, followed by functional bracing and rehabilitation. The use of the boot allows for skin care and adjustment for swelling. To minimize stiffness, patients are encouraged to perform dorsiflexion/plantarflexion range-of-motion exercises once the ankle is comfortable out of the boot.
- Rehabilitation should commence after swelling has resolved and the patient is able to ambulate (in the functional brace) without significant pain. Peroneal strengthening and proprioceptive exercises should be included.
- Reasons for failure of an ankle sprain to improve after appropriate immobilization and rehabilitation include:
  - Missed fracture:
    - Lateral malleolus.
    - Talus.
    - Anterior process of the calcaneus.
    - Base of the fifth metatarsal.
  - Missed subluxation/dislocation:
    - Subtalar.
    - Chopart.
    - Tarsometatarsal.

- Osteochondral lesion of the talus.
- Syndesmotic disruption.
- Subtalar sprain with pain over the sinus tarsi.
- Complex regional pain syndrome.

Syndesmotic Injuries

- Syndesmotic injuries, or "high ankle sprains," are rare but important injuries.
- They are more difficult to diagnose than typical ankle sprains and are often missed.
- Syndesmotic injuries have been reported in 1% to 17% of acute ankle injuries, although complete injuries are rare.
- They are more common in skiers, football players, and athletes participating in "cutting" sports.
- Recovery time from syndesmotic injury was reported to be double that from other ankle sprains in a study of military recruits (Hopkinson et al, 1990).

❑ Mechanisms of Injury
- Proposed mechanisms of injury include foot external rotation, talar eversion, and hyperdorsiflexion.
  - These mechanisms are in contrast to the inversion mechanism of the typical ankle injury.
  - A higher index of suspicion for syndesmotic injury is warranted for ankle injuries with an atypical mechanism.
  - Deltoid ligament injuries are common in the setting of syndesmotic injury.

❑ Physical Examination
- Proper physical examination techniques can be helpful in diagnosing syndesmotic injury.
- Swelling is often absent or mild, especially in comparison with swelling in lateral ankle ligament injuries.
- Tenderness is often present over the anterior inferior tibiofibular ligament (AITFL).
- The *external rotation test* is performed with the patient seated and the affected extremity hanging free:
  - The examiner stabilizes the tibia with one hand and applies external rotation force to the foot with the other.
  - The test is performed with the ankle both in neutral dorsiflexion and in plantarflexion.
  - Pain over the AITFL is suggestive of syndesmotic injury.
  - Pain over the medial ankle is suggestive of deltoid ligament injury.
- The *squeeze test* is performed with the patient in the same position as the external rotation test:
  - The examiner grasps the affected leg at the midcalf.
  - Then the examiner compresses the fibula and tibia by squeezing them together at this level.
  - Pain at the level of the syndesmosis is suggestive of injury.

❑ Imaging
- No consensus exists for the proper radiographic evaluation of suspected syndesmotic injury.
- Plain radiographs are useful to rule out fractures and to evaluate the tibiofibular overlap:
  - Proposed measurements exist for this overlap on AP and mortise views, but there is controversy about their accuracy.
  - Lack of overlap between the tibia and the fibula on the mortise view is highly suggestive of a syndesmotic injury.
- CT is useful to evaluate the position of the fibula within the incisura (Fig. 8–7):
  - The other ankle should be included for comparison.
  - CT is a "nonstress" test and so may miss an injury in which the tibiofibular articulation remains reduced without weight-bearing.
- MRI has been shown to have high sensitivity and specificity for syndesmotic injury.
  - Other pathology, such as lateral ligament injury, deltoid ligament injury, and osteochondral lesion of the talus (OLT), may also be seen on MRI.

❑ Treatment
- Nonoperative treatment is considered only if the tibiofibular articulation remains well-reduced on imaging studies and there is no evidence of a complete syndesmotic disruption:
  - Initial treatment consists of immobilization and restricted weight-bearing for 6 weeks while initial pain and swelling subside.
  - Cast boot treatment is appropriate and allows for skin care and adjustment for swelling.
  - The patient is then allowed to begin partial weight-bearing and light rehabilitation; the patient should have no pain at the syndesmosis.

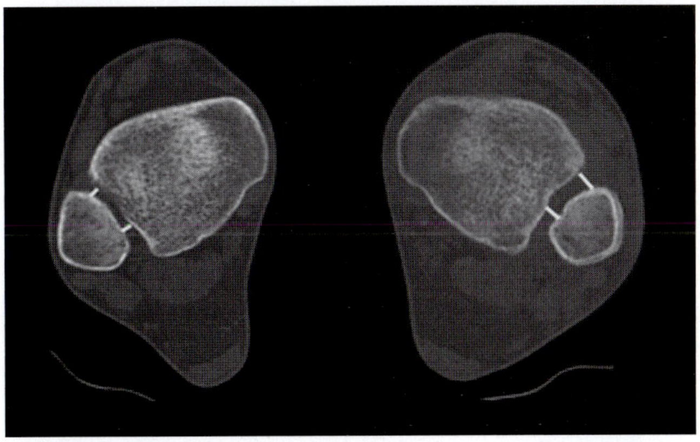

Figure 8–7 Axial computed tomography scan of a patient with a syndesmotic injury. Note the relative increase in the distal tibiofibular space on the left leg (image on the *right*).

- The patient is progressed to full weight-bearing in an ankle stirrup brace and more aggressive rehabilitation when he/she can perform in this manner pain-free.
- Surgical intervention is indicated when there is any evidence of a severe or complete syndesmotic disruption on radiography, CT, or MRI.
  - Reduction of the tibiofibular articulation with screw fixation is the accepted method.
    - The use of suture button fixation for the syndesmosis has shown early promise; however, insufficient evidence exists at this time to recommend its use over screws.
  - Weight-bearing is restricted postoperatively for 6 weeks.
  - The size and number of screws, the number of cortices captured, the period of postoperative weight-bearing restriction, and the need for routine hardware removal remain controversial topics.
  - Our preferred method of treatment is the use of a four-hole plate with two 3.5-mm syndesmotic screws (Fig. 8–8):
    - Prior to syndesmotic screw placement, a large reduction clamp is placed over the widest aspect of the medial and lateral malleolus to reduce the syndesmosis.
    - Postoperatively, the patient is in a non–weight-bearing cast for 6 weeks, followed by weight-bearing in a boot for 6 more weeks.
    - After 3 months, an ankle stirrup orthosis is utilized.
    - Syndesmotic screws are removed 4 to 5 months postoperatively.
    - The use of the plate allows immediate and unrestricted weight-bearing after removal of the screws without risk of fibular fracture.

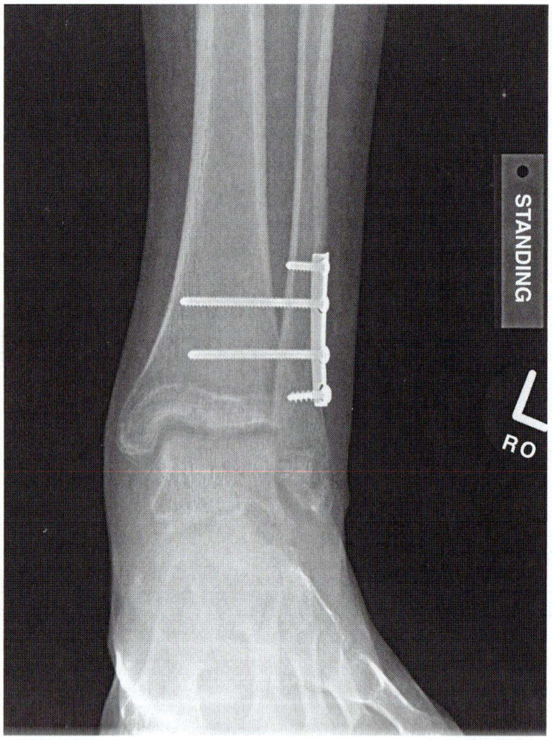

Figure 8–8 Anteroposterior standing radiograph of the ankle demonstrating the use of a four-hole plate with two 3.5-mm syndesmotic screws for the treatment of a syndesmotic disruption.

Acute Sprains Questions

1. A lateral ankle sprain does NOT involve which ligament?
A. Anterior talofibular ligament (ATFL).
B. Calcaneofibular ligament (CFL).
C. Posterior talofibular ligament (PTFL).
D. Anterior inferior tibiofibular ligament (AITFL).

2. A useful clinical test for evaluation for a syndesmotic injury is:
A. Thompson test: Compression of the calf.
B. Squeeze test: Compression of tibia and fibula at the midcalf.
C. Gravity test: Forced internal rotation of the ankle with the foot in neutral.
D. Distraction test: Forced eversion of the hindfoot with the foot in neutral.

3. A complete syndesmotic disruption is most appropriately treated with:
A. Non–weight-bearing cast.
B. Reduction and primary surgical ligamentous repair.
C. Reduction and fixation with two 3.5-mm screws from the fibula to the tibia.
D. Weight-bearing cast.

Ankle Instability

- Chronic ankle instability occurs as a sequela of ankle injury and is often multifactorial.
  - Mechanical factors include varus hindfoot alignment, generalized ligamentous laxity, and attenuation of normal ligaments.
  - Functional factors include muscle weakness, impaired proprioception, and impaired neuromuscular control.
- Repeated episodes of the ankle giving way, repeated ankle sprains, and chronic pain are the presenting symptoms.
  - This condition can be debilitating to athletes in terms of competition but may also significantly affect the activities of daily living in other affected patients.
- A history should include previous injuries, frequency and setting of instability events, location and chronicity of pain, and any prior treatments or therapies.

Physical Examination

- After a general foot and ankle examination, a focused examination should include provocative tests for instability.
- The anterior drawer test is used to evaluate for ankle laxity:
  - Use one hand to stabilize the anterior distal tibia and cup the other around the posterior calcaneus.
  - Translate the heel anteriorly with respect to the tibia, and note any subluxation.
  - Subluxation in neutral dorsiflexion indicates ATFL laxity.
  - Always compare affected and unaffected extremities.
- The inversion test is used to test for CFL laxity:
  - Use one hand to stabilize the distal tibia and the other to grasp the calcaneus.
  - Hold the foot in dorsiflexion, and invert the calcaneus.
  - Always compare affected and unaffected extremities.

Imaging

- Standard plain radiographs are obtained to evaluate for bony injury, evidence of malalignment, and any associated injury, such as an OLT.
- Stress radiographs can be performed to verify the diagnosis (Fig. 8–9).

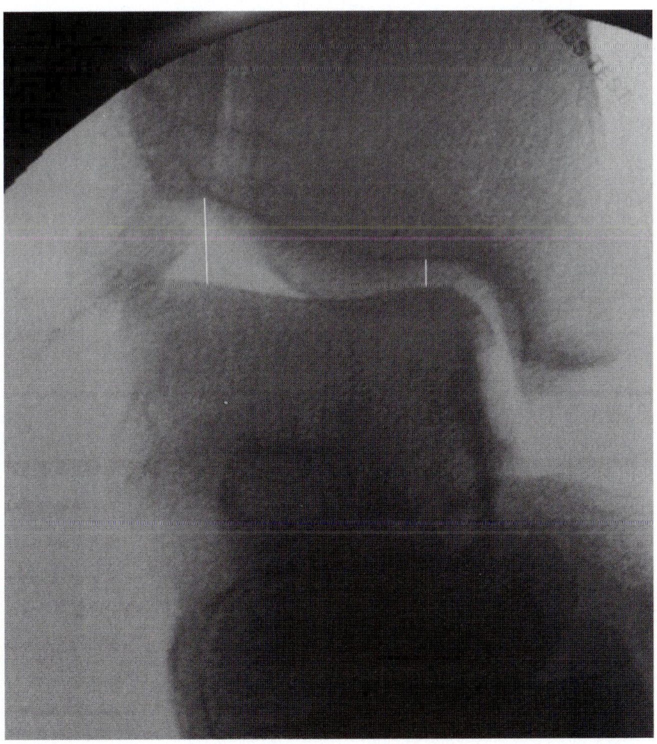

Figure 8–9 Varus stress radiograph of a patient with ankle instability. Note the relative increase in the lateral tibiotalar joint space and the varus tilt of the talus.

Treatment

- Treatment begins with nonsurgical management:
  - Functional bracing should be combined with a focused rehabilitation program.
  - Rehabilitation should include peroneal strengthening and proprioceptive components.

❑ Surgical Treatment

- Operative intervention is considered if nonoperative management fails.
- Presence of ankle pain in addition to instability should prompt the surgeon to consider additional intra-articular pathology:
  - Concomitant ankle arthroscopy is indicated in this setting.
  - Preoperative MRI can be very useful to detect intra-articular pathology for preoperative planning.
- Many techniques for repair and/or reconstruction of the lateral ligaments have been described and investigated.
  - Presence of a varus heel alignment must be assessed prior to surgery.
    - Lateral closing wedge calcaneal osteotomy is required as an adjunctive procedure to prevent failure in this setting.
- Good results have been reported for anatomic repair techniques, such as the Gould modification of the Broström technique (Fig. 8–10):
  - The ATFL and CFL are imbricated to appropriate tension.
  - The Gould modification reinforces this step with a portion of the extensor retinaculum, which is brought to the fibula after imbrication of the ligaments.
    - The modification improves stability of the subtalar joint.
  - The success of any anatomic repair relies on the presence of adequate ligamentous tissue.
- Nonanatomic reconstruction techniques are useful in the setting of failed anatomic repair or long-standing instability, and in patients with generalized ligamentous laxity.
  - Commonly described reconstructions include the Watson-Jones, Evans, and Chrisman-Snook.
  - Many studies have shown a higher rate of complications with nonanatomic reconstructive procedures than with the Broström and modified Broström techniques.
- Anatomic reconstruction techniques using autograft or allograft have been described. Early results are promising, although larger studies with longer follow-up are needed (Fig. 8–11).

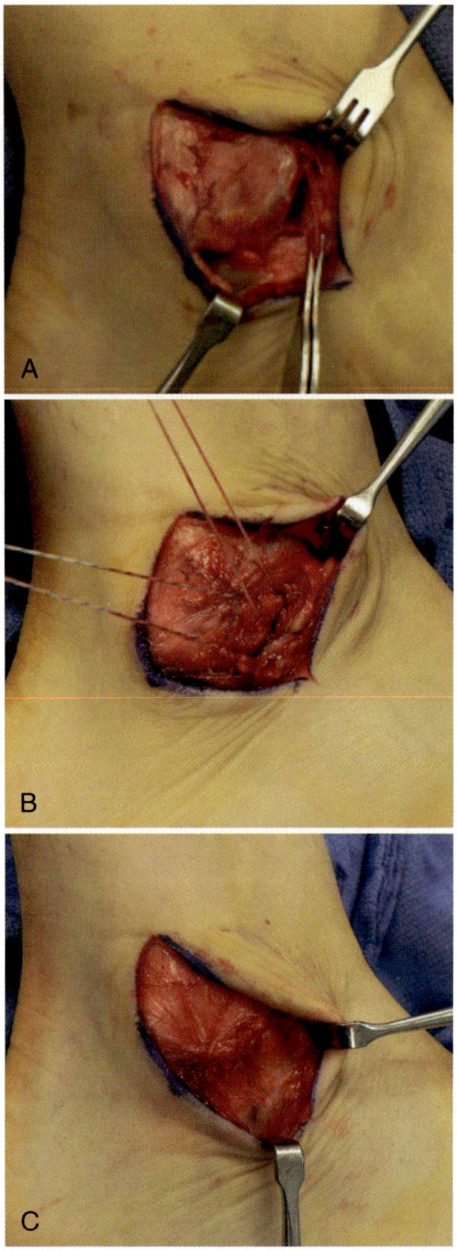

Figure 8–10 Intraoperative photographs of a modified Broström reconstruction. **A,** Incision of the anterior talofibular ligament (ATFL) and calcaneofibular ligament (CFL). **B,** Imbrication of the ATFL and CFL with the use of a suture anchor. **C,** Final construct after the Gould modification.

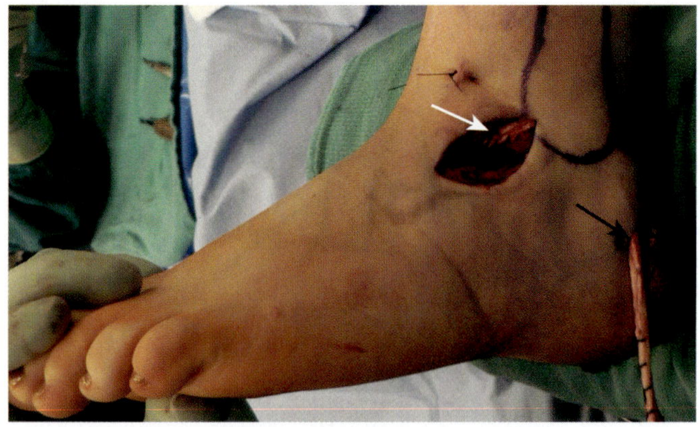

Figure 8–11 Intraoperative photograph of an allograft reconstruction of the lateral collateral ligaments. Near anatomic reconstruction of the anterior talofibular ligament (*white arrow*) and calcaneofibular ligament (*black arrow*) can be achieved with this technique.

Ankle Instability Questions

1. A 25-year-old female runner complains of recurrent ankle instability over the last 6 months. Examination elicits a positive anterior drawer test result and normal motor findings. She has had no previous treatment. The next most appropriate step is:
   A. Modified Broström lateral ligament reconstruction.
   B. MRI.
   C. Anatomic autograft hamstring lateral ligament reconstruction.
   D. Ankle orthosis and physical therapy.

2. A 250-lb football player has complaints of ankle instability for which 6 months of bracing and physical therapy has failed. Examination finds a positive anterior drawer test result, and stress radiographs demonstrated increased tibiotalar tilt. Hindfoot alignment is varus. Surgical intervention should consist of:
   A. Modified Broström technique.
   B. Modified Broström technique with lateral closing wedge calcaneal osteotomy.
   C. Nonanatomic (e.g., Chrisman-Snook) ligament reconstruction.
   D. Nonanatomic (e.g., Chrisman-Snook) ligament reconstruction with lateral closing wedge calcaneal osteotomy.

3. A 40-year-old active man has recurrent ankle instability after having undergone a modified Broström procedure 1 year ago. Hindfoot alignment is physiologic valgus. Objective instability with generalized ligamentous laxity is noted on examination. The most appropriate surgical intervention is:
   A. Repeat modified Broström repair.
   B. Repeat modified Broström repair with lateral closing wedge calcaneal osteotomy.
   C. Nonanatomic (e.g., Chrisman-Snook) ligament reconstruction.
   D. Nonanatomic (e.g., Chrisman-Snook) ligament reconstruction with lateral closing wedge calcaneal osteotomy.

■

Osteochondral Lesions of the Talus

- *Osteochondral lesion of the talus* (OLT) is now used in favor of the *osteochondritis dissecans* for this lesion, because thoughts regarding the etiology of these lesions have changed.
- Most lesions are now thought to be a result of trauma:
  - Often coincide with ankle sprains or fractures (Fig. 8–12).

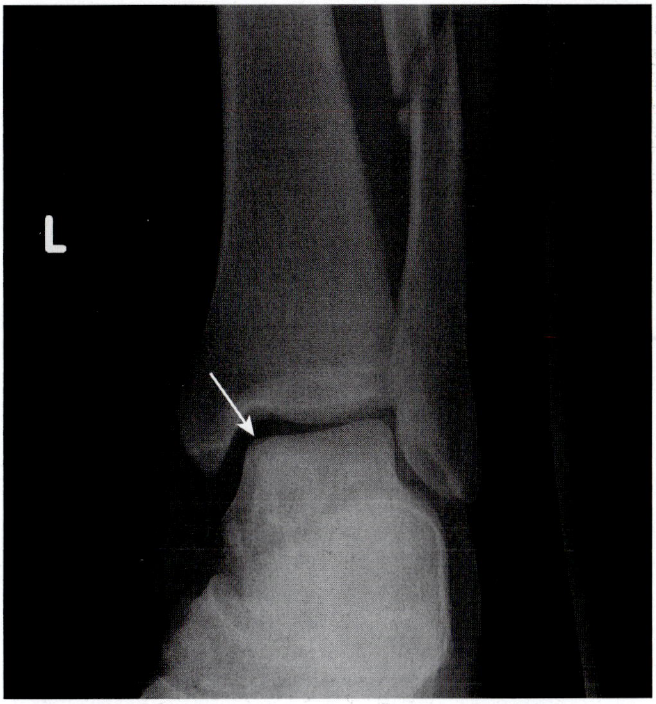

Figure 8–12 Anteroposterior non–weight-bearing radiograph of the ankle of a patient with an acute ankle fracture. Note the medial talar osteochondral lesion (*arrow*).

- Often are not immediately recognized in the setting of such injuries.
- May be the result of a single event or of repeated trauma.
- OLT should be in the differential diagnosis both for a patient with chronic ankle pain after previous trauma and for a patient with ankle pain and no known history of trauma.
- Common mechanical symptoms include:
  - Locking.
  - Clicking.
  - Catching.
  - Giving way.
  - Sensation of pain preceding instability.
- Some studies suggest that medial lesions are more common, although others have found equal rates of medial and lateral injuries:
  - Virtually all lateral lesions are thought to be traumatic.
  - About 80% of medial lesions have a known history of trauma.
- Classification of OLT by Berndt and Harty:
  - Stage I: Area of subchondral compression without full-thickness cartilage lesion.
  - Stage II: Partial detachment of osteochondral fragment.
  - Stage III: Complete detachment but no displacement of fragment.
  - Stage IV: Complete detachment with displacement of fragment.
  - This system has been called into question because the appearance of the OLT during arthroscopy may not correlate with the classification.
- Other classification systems using MRI or arthroscopy have been used.

Physical Examination

- Physical examination should include the usual palpation, range-of-motion, motor, and sensory examinations as well as testing for ankle stability.

Imaging

- Initial imaging studies should include weight-bearing ankle radiographs.
- MRI is recommended for evaluation of suspected OLT in the setting of normal plain radiographic findings.
  - MRI has been shown to correlate with bone scan and arthroscopic findings (Fig. 8–13).
  - Other structures and causes of pain may also be identified on MRI.
- CT is useful for characterizing OLT identified on plain radiographs and for preoperative planning.
  - CT may miss low-grade lesions, which may be visible on other studies. Therefore, CT is not recommended for evaluation of suspected OLT in the setting of normal plain film findings.

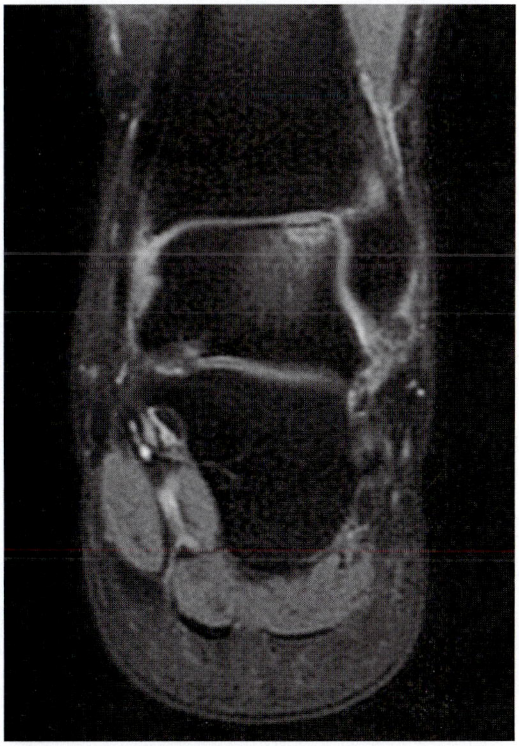

Figure 8–13 Coronal magnetic resonance image of a patient with a lateral talar osteochondral lesion. The fragment has completely detached without any significant displacement. Note the subchondral bone edema.

- Bone scanning has also been shown to be sensitive and specific in identifying OLT but does not evaluate the surrounding soft tissues.

Treatment

- Nonsurgical treatment is successful in many patients (25% to 56%; likely higher in low-grade lesions).
  - Initial period of cast immobilization without weight-bearing, followed by slow return to weight-bearing.
  - The patient should be back to normal ambulation by 12 to 16 weeks.
- Surgical treatment is indicated after failure of nonsurgical treatment, and possibly in displaced OLT without a trial of nonsurgical methods or in patients with mechanical symptoms.
- Excision of the fragment with drilling or microfracture of the subchondral bone has a high rate of success, even for stage III lesions (Fig. 8–14).
- Débridement of the subchondral bone, with fixation of the fragment back to the talus, should be considered in younger patients with large lesions (more than one third of the width of the talar dome).
- Osteochondral autograft and allograft procedures continue to be investigated, with promising early results. Long-term results and specific indications are not yet known.

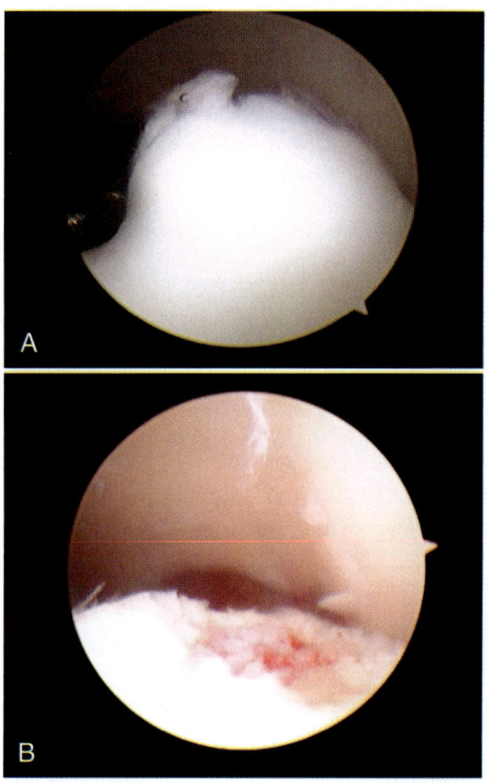

Figure 8–14 A, Intraoperative photographs of an unstable osteochondral lesion, which underwent excision with microfracture (B). Note bleeding at the base of the lesion, which denotes the appropriate depth of microfracture.

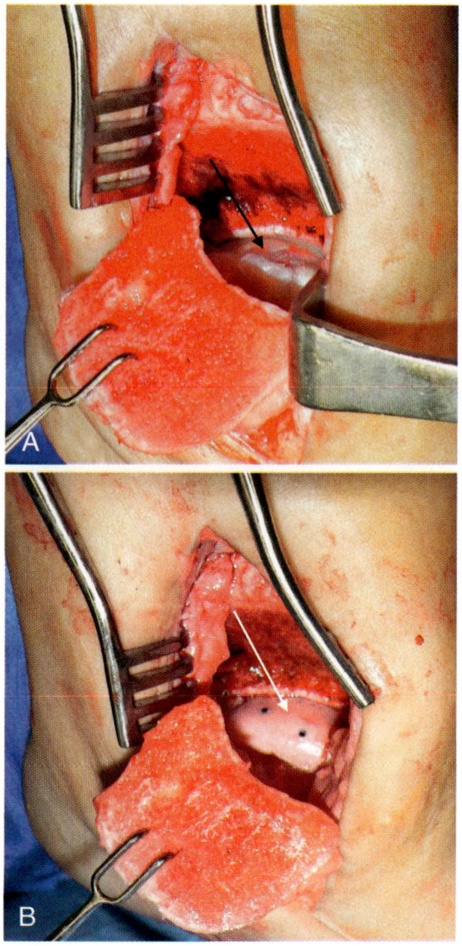

Figure 8–15 Intraoperative photographs of a large medial talar osteochondral lesion. A, Large medial osteochondral lesion (*black arrow*), which underwent allograft osteoarticular reconstruction (B, *white arrow*).

  - Failure of prior arthroscopic débridement is the most common indication.
  - However, later literature has suggested that repeat arthroscopy and débridement can yield satisfactory results and therefore can be performed to avoid a more invasive procedure.
- Lesions larger than 2 cm^2 may be better suited for osteoarticular autograft transplantation as a primary intervention.
- Large lesions involving a significant portion of the shoulder of the talus are best treated by allograft reconstruction in order to restore the anatomy of the medial or lateral gutter (Fig. 8–15).
  - Use of an anterior approach for allograft reconstruction can mitigate the need for medial malleolar or lateral malleolar osteotomy.

Osteochondral Lesion Questions

1. A 30-year-old woman complains of her ankle "giving way" after an ankle sprain 2 years ago. Detailed history reveals that she has pain preceding each episode of instability.

Physical examination demonstrates a normal anterior drawer test result, and there is no radiographic evidence of varus laxity. An MRI shows evidence of a lateral OLT. The most appropriate surgical intervention is:
A. Modified Broström technique.
B. Modified Broström technique and ankle arthroscopy with drilling of the OLT.
C. Ankle arthroscopy with drilling of the OLT.
D. Osteochondral autograft procedure.

2. The modality with the highest sensitivity to evaluate for the presence and location of an osteochondral lesion of talus is:
A. Weight-bearing radiographs.
B. MRI.
C. CT.
D. Bone scanning.

3. A 20-year-old patient presents with history of an ankle sprain 2 months ago and MRI findings of a stable medial osteochondral lesion. Current symptoms include complaints of instability without pain. The patient has not had any prior treatment for the sprain. The next most appropriate step is:
A. Ankle arthroscopy with drilling of the OLT and modified Broström technique.
B. Cast treatment and 6 weeks without weight-bearing.
C. Ankle orthosis and physical therapy.
D. Ankle arthroscopy with drilling of the OLT.

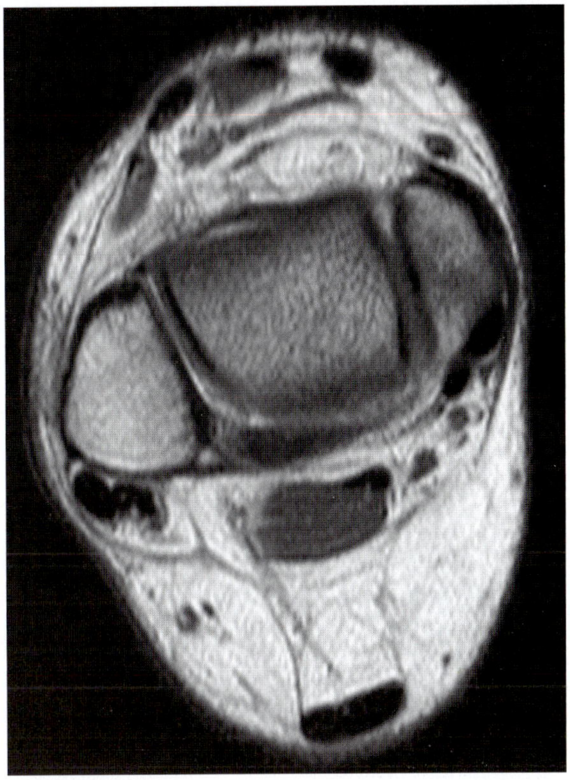

Figure 8–16 Axial T1-weighted magnetic resonance image of the distal leg. Note the shallow fibular groove and a split tear of the peroneus brevis.

Peroneal Tendon Subluxation

- Symptomatic peroneal tendon subluxation is uncommon but is often misdiagnosed and may be the source of significant pain and disability.
- The peroneal tendons curve posteriorly to the lateral malleolus in a groove (Fig. 8–16):
  - This groove is concave in more than 80% of ankles.
  - Shallow, flat, or convex grooves impart a higher risk of subluxation.
  - The tendons are restrained by a combination of the groove and the superior peroneal retinaculum (SPR).
- Chronic peroneal tendon subluxation most often occurs after an acute injury to the SPR.
  - The most common mechanism is forceful contraction of the peroneal tendons with the foot in dorsiflexion.
  - This acute injury is often misdiagnosed as a sprain.
  - Chronic subluxation often manifests as posterolateral ankle pain with or without a feeling of tendon snapping or instability:
    - Pain is usually worse with eversion motions, during which the peroneal tendons are activated.
    - Patients may complain of a lump or mass that occurs with the pain. This is consistent with the subluxation of the tendons out of the groove (Fig. 8–17).

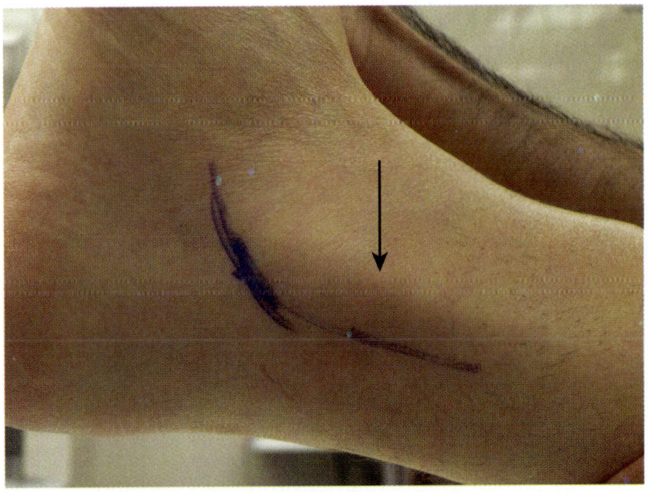

Figure 8–17 Intraoperative photograph of the lateral aspect of the ankle. Note the anteriorly subluxated peroneal tendons (*arrow*) relative to the posterior margin of the fibula (purple skin marking).

Physical Examination

- After a general physical examination of the foot and ankle, the peroneal tendons are evaluated.
- There is often tenderness over the tendons as they pass posterior to the lateral malleolus.
- Resisted dorsiflexion and eversion may reproduce the subluxation.

- Foot alignment and ankle stability should be assessed.
- The patient should also be evaluated for hindfoot varus.

Imaging

- Plain radiographs may rule out other common causes of ankle pain, and may be diagnostic in a small number of acute SPR injuries in which a piece of the lateral malleolus has been avulsed.
- MRI is useful to evaluate the status of the SPR and the peroneal tendons but may miss chronic subluxation, in which the tendons are reduced at rest.
  - Allows preoperative planning to address peroneal tendon tears.
  - Allows evaluation of the shape of the fibular groove.
- Ultrasound has the advantage of enabling a dynamic examination and has been shown to be effective in the evaluation for chronic subluxation.
  - This examination is very useful in establishing the even more rare diagnosis of intrasheath peroneal tendon subluxation.

Treatment

- Acute SPR injuries have traditionally been treated with immobilization.
- Because of the high reported rates of chronic subluxation in patients treated nonoperatively, however, some writers advocate surgical repair of the SPR after acute injury:
  - Small case-series show promising results.
  - Primary repair of the SPR is the treatment of choice in high-level athletes.
- Symptomatic chronic subluxation should be addressed surgically. Several methods have been described, with good results:
  - The peroneal tendons can be rerouted beneath the CFL, which thereafter serves as a new retinaculum.
  - Many SPR reconstructions with local tissue and tendons have been reported.
  - Bony procedures, including groove deepening, have also been successful.
  - Combination procedures with SPR reconstruction and groove deepening have been advocated.
  - Any ankle instability or hindfoot malalignment must be corrected concurrently.

❑ Groove Deepening with Imbrication of the Superior Peroneal Retinaculum

- The patient is positioned supine with a bolster under the ipsilateral hip.
- An extensile posterolateral incision is made.
  - The retinaculum is incised 1 mm posterior to the fibula.

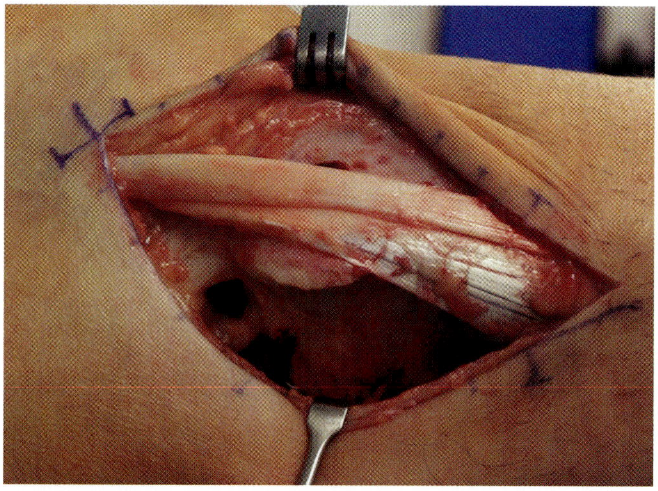

Figure 8–18 Intraoperative photograph of the peroneal tendons after incision of the superior peroneal retinaculum and synovectomy. Note the subluxated position of the tendons and the lack of a concomitant tear.

- Peroneal tendons are examined and synovectomy is performed (Fig. 8–18).
  - Concomitant tears are treated with débridement and tubularization.
- Groove deepening may be performed using one of the following three techniques:
  - Trapdoor technique:
    - A cortical window is made in the posterior fibula.
    - The cancellous bone is removed, and the cortical window is tamped back into place.
  - Bur technique (Fig. 8–19):
    - An oblong bur is utilized to debride the cortical and cancellous bone.
    - Bone wax is applied to create a smooth gliding surface.
  - Intramedullary drill technique:
    - A drill is placed from the tip of the fibula directed superiorly.

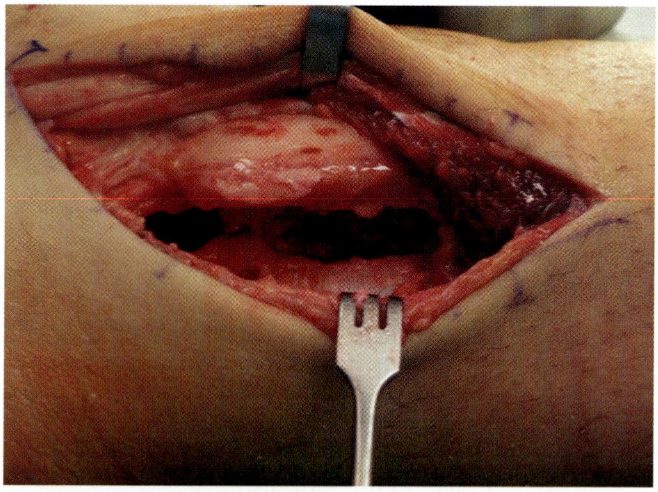

Figure 8–19 Intraoperative photograph of the fibular groove after it has been deepened via the bur technique.

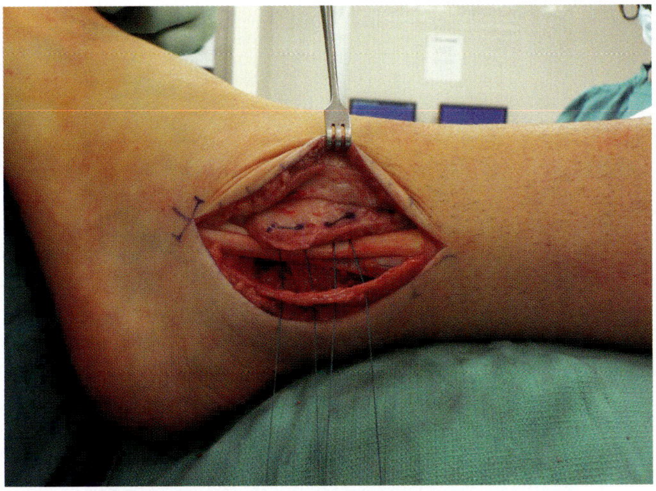

Figure 8–20 Intraoperative photograph demonstrating imbrication of the superior peroneal retinaculum via drill holes in the fibula. Note placement of the knots on the retinaculum to avoid prominence under the skin.

      - A tamp is then used from posterior to anterior to impact the cortical bone into the defect.
- SPR reconstruction:
  - The peroneal tendons are reduced and should be stable within the groove prior to imbrication.
  - The SPR is then repaired through drill holes in the fibula (Fig. 8–20).

Peroneal Subluxation Questions

1. A professional baseball player has an acute injury consistent with a peroneal tendon dislocation. MRI reveals evidence of peroneal tendon dislocation without tear. The next most appropriate step is:
   A. Reduction of the tendons with 6 weeks of cast treatment.
   B. Acute surgical repair of the superior peroneal retinaculum.
   C. Acute surgical repair of the inferior peroneal retinaculum.
   D. Reduction of the tendons with early rehabilitation and use of an ankle orthosis.
2. A 25-year-old patient complains of pain and snapping within the posterolateral aspect of the ankle, directly behind the lateral malleolus. Provocative testing with dorsiflexion and eversion does not produce subluxation of the tendons. The next most appropriate step is:
   A. MRI.
   B. Dynamic ultrasound.
   C. Corticosteroid injection.
   D. Physical therapy.
3. A 40-year-old woman complains of 2 years of recurrent subluxation of the peroneal tendons. Clinical examination confirms the diagnosis. MRI shows a flat fibular groove and no evidence of a peroneal tendon tear. The most appropriate surgical intervention is:
   A. Imbrication of the superior peroneal retinaculum.
   B. Peroneal tendon synovectomy and imbrication of the inferior peroneal retinaculum.
   C. Fibular groove deepening and imbrication of the inferior peroneal retinaculum.
   D. Fibular groove deepening and repair of the superior peroneal retinaculum.

■

Achilles Tendon Rupture

- Occurs most commonly in men during the third or fourth decade of life.
- The most common mechanism is a sudden forced plantarflexion of the foot (most often during sporting activities).
  - May also be sustained from unexpected or violent foot dorsiflexion.
- It is thought that most ruptures occur in previously abnormal, although often asymptomatic tendons.
- Proposed risk factors include Achilles tendinosis, topical or injected corticosteroids, fluoroquinolones, inflammatory arthritis, and mechanical abnormalities of the foot.
- The patient often reports a feeling of sudden "pop" or "snap" in the affected calf:
  - The patient often reports a feeling of being struck in the back of the calf (e.g., by a ball, another player, or a foot).
  - An audible popping sound is not uncommon.
- Pain may be significant initially but often subsides to a mild level relatively quickly.
  - This pattern may contribute to a delay in presentation.

Physical Examination

- Diagnosis is generally confirmed with a physical examination. After a general examination of the foot and ankle, focused examination for suspected achilles tendon rupture should include all of the following:
  - The affected extremity has weak plantarflexion in comparison with the contralateral side.
    - Plantarflexion *weakness* is evaluated in contrast to *ability*, because the ability to plantarflex may be facilitated by the toe flexors, posterior tibialis, or plantaris.
  - A defect in the tendon may often be palpated, although this finding varies with body habitus and swelling:
    - Palpate the length of the substance of the tendon with the foot passively dorsiflexed.
    - Rupture is most common 4 to 5 cm proximal to the insertion of the tendon.
  - The hallmark provocative test is the Thompson test (Fig. 8–21):

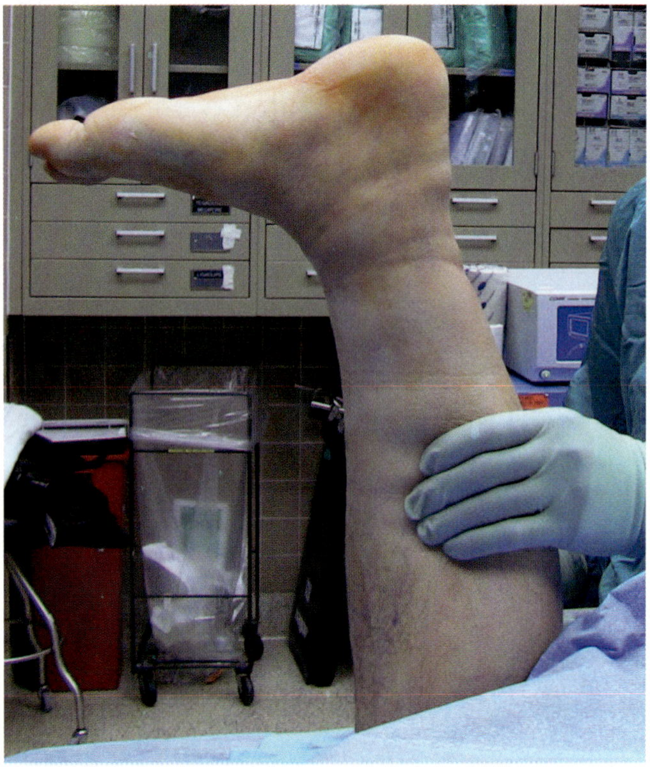

Figure 8–21 Intraoperative photograph demonstrating a positive Thompson test result. Note failure of the foot to plantarflex with compression of the calf.

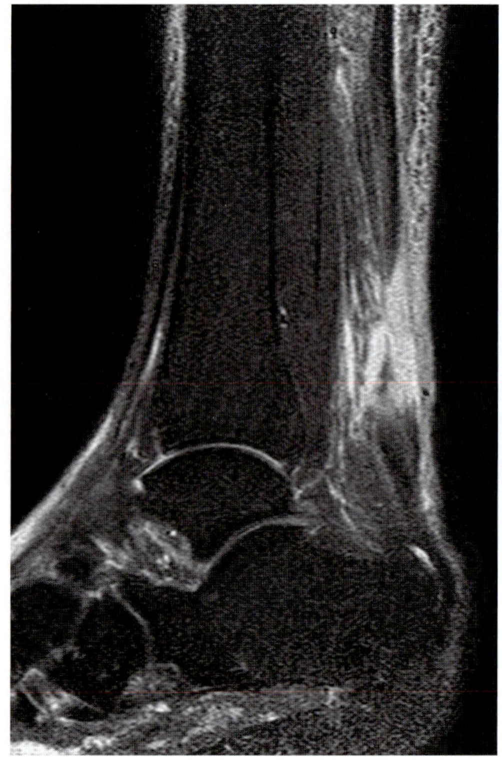

Figure 8–22 Sagittal T2-weighted magnetic resonance image demonstrating an Achilles tendon rupture. Note the lack of continuity of the Achilles tendon, with significant edema in place of the tendon.

- This test is often performed with the patient prone, and the affected knee flexed to 90 degrees. Gravity provides a dorsiflexion force to the foot.
- The examiner grasps the calf at the widest part of the gastroc-soleus complex and provides circumferential force (squeeze).
- The result is positive if there is no plantarflexion of the foot with the squeeze.
- Comparison with the contralateral extremity is helpful.

Imaging

- Plain radiographs should be obtained if there is concern that the rupture is at the insertion of the tendon. A large bony fragment may cause skin necrosis, and urgent surgery is necessary.
- If the diagnosis is in doubt, further imaging may be helpful.
- Ultrasonography has high sensitivity and specificity for Achilles tendon rupture.
  - Dynamic studies may show whether the tendon ends are apposed in appropriate plantarflexion. This demonstration is useful if nonoperative treatment is considered.
- MRI is also a reliable study but is not often used to diagnose acute ruptures (Fig. 8–22).

Treatment

- Many nonoperative and operative treatment strategies have been investigated, and some controversy regarding treatment still exists.
- Nonoperative strategies generally begin with immobilization:
  - Ultrasonographic demonstration of the apposition of the tendon with 20 degrees of plantarflexion has been shown to lead to successful outcomes with nonoperative management.
  - There is little agreement or evidence to guide the need for limited weight-bearing, the amount of plantarflexion, progression to neutral dorsiflexion, or the appropriate duration of casting.
  - Immediate functional bracing has shown to have results comparable with those of casting alone.
  - Functional bracing begins using heel wedges in the brace to attain tendon end apposition. Over the course of weeks, these wedges are removed, bringing the foot to neutral dorsiflexion.
  - Nonoperative methods avoid the risks of surgery, including wound complications and nerve injury.
- Several operative methods have been investigated, and have been shown to yield good functional results.

- Operative treatment has been shown to have a significantly lower rerupture rate in many studies (<5% for surgical treatment vs. 15%-25% for nonsurgical treatment).
- Compared with nonoperative treatment, surgical intervention leads to an earlier return to activities.
- Operative treatment is also believed to result in better recovery of strength than nonoperative treatment, although definitive evidence is lacking in the literature.
- Percutaneous methods have lower risks of wound complications but higher risk of nerve injury than open methods.

❑ Preferred Method

- Open operative intervention is our preferred treatment of choice, especially in the athletic population.
- The patient is typically placed prone, although lateral and supine positioning techniques have been described.
- Incision is made medial to the Achilles tendon and centered over the level of the tear to avoid damage to the sural nerve.
- The paratenon is carefully incised longitudinally to allow for closure at the completion of the procedure.
- Débridement of the ruptured ends of the tendon is kept to a minimum to avoid iatrogenic shortening.
- A locking Krackow stitch is placed into each segment of the Achilles tendon with a No. 2 braided composite suture (FiberWire, Arthrex, Inc., Naples, FL) (Fig. 8–23):
  - The tendon should appose easily without undue tension.
  - Surgically preparing the other leg so that it can be included in the surgical field allows comparison of resting tension levels.
  - A good rule of thumb is that the foot should be in 15 degrees of resting equinus.
- A running "baseball" stitch is then placed with 3-0 nylon to increase the strength of the repair and minimize gapping.
- After closure of the paratenon, the foot is splinted in 20 degrees of plantarflexion to maximize perfusion to the wound (Fig. 8–24).
- After 2 weeks of postoperative splinting, the patient is started on a functional rehabilitation protocol.

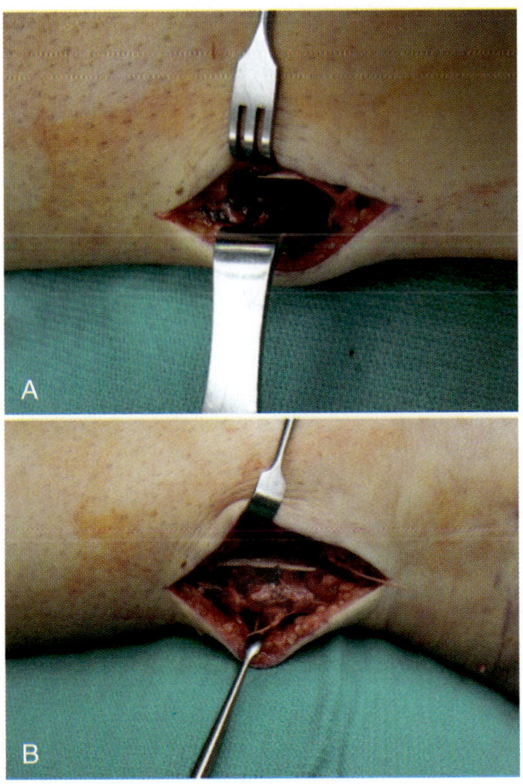

Figure 8–23 Intraoperative photographs of an Achilles tendon rupture with a defect. **A,** Prior to repair. **B,** Complete apposition after repair with sutures.

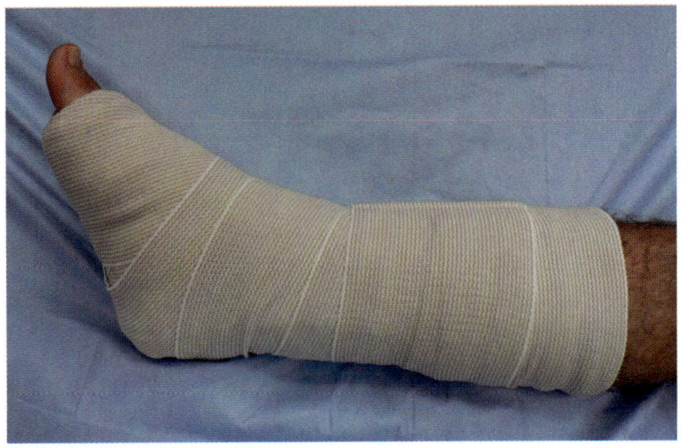

Figure 8–24 Postoperative splint for an Achilles tendon rupture in 20 degrees of plantarflexion. Perfusion to the posterior skin of the ankle is maximized in this position, and all incisions made posteriorly are splinted in this position to minimize wound complications.

Achilles Tendon Rupture Questions

1. A 65-year-old woman with diabetes presents with an acute Achilles tendon rupture. Clinical examination confirms the diagnosis. The next most appropriate step in the management of this patient is:
A. MRI.
B. Dynamic ultrasound
C. Immediate cast treatment in neutral.
D. Percutaneous surgical repair.

2. Compared with nonoperative treatment, open surgical repair of the Achilles tendon results in:
A. Higher rerupture rate, higher wound complication rate, faster return to activities.
B. Lower rerupture rate, lower wound complication rate, slower return to activities.
C. Higher rerupture rate, lower wound complication rate, slower return to activities.
D. Lower rerupture rate, higher wound complication rate, faster return to activities.

3. A 35-year-old active man felt a sudden "pop" in his right calf 5 days ago. At presentation he is ambulatory with minimal pain. Clinical examination reveals

active plantarflexion of the affected leg. The result of Thompson test is positive. The most next appropriate step is:
A. Functional rehabilitation with an ankle orthosis.
B. Cast treatment in neutral.
C. Open surgical repair.
D. Open surgical repair with flexor hallucis longus augmentation.

■

Stress Fractures

- The most common site of lower extremity stress fracture is the tibia. The tarsal bones account for approximately 25% of these stress fractures, and the metatarsals for less than 10%.

Fifth Metatarsal Stress Fractures

- Common in basketball players and most commonly occurs at the proximal diaphysis (Fig. 8–25).
  - This fracture pattern should be distinguished from a fracture extending into the 4 5 intermetatarsal joint (so called Jones fracture).
- Risk factors include a sudden increase in activities, improper training, foot deformities, hormonal factors, systemic diseases, and use of certain medications.

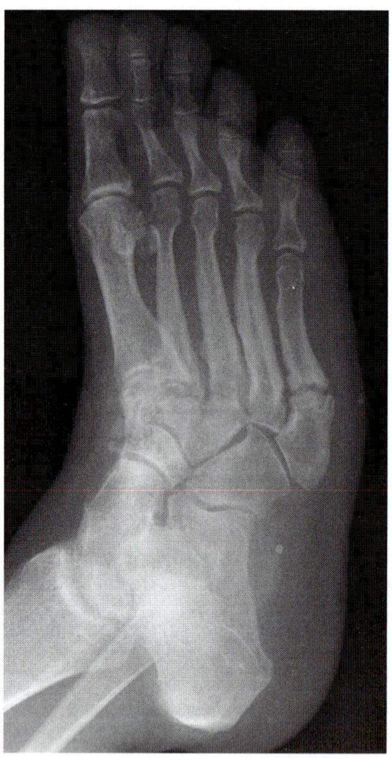

Figure 8–25 Oblique radiograph of the foot demonstrating a stress fracture of the fifth metatarsal. Note the sclerosis at the fracture site.

  - The *female athlete triad,* consisting of amenorrhea, eating disorder, and osteoporosis, has been linked to stress fractures.
- Patients commonly have pain along the lateral border of the foot.
- Physical examination shows tenderness over the fifth metatarsal at the site of the fracture.
  - Pain may be elicited or exacerbated with foot inversion.
- Diagnosis is often confirmed with plain radiographs of the foot (three views).
  - A fracture line is often visualized.
  - Depending on the chronicity of the injury, varying amounts of periosteal reaction and sclerosis may be present.

❑ Treatment
- Many nonoperative treatment regimens have been reported, without adequate evidence to support any single method.
  - Immobilization in a cast or cast boot with no weight-bearing for approximately 4 weeks is reasonable.
  - Protected weight-bearing is initiated, followed by transition to a rehabilitation program when the patient is pain-free and healing is observed on radiographs.
- A custom orthotic or carbon fiber plate should be used during rehabilitation and return to sport.
- Operative intervention should be considered after failure of nonoperative treatment or in high-functioning athletes who require a faster return to activity.
  - Surgery should also be considered as primary treatment for Jones fractures.
  - Multiple surgical techniques have been described with good results.
  - Evidence for effectiveness of these techniques is generally limited to level IV or V.
  - Good results have been reported for intramedullary screw fixation in several studies:
    - 4.5-mm cannulated screw fixation has been shown to be adequate in biomechanical studies.
    - Proper screw placement can be demanding.
  - Complications include improper hardware placement, non-union, infection, and symptomatic hardware.
- If lower extremity deformities (limb length discrepancy, cavus foot, etc.) are present, use of orthotics or even corrective surgery should be considered.
  - Presence or absence of a varus deformity of the hindfoot should be elucidated in every patient.

Navicular Stress Fracture

- The navicular is part of the medial column of the foot, articulating proximally with the talar head and distally with the three cuneiform bones.
  - Talonavicular articulation allows for rotation of the midfoot on the hindfoot during inversion and eversion.
- The vascular supply to the navicular stems from the dorsal pedis artery dorsally and the plantar arteries plantarly.
  - The vascular supply is rich medially and laterally, but there is a watershed area in the central third corresponding to the branching of the peripheral vessels.
- It is thought that any anatomic variation or activity that increases the shear stresses across the navicular raises the risk of stress fracture.
  - A long second metatarsal, a short first metatarsal, a cavus foot, metatarsus adductus, and limited foot motion have been implicated as increasing navicular shear stress.
  - There is little clinical data to correlate these theories with a higher risk of navicular stress fracture.
  - Activities in which the foot strikes in a plantarflexed position (e.g., sprinting, jumping) are also believed to increase this risk.
  - These fractures are most common in sports that require quick changes in direction or push-off, such as football, basketball, rugby, and track-and-field events.
  - They are less common in lower-impact repetitive sports such as distance running.

❑ Physical Examination
- The presentation of navicular stress fractures is variable:
  - Patients may complain of vague foot pain or cramping with activities.
  - Patients may not localize the pain specifically to the navicular. Complaints may consist of vague dorsal pain or pain along the longitudinal arch.
  - Symptoms often have an insidious onset and irregular pattern.
- Physical examination may help localize the complaints. After a general foot and ankle examination, attention should be turned to palpation of the midfoot in patients in whom navicular stress is suspected.
  - There is often tenderness over the dorsal central aspect of the navicular.
  - Pain may be elicited with percussion over the navicular.
  - Hopping on the plantarflexed foot may reproduce the symptoms.
  - Swelling or ecchymosis is generally absent.

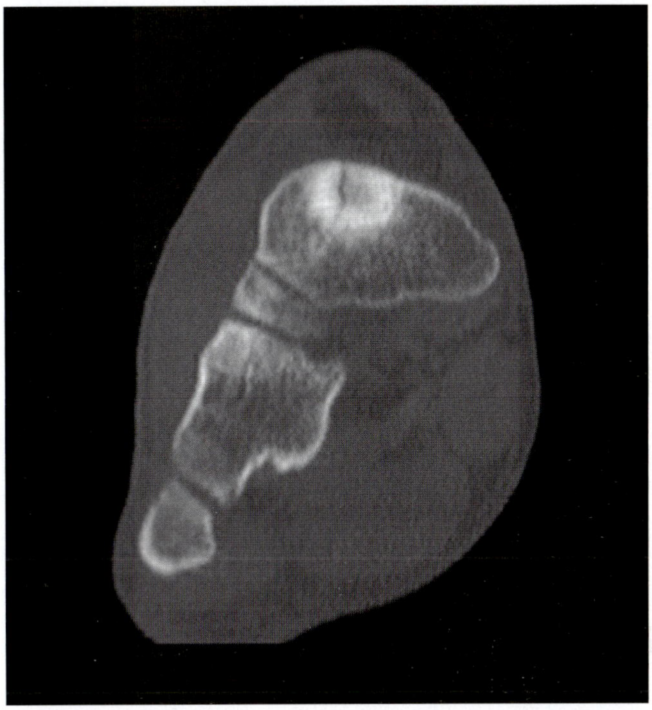

Figure 8–26 Coronal computed tomography scan of a navicular stress fracture. Note the incomplete and nondisplaced fracture pattern. Significant sclerosis is present.

❑ Imaging
- Plain radiographs have a low sensitivity for navicular stress fractures, especially incomplete fractures.
- Bone scanning has a high sensitivity for the evaluation of navicular stress fracture but is not specific to stress fracture and provides no anatomic detail.
- CT has the advantage of better demonstration of the bony anatomy, fracture lines, and extent of comminution (Fig. 8–26).
- MRI may combine the advantages of high sensitivity with the ability to evaluate the fracture anatomy. These are theoretical advantages and have not been scrutinized in the literature.

❑ Treatment
- Navicular stress fractures may be classified as complete or incomplete and as displaced or nondisplaced.
- Because these fractures often occur in high-functioning athletes, treatment must be individualized for the patient.
- Nonoperative management can be successful in patients with nondisplaced or incomplete fractures.
  - Cast immobilization and non–weight-bearing status for 6 to 8 weeks are preferred.
  - Nonoperative methods that include early weight-bearing activities are less successful.
  - When the patient is pain-free, with no tenderness, activity is resumed.

- Surgical intervention should be considered in patients with displaced or comminuted fractures, those in whom conservative treatment fails, and those who cannot tolerate a prolonged treatment and recovery timeline.
  - The central portion of the navicular is exposed through a longitudinal dorsal incision. The proximal and distal articulations need not be violated.
  - The fracture is identified with direct visualization and fluoroscopy.
  - Autologous or allogenic bone graft may be applied to the fracture site.
  - Correction of forefoot or midfoot deformity should also be considered.
  - Screw fixation providing compression across the fracture site is optimal:
    - Directing the screws from lateral to medial provides better bone purchase (Fig. 8–27).
    - A percutaneous technique may be used to minimize the necessary dissection.
- Postsurgical rehabilitation begins with 4 to 6 weeks of no weight-bearing in a cast.
  - Progression to protected weight-bearing in a cast or cast boot varies according to the severity of the fracture and quality of the fixation.
  - Progression to athletic activity begins when the patient can ambulate without pain.

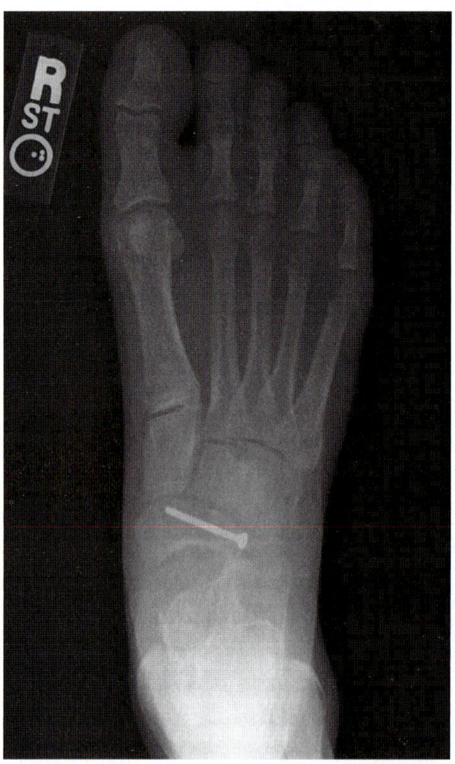

Figure 8–27 Postoperative anteroposterior standing radiograph of a patient who underwent open reduction with internal fixation of a navicular stress fracture. Note the placement of the screw from lateral to medial.

    - A custom orthotic or carbon fiber plate should be used during this period of return to sport.
  - Patient can typically begin to run 12 to 16 weeks postoperatively.

❑ Complications
- Delayed union and non-union are the most common complications of nonoperative and operative treatment of stress fractures.
- They are signaled by continued symptoms and tenderness.
- The optimal treatment of these difficult cases is unknown.
- Revision surgical fixation with grafting is reasonable.
- Refractory cases may require arthrodesis.
- Osteotomy for correction of deformity should be considered.

Stress Fracture Questions

1. A 17-year-old female track-and-field athlete presents with pain over the dorsal midfoot. Examination findings are consistent with a stress fracture of the navicular. In addition to a CT to delineate the injury, the next most appropriate step is:
A. Prescription of a bone stimulator.
B. Weight-bearing cast treatment.
C. Detailed history to review dietary habits and menstruation cycle.
D. DEXA scan.

2. A professional basketball player presents with a stress fracture of the fifth metatarsal. The patient has a history of prodromal pain with radiographic evidence of a stress fracture with sclerosis. Hindfoot alignment is varus. The most appropriate treatment is:
A. 6 weeks of no weight-bearing with the foot in a cast followed by weight-bearing with the foot in a boot.
B. ORIF with a plate and screws.
C. ORIF with an intramedullary screw.
D. ORIF with an intramedullary screw and lateral closing wedge calcaneal osteotomy.

3. The most common location for a navicular stress fracture is:
A. Medial third.
B. Lateral third.
C. Central third.
D. Plantar third.

Turf Toe

- Turf toe injuries involve traumatic capsuloligamentous disruption of the first metatarsophalangeal (MTP) joint of variable severity.
- Mechanism of injury is great toe MTP hyperextension with an axial load.

- The plantar joint capsule, or components of the plantar plate complex, may sustain damage.
- Postulated predisposing factors include flexible shoes, hardness of playing surface, and patient factors such as body weight, MTP joint morphology, and adjacent joint flexibility.
- Patients typically present after an athletic injury with complaints of pain with weight-bearing, especially at toe-off.

Physical Examination

- Clinical manifestations vary from short-lived pain with push-off in sports activities to chronic pain and weakness, post-traumatic hallux rigidus, hallux valgus, or hallucal cock-up deformity.
- After a general foot and ankle physical examination, the alignment of the hallux, including clinical MTP joint reduction, should be evaluated:
  - Palpate the plantar (including individual sesamoids), lateral, and dorsal structures for focal tenderness.
  - Evaluate hypermobility or a mechanical block at the MTP in comparison with the contralateral side.

Imaging

- Imaging should include weight-bearing AP and lateral views, a medial oblique view, and an axial sesamoid view to assess for joint reduction, impaction fractures, sesamoid bipartition or fractures, as well as proximal migration of the sesamoids that would suggest a complete plantar plate disruption.
  - Dorsoplantar drawer and varus/valgus stress radiographs may be useful to detect injuries to the plantar plate complex and collateral ligaments, if there is sufficient clinical concern about these possibilities.

Grading

- Turf toe may be graded as follows:
  - Grade 1: An incomplete tear of the capsule, which is associated with mild swelling and localized plantar or medial tenderness and generally heals with rapid return to sport and minimal loss of playing time.
  - Grade 2: Involves a more extensive capsular tear, moderate swelling, ecchymosis, more diffuse tenderness, and some initial loss of range of motion.
    - Typically, athletes with grade 2 injury are unable to play for 3 to 14 days and recover fully with symptomatic management.
- Grade 3: Complete capsuloligamentous disruption, attended by marked swelling, ecchymosis, and inability to bear weight; may require 4 to 6 weeks of treatment before return to play.

Treatment

- Treatment generally begins with nonsurgical management.
  - Grade 1 and 2 injuries typically respond to an initial program of rest, ice, and elevation coupled with anti-inflammatory and analgesic agents to control symptoms.
    - Athletes may benefit from taping or a shoe insert to prevent dorsiflexion when returning to play.
  - Grade 3 injuries may require a period of 4 to 6 weeks of immobilization with a walker boot or short-leg cast with a toe extension.
    - As a rule in these cases, 50 to 60 degrees of painless dorsiflexion at the MTP joint is advocated before the athlete returns to competitive sport.
- Surgical indications include intra-articular loose bodies and chondral flaps, displaced sesamoid fractures, bipartite sesamoids with diastasis, proximal retraction of the sesamoids, and traumatic hallux valgus.
  - In severe, repetitive or untreated cases, persistent instability may lead to chronic synovitis and pain, or progression to degenerative arthrosis/hallux rigidus.
  - Surgical procedure is based on the specific pathology.
  - If there is disruption of the plantar plate complex and proximal migration of both the tibial and fibular sesamoids, operative repair is indicated to prevent chronic instability.

Turf Toe Questions

1. Treatment of a grade 3 turf toe is:
A. Immediate return to play with taping of the toe.
B. 1 week of rest with return to play with a shoe insert.
C. 4 to 6 weeks of immobilization in a cast boot with return to play once three is 60 degrees of painless dorsiflexion.
D. Surgical intervention to repair the capsuloligamentous disruption.

2. Surgical intervention for turf toe is indicated if:
A. Patient is a professional athlete requiring return to play with a grade 2 injury.
B. Patient has continued pain despite 6 weeks of taping.
C. Patient has pain with dorsiflexion of the great toe past 40 degrees.
D. There is retraction of both sesamoids.

3. The mechanism that results in a turf toe is:
A. Dorsiflexion with axial load.
B. Plantarflexion with axial load.
C. Valgus with axial load.
D. Varus with axial load.

Resources

Boden, B.P., Osbahr, D.C., 2000. High-risk stress fractures: Evaluation and treatment. J. Am. Acad. Orthop. Surg. 8, 344–353.

Boss, A.P., Hintermann, B., 2002. Anatomical study of the medial ankle ligament complex. Foot Ankle Int. 23, 547–553.

Chiodo, C.P., Wilson, M.G., 2006. Current concepts review: Acute ruptures of the Achilles tendon. Foot Ankle Int. 27, 305–313.

Dattani, R., Patnaik, S., Kantak, A., et al., 2008. Injuries to the tibiofibular syndesmosis. J. Bone Joint Surg. Br. 90, 405–410.

Gehrmann, R.M., Renard, R.L., 2006. Current concepts review: Stress fractures of the foot. Foot Ankle Int. 27, 750–757.

Goodwin, R.C., Sferra, J.J., 2004. Physical Examination and Orthotics: Foot & Ankle. Lippincott Williams & Wilkins, Philadelphia.

Gray, H., Lewis, W.H. (Eds.), 2000. Anatomy of the Human Body, twentieth ed. Bartleby.com, New York.

Hopkinson, W.J., St. Pierre, P., Ryan, J.B., Wheeler, J.H., 1990. Syndesmosis sprains of the ankle. Foot Ankle 10, 325–330.

Khan, R.J., Fick, D., Keogh, A., et al., 2005. Treatment of acute Achilles tendon ruptures: A meta-analysis of randomized, controlled trials. J. Bone Joint Surg. Am. 87, 2202–2210.

Leddy, J.J., Smolinski, R.J., Lawrence, J., et al., 1998. Prospective evaluation of the Ottawa Ankle Rules in a university sports medicine center: With a modification to increase specificity for identifying malleolar fractures. Am. J. Sports Med. 26, 158–165.

Lee, S., Anderson, R.B., 2004. Stress fractures of the tarsal navicular. Foot Ankle Clin. North Am. 9, 85–104.

Lin, C.F., Gross, M.T., Weinhold, P., 2006. Ankle syndesmosis injuries: Anatomy, biomechanics, mechanism of injury, and clinical guidelines for diagnosis and intervention. J. Orthop. Sports Phys. Ther. 36, 372–384.

Maffulli, N., Ferran, N.A., 2008. Management of acute and chronic ankle instability. J. Am. Acad. Orthop. Surg. 16, 608–615.

Niek van Dijk, C., van Bergen, C.J., 2008. Advancements in ankle arthroscopy. J. Am. Acad. Orthop. Surg. 16, 635–646.

Schachter, A.K., Chen, A.L., Reddy, P.D., Tejwani, N.C., 2005. Osteochondral lesions of the talus. J. Am. Acad. Orthop. Surg. 13, 152–158.

Wonga, Y., Kimb, W., Ying, N., 2005. Passive motion characteristics of the talocrural and the subtalar joint by dual Euler angles. J. Biomech. 38, 2480–2485.

CHAPTER 9

Head and Spine

SANJITPAL S. GILL AND KATHRYN A. DORWEILER

Anatomy of the Spinal Column

Spinal Cord and Nerves

- The spinal cord is a soft bundle of nerves that is a continuation from the medulla and ends at the conus medullaris around level L1-L2.
- Continues as the cauda equina.
- The three coverings over the spinal cord, called meninges, are the dura mater, arachnoid, and pia mater.
- Spinal cord consists of gray matter and white matter.
- Gray matter: Cell bodies of efferent neurons that help with motor and sensory function.
- White matter: Nerve fibers and glia; and is divided into anterior, posterior, and lateral columns.
- 31 spinal nerves (8 cervical, 12 thoracic, 5 lumbar, 5 sacral, 1 coccygeal).

Cervical Spine

- 7 cervical vertebrae (Fig. 9–1).
- Atlas (C1) and axis (C2).
- Spinal canal is triangular configuration.
- Lordotic curve.

Thoracic Spine

- 12 thoracic vertebrae.
- Less mobile than the cervical spine vertebrae because of rib attachments.
- The vertebral bodies are heart shaped.
- Spinal canal is circular configuration and smaller in diameter than cervical and lumbar regions.
- Kyphotic curve.

Lumbar Spine

- Five lumbar vertebrae.
- The vertebral bodies are kidney bean shaped.
- Spinal canal has a triangular configuration.
- Lordotic curve.

Head Injuries

Diffuse Brain Injuries

❑ Mild Cerebral Concussion

- Neurologic dysfunction WITHOUT loss of consciousness (Table 9–1).
- Most frequently occurring concussion, at a rate of 85%.
- Grade 1: confusion and disorientation without amnesia (can also be called simple concussion)
- Grade 2: retrograde amnesia after the injury
- Grade 3: amnesia from time of impact and after injury

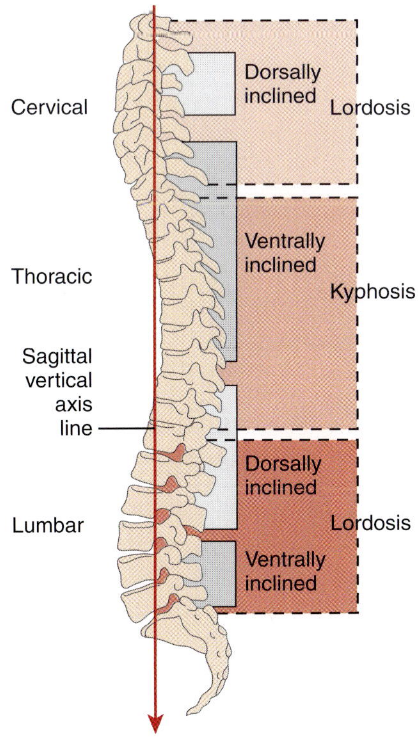

Figure 9–1 Sagittal contour balance of the spine.

Table 9–1 Concussion Management

Classification	Grade	Signs/Symptoms	1st Concussion	2nd Concussion	3rd Concussion
Colorado Medical Society	I	(+) Confusion (−) Amnesia (−) LOC	Return to play if symptoms resolve within 20 min	Terminate contest Return to play if without symptoms for 1 wk	Terminate contest Return to play if without symptoms for 3 mos
	II	(+) Confusion (+) Amnesia (−) LOC	Terminate contest Return to play if without symptoms for 1 wk	Terminate contest Return to play if without symptoms for 1 wk	Terminate season Return to play if without symptoms next season
	III	(+) LOC	Terminate contest Hospital evaluation Return to play in 1 mo after 2 consecutive wks without symptoms	Terminate season Return to play if without symptoms next season	Terminate season Hospital evaluation Strongly discourage return to contact or collision sports
Cantu grading	I	(+) Amnesia < 30-min duration (−) LOC	Return to play if asymptomatic for 1 wk*	Return to play in 2 wks after 1 wk without symptoms	Terminate season Return to play next season if asymptomatic
	II	(+) LOC < 5-min duration OR (+) Amnesia > 30-min but < 24-hr duration	Return to play if asymptomatic for 2 wks*	Return to play in 1 mo (consider season) after 1 wk without symptoms	Terminate season Return to play next season if asymptomatic
	III	(+) LOC > 5-min duration OR (+) Amnesia > 24-hr duration	Return to play in 1 mo after 1 wk without symptoms*	Terminate season Return to play next season if asymptomatic	Consider no further contact sports
American Academy of Neurology	I	(+) Transient confusion (−) LOC Symptoms < 15-min duration*	May return to play if symptoms clear within 15 min	Terminate contest May return to play if without symptoms on exertion for 1 wk	
	II	(+) Transient confusion (−) LOC Symptoms > 15-min duration*	Terminate contest May return to play if without symptoms on exertion for 1 wk	Terminate contest May return to play if without symptoms on exertion for 2 wk Terminate season if any abnormalities on computed tomography or magnetic resonance imaging	
	III	(+) LOC	Terminate contest Hospital evaluation if LOC persists or neurologic abnormality IF LOC brief, return to play in 1 wk if no symptoms on exertion If LOC prolonged (>1 min), return to play in 2 wk if no symptoms on exertion	Terminate contest Return to play after 1 mo without symptoms*	

LOC, Loss of consciousness; (+), presence of; (−), absence of.
*CT or MRI should be performed if signs or symptoms persist.
Modified from Asthagiri AR, Dumont AS, Sheehan JM: Acute and long-term management of sports-related closed head injuries. Clin Sports Med 2003;22:559-576; data from Bailes JE, Cantu RC: Head injuries in athletes. Neurosurgery 2001;48:26-46.

- CT: usually no radiographic findings
- Post-concussion syndrome: persistent headaches, difficulty concentrating, irritability.
  - Return to play: Players with post-concussion syndrome should not return to play until 1 week after symptoms have resolved for; newer data suggest use of ImPACT testing to determine normalization for return to play (Schatz et al, 2006).

❑ Classic Cerebral Concussion
- Can also be called complex concussion.
- Loss of consciousness (LOC) for a brief period of time after injury.
- Consider status of the airway and cervical spine with these injuries.
- Computed tomography (CT) and 24-hour observation
- Return to play: Athlete should not return to play that day, and if LOC exceeded 5 minutes, athlete should not return to play for at least 1 week, perhaps for 1 month, or should be out of play for the season for a recurrent classic cerebral concussion.

❑ Diffuse Axonal Injury
- Second impact syndrome when player returns to play before complete resolution of concussion.
- Prolonged LOLC and neurologic impairment.
- CT: widespread axonal damage, hemorrhagic necrosis of corpus callosum and brain stem.
- Intensive care unit with intubation.
- Life-threatening injury.

Cerebral Contusion

- Bruised cortical area.
- Common in frontal and temporal lobes.
- Coup and countercoup impacts.
- CT: high- or low-density areas without mass effect.
- Can cause increased intracranial pressure.
- Surgical decompression if herniation is possible.
- Return to play. Patients are unable to return to play after intracranial surgery.

Intracranial Vascular Injuries

❑ Subdural Hematoma
- Due to trauma to the veins between the cortical surface and the dura matter.
- CT: Concave appearance.
- Acute, subacute (days to 3 weeks), and chronic (over 3 weeks).
- Monitor with serial CT scans; anti-epileptic medications may be required.
- A hematoma causing mass effect or neurologic deficits must be surgically evacuated.

❑ Epidural Hematoma
- Due to a tear of the middle meningeal artery.
- Usually occurs with a temporal bone fracture.
- CT: Lentiform density.
- Life-threatening injury because patient's mental status can deteriorate quickly after "lucid interval."

❑ Subarachnoid Hemorrhage
- Traumatic versus aneurysmal.
- CT: Serpiginous density.
- Common after head injury.

❑ Return to Play for Intracranial Vascular Injuries
- Patients are unable to return to play after intracranial surgery.

Second Impact Syndrome

- Occurs when an athlete who has had one head trauma sustains a second injury before symptoms associated with the first have resolved.
- Usually occurs 1 week after initial injury.
- Can occur without LOC after either traumatic event.
- Involves rapid brain swelling and herniation because the brain has lost autoregulation of its blood supply.
- Brain stem failure develops in 2 to 5 minutes.
- Physical examination: Rapidly dilating pupils, loss of eye movement, respiratory failure, coma.
- On-field management: Removal of helmet and pads for rapid intubation.
- Mortality is 50%; morbidity is 100%.

Head Injuries Questions

1. A 19-year-old basketball player is fouled during a layup and hits his head. There is no LOC, and the player walks to the appropriate side and sits on the bench. He is disoriented at first, responds appropriately after a few minutes, and has no headache. You use the Standardized Assessment of Concussion (SAC) instrument to evaluate him and note that his score is similar to his baseline scores obtained during pre-season. The coach is asking whether the player can return to the game. What is the next step in his management?

A. Observe for additional 15 minutes before return to play.
B. Observe on sideline for the remainder of the game.
C. Transport to an ER.
D. Have patient perform aerobic exercise and repeat the SAC assessment.
E. Allow his immediate return to play.

2. A 17-year-old middle linebacker is involved in a tackle during a high school football game. After clearing of the play, the player remains down and motionless. You, the team physician, run onto the field and evaluate the patient. What is the first thing you do?

A. Remove the player's helmet.
B. Assess the player's breathing.
C. Assess the player's circulation.
D. Assess the player's airway.
E. Stabilize the player's head and C-spine and transport him on a rigid backboard to the sidelines.

Cervical Spine

Burners/Stingers

- Injuries to the brachial plexus resulting from compression, traction, or direct trauma (Fig. 9–2).
- One of the most common cervical spine injuries, reported as occurring in 49% to 65% of collegiate football players.
- C5-C6 most commonly affected, affecting the deltoid, biceps, and rotator cuff.
- Unilateral upper extremity pain, radiculopathy, and weakness that is reversible.
- Radiography: Evaluate coronal alignment, cervical foramina, and stability (Fig. 9–3).
- Magnetic resonance imaging (MRI): Evaluate for suspected spinal cord or nerve root injury, canal or foraminal stenosis, and herniated cervical disc.
- Electromyography: Controversial; can be considered if symptoms persist for 2 to 4 weeks after injury.
- Upper arm sling until symptoms resolved.
- Return to play: Patient may return to full activity when he or she has pain-free range of motion (ROM) and full strength of the upper extremity; consider protective equipment such as a cowboy collar or neck roll.

Cervical Sprains and Strains

- "Whiplash injury."
- *Strains* are muscle-tendon injuries.
- *Sprains* are ligamentous injuries.
- Neck pain, headaches, shoulder and scapular pain, swelling in the area.
- Muscle spasms, decreased range of motion.
- Radiography: Evaluate coronal alignment, cervical foramina, stability.

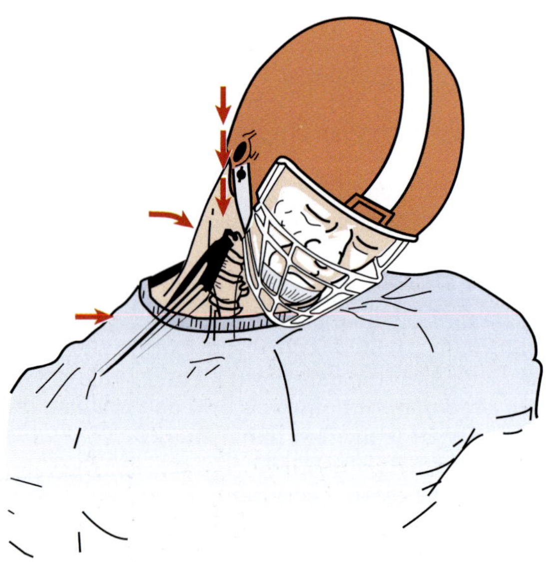

Figure 9–2 Burners and stingers of the cervical spine. *(From Warren WL, Bailes JE: On the field evaluation of athletic neck injury. Clin Sports Med 1998;17:99-110.)*

- MRI: Evaluate for suspected spinal cord or nerve root injury, canal or foraminal stenosis, and herniated cervical disc.
- CT: Evaluation of bony details such as fracture and instability.
- Physical therapy program, nonsteroidal anti-inflammatory drugs (NSAIDs), muscle relaxants, and rest.
- Surgical treatment is not usually required.
- Return to play: Only with pain-free range of motion and normal neurologic findings.

Fractures and Dislocations

- Cervical spine immobilization, airway support, and safe transportation are crucial for on-field management.
- Flexion/extension radiographs to evaluate instability.
- Unstable fractures: More than 3.5 mm of displacement, more than 11 degrees of angulation, and destruction of the anterior or posterior ligaments (Fig. 9–4).
- Unstable fractures: Treated with surgical fusion.
- Stable compression fractures: Treated with cervical collar.
- Occipital condyle fractures: Rare; manifest as cranial nerve palsies. CT to help classify fracture and determine treatment.
- Atlanto-occipital dislocation: Results from hyperextension, translation, and/or rotation; causes severe nerve injury.
- Hangman's fracture (axis isthmus fracture):
  - Hyperextension, axial load, and rebound flexion injury.
  - Type I: Vertical fracture with less than 3 mm of displacement, no angulation; treated with rigid orthosis for 2 to 3 months.
  - Type II: Fractures with more than 3 mm of anterolisthesis and angulation; treated with traction reduction and halo immobilization.
  - Type IIa: Angulation and no anterior translation; suggests disruption of the posterior longitudinal ligament and intervening disc; do not use traction in these injuries.
  - Type III: Vertical fracture with significant anterolisthesis; treated often with open reduction and stabilization because of the increased risk of neurologic deficit.
- Odontoid fracture: Results from flexion injury:
  - Type I: Distal tip fracture; stable if less than 2 mm of displacement; treated with hard cervical collar and monitored with flexion/extension radiographs.
  - Type II: Base of the dens fracture; most common; treated with halo immobilization or surgical intervention.
  - Type III: Fracture extending into the body of the axis; treated with closed reduction and halo immobilization.

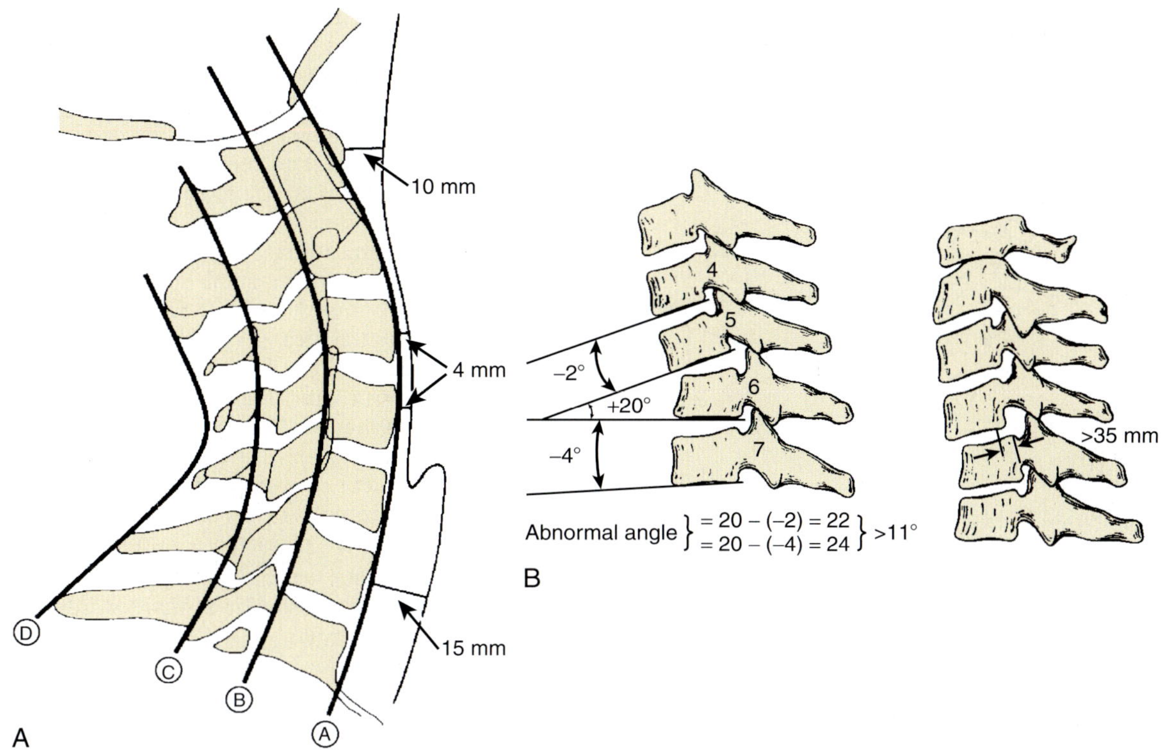

Figure 9–3 Radiographic assessment of cervical spine alignment. **A,** The anterior vertebral line, posterior vertebral line, spinolaminar line, and spinous process line should be smooth and continuous without step-off. **B,** Sagittal displacement greater than 3.5 mm or angular deformity greater than 11 degrees indicates an unstable injury of the cervical spine. *(From Crowl A, Kang J: Cervical spine. In Johnson DL, Mair SD [eds]: Clinical Sports Medicine. Philadelphia, Mosby, 2006, p 145.)*

- Facet dislocations: Treated with surgical reduction and stabilization.
- Return to play: Patients with stable compression fractures can return to play once healed, which is defined as having pain-free ROM and normal neurologic findings.

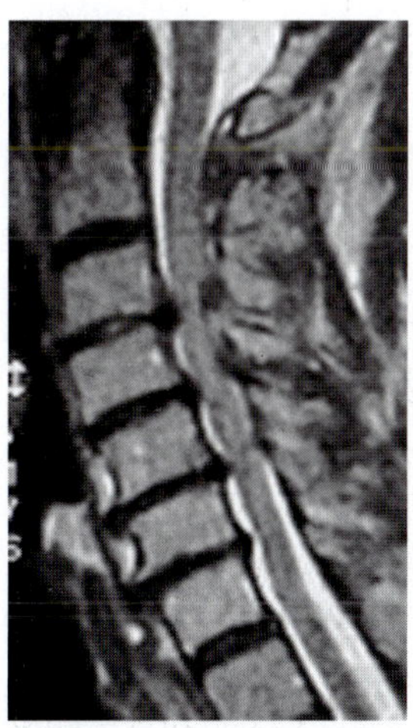

Figure 9–4 Spear tacklers in the cervical spine. Identify athletes with increased risk of permanent injury such as developmental stenosis, loss of cervical lordosis, spondylosis, old compression fractures, instability. "Spearing" refers to tackle when top of the head has an axial load onto a straightened cervical spine which can cause a spinal cord injury. Athletes with these predisposed conditions should withhold from contact activities. *(From Crowl A, Kang J: Cervical spine. In Johnson DL, Mair SD [eds]: Clinical Sports Medicine. Philadelphia, Mosby, 2006, p 146.)*

Cervical Stenosis

- Narrowing of the anteroposterior (AP) diameter of the cervical spine.
- Neurapraxia or transient neurapraxia can occur.
- Numbness, tingling, or burning sensation.
- Radiography:
  - Lateral views to evaluate stenosis.
  - Torg-Pavlov ratio should be determined on radiographs (Fig. 9–5):
    - Ratio of the AP diameters of the canal and vertebral body.
    - Used to assess stenosis and to determine whether the patient is predisposed to cervical neurapraxia.
    - Normal canal diameter on lateral radiograph: 14 to 23 mm.
    - Torg-Pavlov ratio less than 0.8 suggests congenital stenosis.
    - Disc spaces with greatest degeneration correlate to greatest stenosis and cord compression.
- Usually, with mild stenosis, symptoms resolve and there is full recovery.
- MRI: Confirms spinal cord compression:
  - Signal changes in the spinal cord suggest severe compression.
  - Compression ratio: Ratio of the smallest sagittal cord diameter to the largest transverse cord diameter at the same level.
  - Compression ratio less than 0.4 carries a poor prognosis.

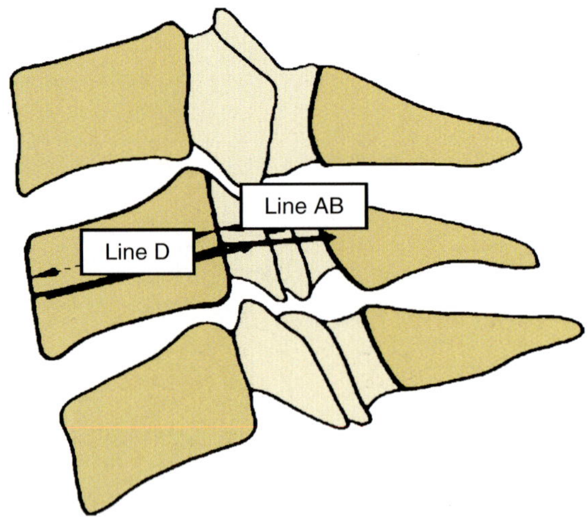

Figure 9–5 Torg-Pavlov ratio of spinal canal to vertebral body. *(From Weinberg J, Rokito S, Silber JS: Etiology, treatment, and prevention of athletic "stingers." Clin Sports Med 2003;22:493-500.)*

- CT: Gives more information on bony anatomy.
- Treatment: Depends on severity of stenosis and findings of advanced imaging studies.
  - Surgical decompression and stabilization versus conservative treatment (injections, physical therapy).
- Return to play: Return to play of an athlete with cervical stenosis is controversial; the athlete should be evaluated for concurrent instability and degenerative changes.

Spinal Cord Injuries

- Due to compression or contusion.
- Classified according to the American Spine Injury Association (ASIA) impairment scale (Fig. 9–6).
- Central cord syndrome: Most common cord injury; upper extremity motor and sensory loss in comparison with lower extremity.
- Anterior cord syndrome: Second most common cord injury; motor loss below the affected level but preservation of proprioception, deep pressure sensation, and vibration; worst prognosis (Fig. 9–7).
- Brown-Séquard syndrome: Ipsilateral motor and proprioception loss and contralateral pain and temperature loss; best prognosis.
- Posterior cord syndrome: Loss of proprioception, vibration, and deep pressure sensation but preservation of motor function; very rare injury.
- Treatment: Stabilize cervical spine with a hard cervical collar; control any signs or symptoms of neurogenic shock with fluids and vasopressors.

❑ Transient Quadriplegia

- Hyperextension injury or axial loading of the neck.
- Occurs in 7 per 10,000 collegiate football athletes.
- Players may have underlying cervical spinal stenosis or disc protrusion.
- Bilateral burning or tingling pain, with loss of strength and sensation in the arms and legs.
- Symptoms are transient, lasting 15 minutes to 36 hours.
- Immobilize the head and neck; arrange for evaluation by a spine specialist.
- Radiography and CT: Evaluate for cervical spine fracture.
- MRI: Evaluate for herniated disc, spinal stenosis, spinal cord contusion/edema.
- Treatment is focused on regaining strength.
- Return to play: The recurrence rate for transient quadriplegia is higher than 50% with return to play and is inversely correlated with canal diameter.

❑ Permanent Quadriplegia

- Mechanism similar to that for transient quadriplegia.
- Spinal injury level can be localized according to ASIA guidelines (see Fig. 9–6).
- Incomplete cord injuries include anterior cord syndrome, central cord syndrome, posterior cord syndrome, and Brown Sequard syndrome.
- Evaluate airway, breathing, and circulation (ABCs): Remove the face mask and evaluate the ability to maintain the airway while leaving the helmet itself in place. The helmet and shoulder pads should be removed together as a unit in the controlled setting of the emergency department.
- Neurogenic shock can cause hypotension and bradycardia; increase mean arterial blood pressure.
- Immobilize the head and neck, and transfer the patient on a spinal board for further evaluation in a hospital setting.
- Treatment focuses on spinal cord decompression and spinal column stability.
- Return to play: A patient who has permanent quadriplegia may participate in adaptive sports, depending on the level of spinal cord injury (Sit-Ski [CH Dye, Inc., Drigg, ID], wheelchair sports such as basketball).

Cervical Spine Questions

1. A 17-year-old high school football player sustains a burner or stinger after tackling another player. Examination immediately following the injury will most likely reveal weakness of the:

A. Infraspinatus, teres minor, and trapezius muscles.
B. Deltoid, biceps, and spinatus muscles.
C. Triceps, wrist, and finger extension muscles.
D. Latissimus dorsi and rhomboid muscles.
E. Finger flexor and interossei muscles.

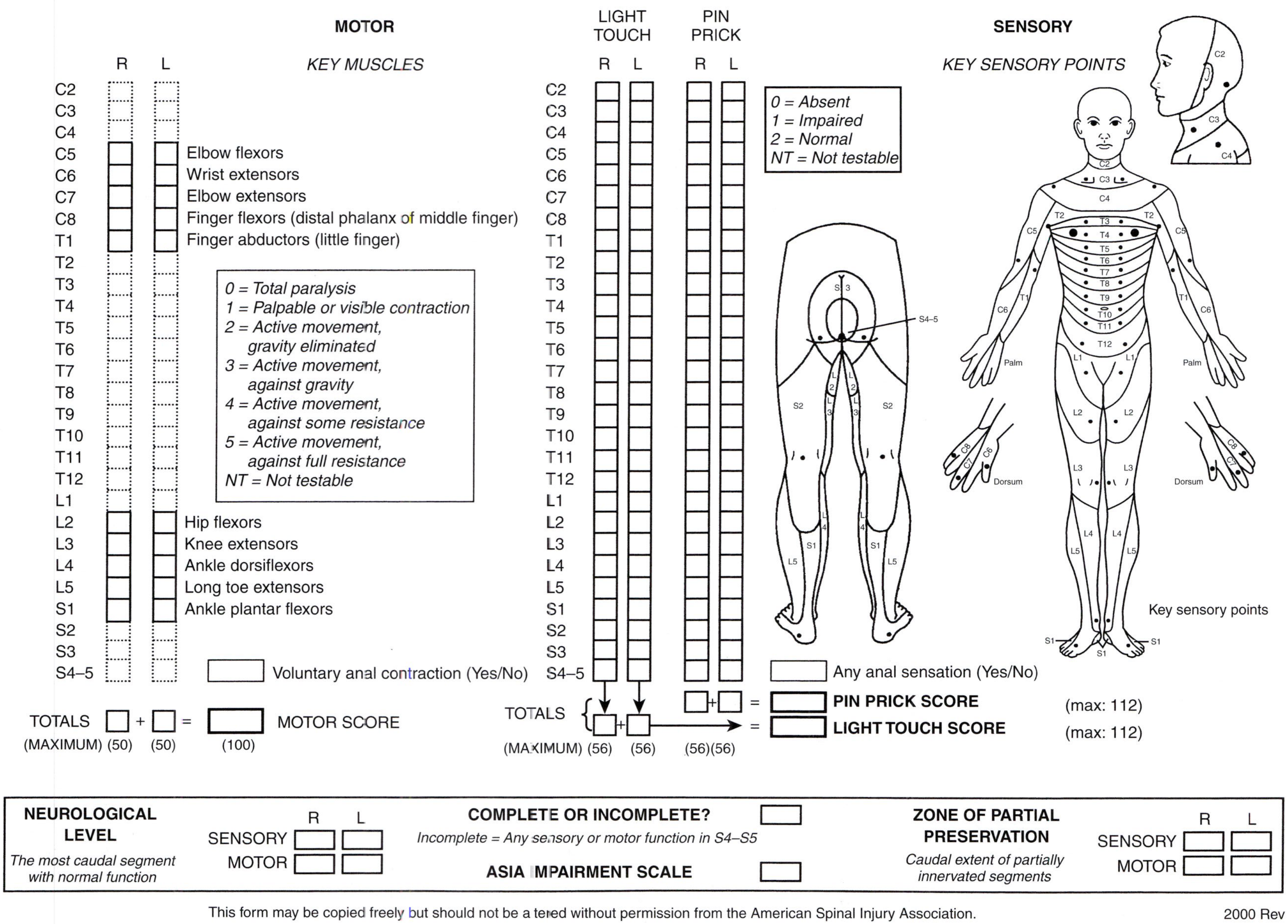

Figure 9–6 American Spine Injury Association standard neurologic classification of spinal cord injury. *(From American Spinal Injury Association: International standards for neurological and functional classification of spinal cord injury. Chicago, American Spinal Injury Association, 2002.)*

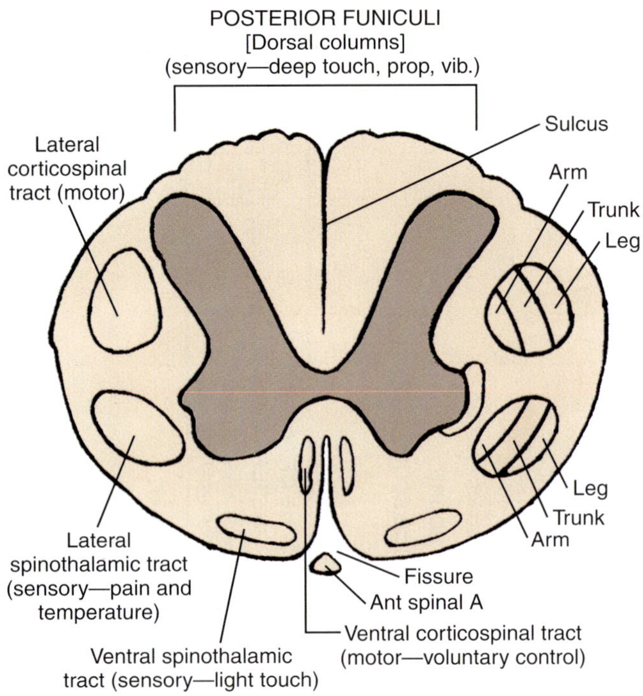

Figure 9–7 Cross-section of the spinal cord. Prop, proprioception; Vib, vibratory sense. *(From Shuler FD: Anatomy. In Miller MD [ed]: Review of Orthopaedics, 4th ed. Philadelphia, Saunders, 2004.)*

2. The mechanism of injury that accounts for the majority of cervical spine fractures or dislocations in football is:
A. Flexion rotation.
B. Posterior compression.
C. Axial loading.
D. Hyperflexion.
E. Hyperextension.

3. A 22-year-old man has burning from the supraclavicular area to the tips of his fingers while playing football. This had occurred twice before in a previous game, followed by a complete resolution of symptoms within 15 minutes and no residual pain or weakness. Appropriate management should consist of which of the following?
A. Re-examination in 20 minutes and assessment for a return to play.
B. Prescribe physical therapy (PT) and allow the patient to play the next game.
C. Monitor deltoid and biceps strength and allow return to play when strength is normal.
D. Restrict the patient from further play in this game, and obtain radiographs of the clavicle and shoulder after the game.
E. Restrict the patient from further play in this game, and obtain radiographs of the cervical spine prior to allowing him return to playing.

■

Lumbar Spine

Mechanical Low Back Pain

- Very common.
- Lower back pain, muscle spasms; usually does not cause radiculopathy.
- Radiography: Evaluate for degenerative changes, fractures, and congenital abnormalities; radiographs may not be needed in the initial workup.
- Activity modification, physical therapy program, and NSAIDs can help.

Lumbar Sprain or Strain

- Ligaments and tendons are abnormally stretched or torn.
- Large paraspinal muscles support the spinal column.
- Lower back and upper buttock pain; neurologic findings normal.
- Pain is associated with activity and usually relieved with rest.
- Radiography: Evaluate for degenerative changes, fractures, and congenital abnormalities.
- Treatment with rest, NSAIDs, and physical therapy.
- Further evaluation with MRI or CT if symptoms persist.
- Return to play: Allowed when symptoms have resolved.

Scoliosis

- Abnormal curvature of the spine.
- Uneven shoulders, one shoulder blade more prominent than the other, uneven waist, leaning to one side, one hip higher than the other.
- May be idiopathic or congenital.
- Can cause chronic low back pain.
- Radiography: Evaluate for C- or S-shaped curves, location of curve, direction of curve, and angle of curve:
  - Mild curve (<20 degrees): Physical therapy, radiographic monitoring.
  - Moderate curve (25-45 degrees) in a growing child: Bracing, radiographic monitoring.
  - Curves more than 45-50 degrees or in a mature skeleton: Scoliosis surgery involving fusion.
- Return to play: Depends on number of levels fused. Newer techniques allow shorter levels of fusion and relatively maintained ROM, and patients can return to play if pain-free and neurologically normal.

Spondylolysis

- Defect in the pars interarticularis of the spine.
- Repetitive hyperextension of the lumbar spine.
- Most common in football interior linemen, gymnasts, and divers (hyperextension sports).

- Physical examination can reproduce pain with provocative hyperextension as well as tightening of the hamstrings.
- Radiography: Oblique and lateral views for "scotty dog" picture.
- CT: Evaluate the pars defect.
- Single-photon emission CT can elucidate the acuity of the lesion (i.e., whether the pars is metabolically active).
- Conservative treatment with bracing and rest.
- Return to play: Possible when patient has pain-free ROM, especially in hyperextension, is neurologically normal, and has supple hamstrings and iliopsoas muscles.

Spondylolisthesis

- Anterior displacement of one vertebral body over another.
- Most common at L4-L5 and L5-S1 vertebral levels.
- Graded I through V according to the severity of the slip (Fig. 9–8).
- Types: Dysplastic, isthmic, degenerative, traumatic, pathologic, and postsurgical:
  - Isthmic is the most common, occurring in patients from 5 to 50 years old; associated with a predisposition to fracture of the pars (L5-S1).
- Physical examination: Hamstring tightness, waddle gait, postural abnormalities.
- Treatment: Flexion exercises, braces, and physical therapy program.
- Surgical treatment consisting of decompression and fusion stabilization should be performed if symptoms persist or neurologic deficits occur.
- Return to play:
  - Stability of slip predicts return to play ability; classically, stability is defined as less than 4 degrees of motion and less than 12 degrees of change in disc angulation on flexion/extension films.
  - Also, patients with stable grade 1 (0%-25%) and grade 2 (26%-50%) slips are cleared for sports if neurologically normal, and those with grade 3 (51%-75%) and grade 4 (76%-100%) slips are withheld from sports and contact activities.

Herniated Disc

- The intervertebral disc is composed of the annulus fibrosus (AF), the cartilage endplate (CE), and the nucleus pulposus (NP) (Fig. 9–9).
- Contact sports and weight lifting can increase the incidence of disc herniation (Fig. 9–9).
- May be from a traumatic event and have an acute onset of symptoms.
- Disc herniation is associated with lower extremity radiculopathy.
- Patient has more pain when sitting in a flexed position because disc pressure is highest then; pain is relieved with lying supine.
- Physical examination: Decreased range of motion, paraspinous tenderness secondary to muscle spasms.

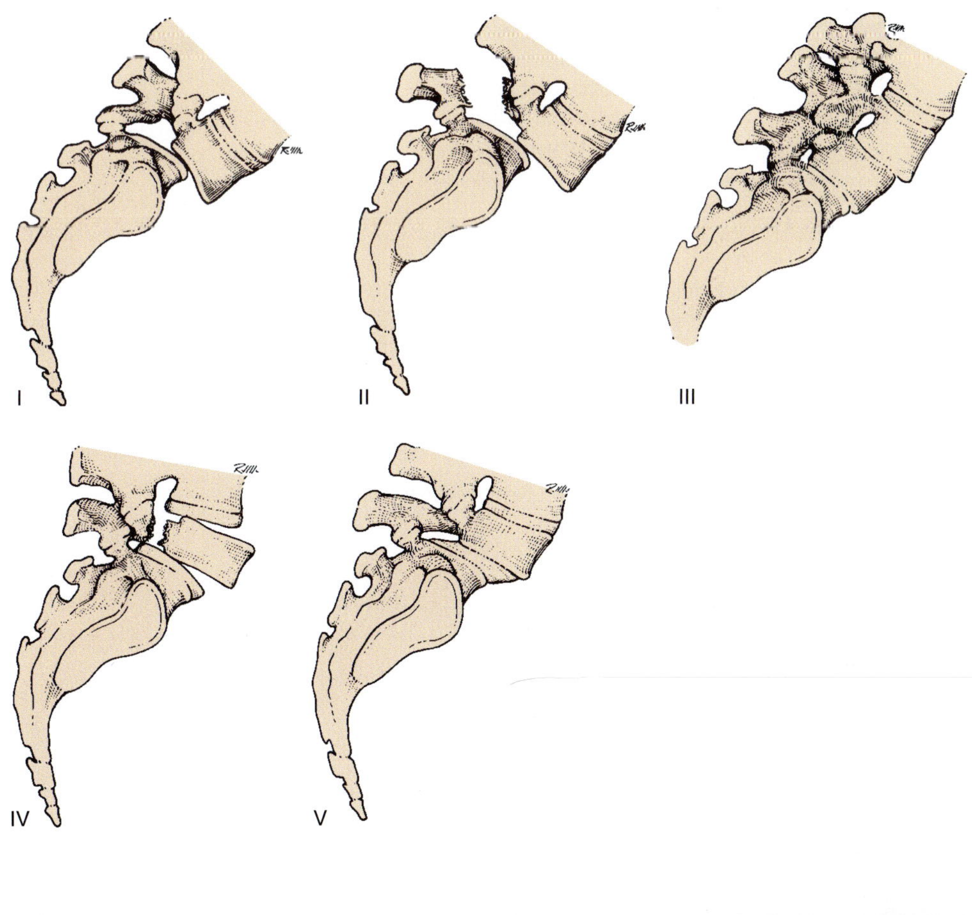

Figure 9–8 Five types of spondylolisthesis. I, dysplastic; II, isthmic; III, degenerative; IV, traumatic; V, pathologic. *(From Freeman BL III: Scoliosis and kyphosis. In Canale ST [ed]: Campbell's Operative Orthopaedics, 10th ed. Philadelphia, Mosby, 2003.)*

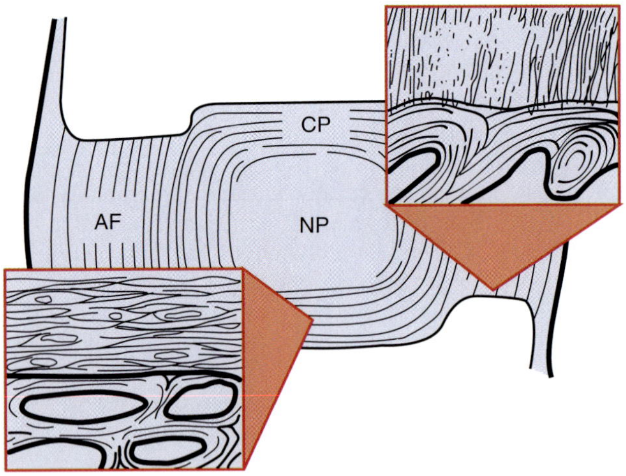

Figure 9–9 Schematic representation of orientation of fibers in disc and endplate. AF, annulus fibrosus; CP, cartilaginous endplate; NP, nucleus pulposus.

- Signs and symptoms are specific to the nerve level involved.
- Herniated discs most common at L4-L5, followed by L5-S1.
- Posterolateral herniations are most common because the posterior longitudinal ligament is the weakest.
- Physical therapy program, bracing, and possible epidural corticosteroid injection.
- MRI: Evaluate for disc herniation, degenerative disc disease, and nerve compression.
- Cauda equina syndrome: Bowel or bladder dysfunction, saddle anesthesia, and bilateral lower extremity symptoms.
  - Requires urgent surgery to prevent permanent neurologic damage.
- Surgical treatment is discectomy.
- Return to play: After formal physical and aquatic therapy, patients with normal neurologic findings and pain-free ROM may resume sports.

Disc Degeneration

- In disc degeneration, an intervertebral disc dehydrates and the amount of fibrous tissue increases.
- Process begins with annular tears and ligament stretching, proceeds to further tearing and laxity, and ends with loss of disc height.
- Genetic predisposition and repeated trauma can accelerate degeneration.
- MRI: Decreased signal within the disc space (dark disc) on T2-weighted images can represent disc degeneration or dehydration.
- Discograms: Correlate MRI findings with clinical symptoms by determining the disc is the pain generator.
- Return to play: After formal physical and aquatic therapy, a patient with normal neurologic findings and pain-free ROM may resume sports.

Lumbar Spine Questions

1. A 15-year-old dancer who has had brief episodes of back pain over the past 2 years now reports a 3-month history of low back pain and a decreased tolerance for dance. Radiographs demonstrate spondylolysis at L5, but no spondylolisthesis. The patient reports no leg pain and no bowel or bladder difficulties. Management should now consist of:
A. Posterior spinal fusion from L5 to S1.
B. Primary repair with an iliac crest bone graft.
C. Posterior spinal fusion of L4-L5.
D. A pantaloon body cast and 6 weeks of bed rest.
E. Rest, NSAIDs, and limited dancing.

2. Examination of the radiographs of a 15-year-old football player that were obtained to rule out scoliosis reveals an isthmic spondylolisthesis. The studies show a 10-degree lumbar scoliosis, along with a 26% forward slip of L5 on S1 because of a pars defect in L5. The patient reports no pain, and neurologic findings are normal. Management should include:
A. Posterior spinal fusion of L5 to S1.
B. Repair of the pars defects, without fusing to an adjacent level.
C. Brace treatment until the patient reaches maturity.
D. No further participation in football or contact sports.
E. No treatment or restrictions unless symptoms develop.

3. A 15-year-old female swimmer presents for evaluation of scoliosis. She has a mild right-sided rib prominence. Which clinical symptom or sign should alert the clinician that this problem is not idiopathic scoliosis?
A. Back pain.
B. Normal neurologic findings.
C. Flexible left lumbar curve.
D. Normal pulmonary function.
E. Presentation during adolescence.

4. While covering a club swim meet, you are approached by a 13 year-old female diver who states that she has had chronic low back pain and very tight hamstrings over 6 months. What condition is likely?
A. Congenital hip dysplasia.
B. Leg length discrepancy.
C. Transitional vertebrae.
D. Lumbar disc protrusion.
E. Spondylolysis.

References and Resources

Bailes, J.E., Hadley, M.N., Quigley, M.R., et al., 1991. Management of athletic injuries of the cervical spine and spinal cord. Neurosurgery 29, 491.

Coumans, J.V., Lauerman, W.C., 2002. Head and spine. In: Miller, M.D., Cooper, D.E., Warner J.J.P., (Eds.), Review of Sports Medicine and Arthroscopy, second ed. Philadelphia: Harcourt Health Sciences, pp. 262–269.

Fazio, V.C., Lovell, M.R., Pardini, J.E., Collins, M.W., 2007. The relation between post concussion symptoms and neurocognitive performance in concussed athletes. NeuroRehabilitation 22, 207–216.

Gill, S.S., Townsend, M.A., 2009. Burners/stingers—brachial plexopathy. In: Miller, M.D., MacKnight, J. (Eds.), Essential Orthopaedics. Elsevier, Philadelphia, pp. 116-1–116-4.

Greenberg, M.S., 2001. Handbook of Neurosurgery, fifth ed. Springer, Berlin, pp. 626–631, 717–719.

Ladd, A., Scranton, P.E., 1986. Congenital cervical stenosis presenting as transient quadriplegia in athletes. J. Bone Joint Surg. Am. 68, 1371.

Rhee, J.M., Riew, K.D., 2006. Cervical spondylotic myelopathy: Including ossification of the posterior longitudinal ligament. In: Spivak, J.M., Connolly, P. (Eds.), Orthopaedic Knowledge Update: Spine 3. American Academy of Orthopaedic Surgeons, pp. 235–246. Rosemont, IL.

Schatz, P., Pardini, J.E., Lovell, M.R., et al., 2006. Sensitivity and specificity of the ImPACT Test Battery for concussion in athletes. Arch. Clin. Neuropyschol. 21, 91–99.

Torg, J.S., 1985. Epidemiology, pathomechanics, and prevention of athletic injuries to the cervical spine. Med. Sci. Sports Exerc. 17, 295.

CHAPTER 10

Sports Medicine Research and Statistics

JOSEPH M. HART

Common Research Designs

- Clinical research studies can be *prospective* or *retrospective*.
  - Retrospective studies start by identifying a patient population and making observations backwards in time via medical record or other historical review.
  - Conversely, studies that are prospective make observations forward in time.
  - *Longitudinal* studies make repeated observations of the same variables/items over time.
- *Observational* or *descriptive* research studies can be retrospective or prospective. This type of study is not designed to allocate a treatment or other intervention and cannot establish cause-effect relationships. Descriptive/observational studies are inexpensive and less time-consuming and can generate hypotheses from which larger-scale experimental studies can develop. These study designs may help the understanding of relationships between disease/injury and other specific variables.

Observational Research Designs

- *Case reports* are descriptions of a unique injury or disease in one patient. There are no attempts at data analysis with case reports.
- *Case series* involve a *cohort* of patients, which is defined as a group of patients who have a common disease, injury, or other characteristic of interest. Case reports and case series do not have any control group and are typically not designed to provide information about frequency or distribution of injury or disease.
- *Cohort studies* identify a group of patients with similar characteristics. Data can be collected retrospectively or prospectively. Data often include *subjective* (patient-reported) and/or *objective* (clinician-measured) outcomes after disease, injury, surgery, and so on. Specific study cohorts can be defined on the basis of study inclusion and exclusion criteria. Associations and differences among study groups can be made with the use of statistical tests and may be interpreted to determine clinical importance.
- *Case-control studies* are a form of a cohort study whereby patients are selected on the basis of their injury or disease status. Observations can be made prospectively or retrospectively. There is no intervention or treatment allocation, but data from the study cohort of interest are compared with those of a control group.
- *Cross-sectional studies* involve data observations of a particular cohort of patients at one point in time with no follow-up. These studies are described as being "snap-shots" that are useful for describing the frequency and distribution of a disease, injury, or characteristic within a population in order to make associations with other variables at that moment in time.

Experimental Research Designs

- Experimental studies involve the allocation of an intervention or treatment to a cohort of patients in order to test a specific hypothesis.

Data are measured prospectively to determine cause-effect relationships. Clinical studies that are experimental are called *clinical trials*.

- A study in which patients receive both interventions in sequence has a *crossover* design. Crossover studies do not have a comparison group because each study patient or participant receives both (all) interventions one after the other. In *parallel* design, independent groups of patients are randomly (or nonrandomly) assigned to receive one of the treatments; each subject/participant receives only one treatment.
- The "gold standard" regarding the ability to establish cause-effect relationships is the *randomized controlled trial* (RCT). This is a clinical trial that is designed to provide maximum protection against common threats to the *internal validity* (ability to attribute differences in outcomes to allocated treatment) and *external validity* (ability to generalize to a population of interest) of an experimental research design.

Common Research Design Terms

- Most research designs contain a variable that is being measured (*dependent variable*) and a variable that is being manipulated (*independent variable*).
- The independent variable is the factor that is being manipulated or controlled. The dependent variable is what is measured. The researcher develops a hypothesis that changes in the dependent variable will be due to manipulation of the independent variable. Intervention is an example of an independent variable and may have two or more levels, such as treatment A, treatment B, and control or no treatment.
- Time is also an example of an independent variable (baseline, 1 year post surgery, 2 years post surgery). Various time points can be selected during the design of an experiment. Dependent variables are measured for patients in each group and at each point in time and may include patient-reported (subjective) outcomes or other quantitative outcomes that are measured from clinical, laboratory, or other medical tests (objective).

Common Threats to Research Designs

- Several issues will commonly threaten the validity of conclusions drawn from the results of a research study. Despite the fact that these issues are unintentionally introduced, they are inherent to research study designs and must be acknowledged and addressed appropriately.
- *Confounding variables* are extraneous factors to a study design that influence both the independent variable (grouping factor) and the dependent variable (measurement/outcome). Confounding is a major threat to the internal validity of a study, because cause-effect relationships resulting from the study may be due to the independent variable(s) or to the confounding factors.
- *Bias* is typically unintentional, systematic error that is nonrandom and will corrupt and threaten the validity of a research study. Bias can occur when specific patient populations are identified for sampling (*selection bias*), when patients are lost to follow-up (*nonresponder bias*), when outcomes are being measured subjectively (*recall bias*) or objectively (*observer/interviewer bias*), and so on. Regardless of the source of bias, there are several considerations essential to designing a study that contains safeguards against the common threats to validity.

Designing a Strong Research Study

- Random allocation of patients into study groups ensures that bias and confounding factors will be equally distributed among study groups. Typically, a random number generator is used to assign each patient to a given treatment or intervention group. In truly randomized designs, each patient has an equal chance of being assigned to any of the included study interventions/groups.
- *Blinding* is a method to keep either the study subjects or observers (*single-blind*) or both the subjects and observers (*double-blind*) from knowing the identities of the treatment or intervention groups. This approach minimizes several forms of bias inherent to reporting or evaluating study outcomes.
- Matching subjects between groups on the basis of specific characteristics helps control for confounding factors. For example, it may be necessary to match subjects according to gender, age, or activity level to ensure that these potentially confounding factors are equally distributed among the study groups. Study designs may also match right and left limbs of the same subject or the same specimen donor to control for confounding factors.
- *A control group* is important because it allows the researchers to describe an outcome measure in a group that receives no

intervention. It provides an essential comparison with outcomes of interventions and treatments. Control subjects can be included concurrent with a study design (*randomized designs*), can be collected sequentially (*crossover designs*), or can be collected in the past (*historical controls*). Control groups may also receive a placebo, or sham intervention, that is intended to control for the *placebo effect*—bias arising from the apparent efficacy of a study intervention that is actually due to the simple act of treatment and not to the treatment itself.

- The clinical trial providing the highest level of evidence is randomized, double-blinded, and prospective with concurrent controls.

Levels of Evidence

- Evidence-based medicine guidelines apply findings from research studies that influence clinical practice and decision-making. Greater influence on clinical recommendations is based on findings from well-designed studies that have the highest level of validity (Table 10–1).
- The level of evidence is based on the quality of the research design with respect to potential threats to validity, which would thereby influence any cause-effect relationships derived from research findings. Level 1 is reserved for the highest-quality, most influential studies, and level 5 for the lowest-quality, lowest-impact research studies (see Table 10–1). Levels of evidence ratings have been identified for *therapeutic studies* (investigating the outcomes from a study treatment), *prognostic studies* (reports of the effect of a patient characteristic on the outcome of a disease), *diagnostic studies* (assessments of diagnostic tools), and *economic studies* (development of economic or decision models).
- The level of evidence determines the strength and impact of research findings in guiding clinical care of patients.

Table 10–1 Levels of Evidence Guidelines for Therapeutic Studies*

	Description of Study Design
Level I	
a	Systematic reviews of randomized controlled trials (RCTs)
b	Individual RCTs
c	All-or-none studies (studies in which all patients die when treatment is not available and no patients die when treatment is available)
Level II	
a	Systematic reviews of cohort studies
b	Individual cohort studies
	Low-quality RCTs
c	Outcomes research
Level III	
a	Systematic reviews of case-control studies
b	Individual case-control studies
Level IV	Case series
	Poor-quality cohort and case-control studies
Level V	Expert opinion

*According to the Oxford Centre for Evidence-Based Medicine as of March 2009; see the Centre's website: www.cebm.net.

Epidemiology and Biostatistics

- *Epidemiology* involves the study of the distribution, frequency, associations and determinants of injury or disease. Common measures of frequency include prevalence and incidence; common measures of association include relative risks and odds ratios (Table 10–2).
- *Prevalence* is the proportion of individuals within a population who have an outcome of interest now or at a particular point in time. Prevalence values are calculated as the number of existing cases of disease or injury divided by the total population who are identified to be at risk for it. Prevalence is interpreted as the percentage of patients who have an injury or disease at that moment in time.
- *Incidence* is the proportion of new cases of an outcome or disease within a specific interval. Therefore, to calculate incidence, a follow-up period or interval is required. Incidence is calculated as the number of new cases of disease or injury divided by the total population at risk for it. It is interpreted as the occurrence of new cases over a particular period.
- *Incidence rates* are calculated with respect to exposures to risk.
  - For example, if 100 athletes participated in 10 games and 20 practices in a single season, then each athlete would be exposed to risk for injury on 30 occasions, totaling 3000 exposures for the 100 athletes.
- The *absolute risk* is an incidence in which the number of new occurrences of disease or injury over a particular period is divided by the total number of patients at risk for it.
  - For example, if 10 of 1000 patients undergoing anterior cruciate ligament (ACL) reconstruction experience a postoperative infection within a week following surgery, the absolute risk for infection is 1% (10/1000).

Table 10–2 Common Epidemiologic Measures and Their Interpretation

Measure	Calculation	Interpretation
Prevalence	$\frac{\text{No. existing instances of outcome}}{\text{Total population at risk}}$	The proportion of individuals within a population who exhibit an outcome of interest
Incidence	$\frac{\text{No. new instances of outcome}}{\text{Total population at risk}}$	The proportion of new instances of an outcome of interest within a specific time interval
Absolute risk	$\frac{\text{No. new outcomes (incidence)}}{\text{Total population at risk}}$	The proportion of the population of interest that are at risk for development of the outcome of interest
Relative risk	$\frac{\text{Incidence in an exposed group}}{\text{Incidence in an unexposed group}}$	1.0: Risk/odds of outcome are identical between groups
Odds ratio	$\frac{\text{Probability of outcome in an exposed group}}{\text{Probability of an outcome in an unexposed group}}$	>1.0: Risk/odds of outcome is greater in exposed group than in unexposed group <1.0: Risk/odds of outcome is less in exposed group than in unexposed group
Specificity	$\frac{\text{True negatives}}{\text{Total patients without disease}}$	Of all patients who DO NOT have the disease or outcome of interest, the proportion who tested negative. Specific clinical tests have high true-negative and low false-positive rates.
Sensitivity	$\frac{\text{True positives}}{\text{Total patients with disease}}$	Of all patients who have the disease or outcome of interest, the proportion who tested positive. Sensitive clinical tests have high true-positive and low false-negative rates
Positive predictive value	$\frac{\text{True positives}}{\text{Total patients testing positive}}$	Proportion of patients with a positive test result who were correctly diagnosed
Negative predictive value	$\frac{\text{True negatives}}{\text{Total patients testing negative}}$	Proportion of patients with a negative test result who were correctly diagnosed
Positive likelihood ratio	$\frac{\text{Sensitivity}}{(1 - \text{Specificity})}$	For example, (+)LR = 5 means that a positive test result indicates that the patient is five times more likely to have the outcome of interest than a patient with a negative result
Negative likelihood ratio	$\frac{(1 - \text{Sensitivity})}{\text{Specificity}}$	For example, (–)LR = 0.2 means that a negative test result will be present in only 2 out of every 10 patients who actually have the outcome of interest.

- *Relative risk (RR)* is used to determine associations between the incidence of injury or disease in two cohorts. RR is calculated as the incidence of injury or disease in one group divided by the incidence of injury or disease in another group. Groups can be defined as a cohort of patients who were exposed to risk or to an intervention. RR values range from 0 to infinity and are interpreted relative to a value of 1.0:
  - *RR = 1.0* indicates that the incidence of the outcome of interest is identical in the (exposed and unexposed) groups.
  - *RR < 1* indicates an inverse relationship, or a decreased risk in the exposed group.
  - *RR > 1* indicates increased risk among patients in the exposed group (group presented in the numerator of the RR calculation).
  - In the comparison of a treatment (exposed) group with a control group for a particular outcome of interest, an RR value of 0.5 would indicate that treated patients have half the risk that the untreated patients do for experiencing the outcome of interest; an RR value of 2.5 would indicate that treated patients have a 2½ times higher risk than the untreated patients for experiencing the outcome of interest.
- *Odds* can be calculated as the percentage of new cases or instances in a given population (i.e., risk) divided by the proportion of the population that remained healthy during the same period. *Odds ratios* are more commonly used in retrospective studies and are calculated as the probability of injury or disease in an exposed group divided by the probability of injury or disease in an unexposed group. Interpretation of odds ratios is similar to interpretation of RR.

Effectiveness of Diagnostic Tools

- Effectiveness of diagnostic tools can be measured by constructing a 2×2 *contingency table* (Table 10–3) that compares the outcome of a specific diagnostic test with a gold standard:
  - In a person who does have the disease or outcome of interest:
    - A positive diagnostic test result is a *true-positive* result.

Table 10–3 Calculations of Specificity, Sensitivity, Positive and Negative Predictive Values*

	Disease Present (+)	Disease Absent (–)		
Diagnostic Test (+)	True positives	False positives	Total patients with positive diagnostic Test = True positives + False negatives	Positive predictive value = True positives ÷ Total patients with positive test result
Diagnostic Test (–)	False negatives	True negatives	Total patients with Negative diagnostic test = False negatives + True negatives	Negative predictive value = True negatives ÷ Total patients with negative test result
	Total patients with disease = True positives + False negatives	Total without disease = False positives + True negatives		
	Sensitivity = True positives ÷ Total patients with disease	Specificity = True negatives ÷ Total patients without disease		

*Presented in relation to a 2×2 contingency table. All patients (N) can be calculated by summing the 4 boxes in the contingency table. Prevalence can be calculated as Total patients with disease ÷ N.

- A negative diagnostic test result is a *false-negative* result.
- In a person who does *not* have the disease or outcome of interest:
  - A positive test result is a *false-positive* result.
  - A negative diagnostic test result is a *true-negative* result.
- *Accuracy* describes the ability of a test or measure to differentiate between positive (+) and negative (–) diagnoses. Therefore, accuracy can be calculated as a percentage by dividing the number of patients with true-positive and true-negative results by the total number of patients in a given study. Similarly, *validity* describes the ability of a measure, test, or instrument to effectively represent truth and reality.
- *Precision* describes the repeatability of a test result with multiple testing; that is, the ability of test to yield similar scores or results when the same specimen or patient is tested on multiple occasions. Analogous to precision is *reliability* which describes the reproducibility of a measure.
- One method of establishing reliability is the use of an *intraclass correlation coefficient* (ICC). This measure ranges from 0 to 1.0, and 1.0 describes a perfectly reliable and repeatable test. This test can be used to compare examination findings between two examiners or the findings of the same examiner over multiple trials.
- Sensitivity, specificity, and positive and negative predictive values can be calculated from a contingency table (see Table 10–3).
  - *Sensitivity* describes the ability to detect true-positive test results.
  - *Specificity* describes the ability to detect true-negative test results (see Table 10–2).
  - When the result of a highly sensitive (Sn) test is negative (high sensitivity = few false-negative results), it is good for ruling OUT an injury. (Pneumonic: SnOUT.)
  - When the result of a highly specific (Sp) test is positive (high specificity = few false-positive results), it is good for ruling IN an injury or disease. (Pneumonic: SpIN.)
  - The positive predictive value of a particular diagnostic test describes the proportion of patients with a positive test result and who were correctly diagnosed (actually have the disease of interest). Conversely, the negative predictive value describes the proportion of

patients with a negative test result and who were correctly diagnosed.

- Likelihood ratios (LRs) are calculated from sensitivity and specificity:
- *Positive likelihood ratios* describe the impact of a positive examination finding (clinical test result) on the probability that a disease exists:

$$(+)\text{LR} = \frac{\text{sensitivity}}{(1 - \text{specificity})}$$

- *Negative likelihood ratios* describe the impact of a negative clinical test on the probability that the disease is present:

$$(-)\text{LR} = \frac{(1 - \text{sensitivity})}{\text{specificity}}$$

- *Receiver operating characteristic curves* are graphical representations of the relationships between sensitivity and specificity whereby the sensitivity value is plotted on the vertical axis and 1 – specificity is plotted on the horizontal axis. The area under this curve is represents the overall diagnostic value of a given test result. A value of 1.0 indicates a perfectly accurate diagnostic test; a value of 0.5 indicates a diagnostic test that is no better than a random guess.

Descriptive and Inferential Statistics

Basic Terminology

- A *population* of patients has a common characteristic of clinical or scientific interest.
- Because it is impossible to observe the entire population, we take a smaller *sample* of patients or specimens that we assume is representative of the entire population of interest.
- *Random sampling* gives all members of an entire population an equal chance of being selected for observation or experimentation. This is typically not possible for most research designs and an unavoidable limitation to most of them.

Types of Data

- Data collected from a patient, subject, or specimen can be classified as continuous or categorical:
  - *Continuous data,* such as height, weight, time, and age, have an infinite number of possible values.
  - *Categorical or discrete data* have a limited number of possible values:
  - Binary (Yes/No, Failure/Success, Satisfactory/Unsatisfactory, gender).
  - Ordered (severities—mild, moderate, severe; outcome—excellent, good, fair, poor).
  - Unordered (race).
- Data can be plotted in *frequency distributions* to summarize or describe important characteristics of the study patient sample. Frequency distributions are histograms that plot the frequency of occurrences of each possible outcome (Fig. 10–1).

Descriptive Statistics

- Descriptive statistics, such as mean, median, and mode, are collectively termed *measures of central tendency* and are used to characterize the basic features of study data distributions. The dispersion of a data distribution is characterized by standard deviation, range, and percentiles.
- The *mean* is an average calculated as the sum of all scores from a sample, divided by the number of subjects (n) from that sample.
- The *median* is the value that divides the data set into two equal halves. Half of the values in a data set are greater than the median, and half of the values in a data set are less than the median.
- The *mode* is the most frequently occurring data point in the frequency distribution.
- The *standard deviation* describes how spread out the values are in a data set. A higher standard deviation means that the variability among the data are greater and the data points span a wider range.

Characterizing the Data Frequency Distribution

- A *normal* or *gaussian distribution* is a data set that clusters evenly around the mean. The mean, median, and mode of a gaussian distribution are the same value.
- In a normal distribution, 68% of the values are within 1 standard deviation above and below the mean, and 95% of the values are within 2 standard deviations above and below the mean (Fig. 10–2).
- *Skewness* is a measure of the symmetry of a data distribution (histogram). Data distributions can be skewed to the left (*negative skew*) or the right (*positive skew*). If one or more data values are far from the rest of the values (i.e., most of the scores are close to 100 units, and 1 score is 950 units) the distribution is *skewed positively* (if the outlier value [see definition in later section] is excessively high) or *negatively* (if the outlier value is excessively low) (see Fig. 10–1).
- *Kurtosis* describes the peak of the data distribution and whether it is excessively high or flat (see Fig. 10–1). This measure describes the relative concentration of data points at the center or in the peripheral areas (tails) of the data distribution.

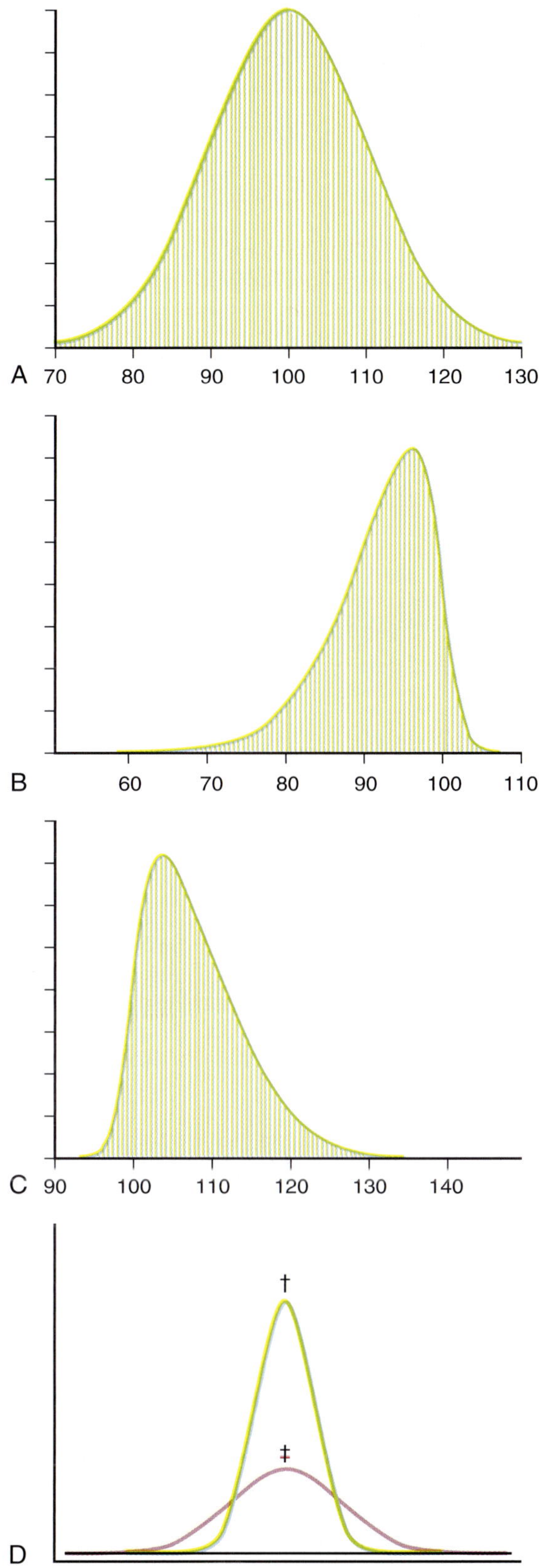

Figure 10–1 Examples of normally distributed data (**A**) and of data distributions that are skewed to the left (negative skew) (**B**), that are skewed to the right (positive skew) (**C**), and that exhibit high (†) and low (‡) kurtosis (**D**).

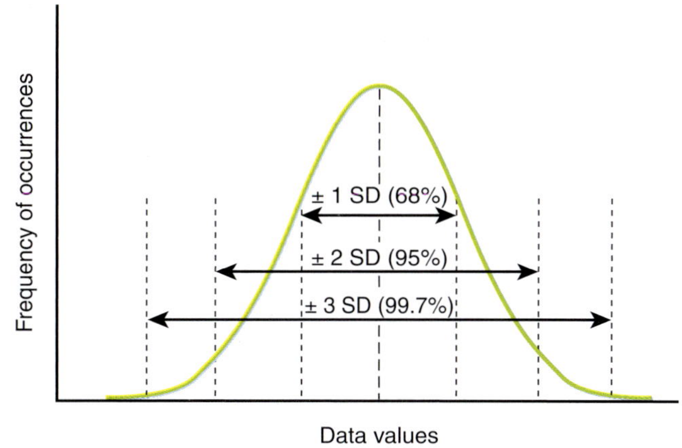

Figure 10–2 Graphical representation of the calculation of 95% confidence intervals, which are based on the assumption that the data are distributed normally. Note that 68% of the data is contained within an area ±1 standard deviations, 95% within ± 2 standard deviations, and 99.7% within ± 3 standard deviations from the mean.

Inferential Statistics

- Inferential statistics attempt to generalize data collected from a representative sample to the entire population. Inferential statistics can be used to test a hypothesis about the differences between groups of data or the associations between groups of data using specific statistical tests (Table 10–4).
- Inferential statistics can be divided into *parametric statistics* and *nonparametric statistics* (see next section for definitions). Because the ultimate goal of inferential statistics is to estimate parameters (descriptors of the entire population), thereby generalizing study findings to the population of interest, default statistical tests should be parametric.
- However, parametric statistics are valid only if certain assumptions are met. Most important is the assumption that the data collected are normally distributed (resemble a gaussian distribution). This can be tested by observing the shape (skewness and kurtosis) of a data distribution (see Fig. 10–1). If the basic assumptions of a statistical test are violated, the test may no longer be valid.

Parametric and Nonparametric Tests

- *Parametric statistical tests* use the mean and standard deviations to compare groups or identify associations.
- *Nonparametric statistical tests* use medians and ranks and are therefore more powerful than parametric tests because they are less sensitive to *outliers* (data points that are considerably different from the rest of the data set), and therefore are said to be more *robust.*

Table 10–4 Basic Decision-Making for Statistical Tests

	Parametric Statistics[1]	Non-parametric Statistics[1]
Descriptive statistic	Mean and standard deviations	Median, ranks, range
Two groups[2]:		
Paired		Wilcoxon signed-rank test
Unpaired	Dependent (paired) sample t-test	Mann-Whitney U test
	Independent samples t-test	
Three or more groups[3]:		
1 dependent variable	Analysis of variance (ANOVA)	Kruskal-Wallis Test
Multiple dependent variables	Multivariate analysis of variance (MANOVA)	
Analysis including a covariate	Analysis of covariance (ANCOVA)	
Repeated observations in the same patient	Repeated measures ANOVA	
Relationship/association	Pearson product-moment correlation coefficient	Spearman rank correlation coefficient
Prediction:		
From 1 predictor variable	Simple regression	Logistic regression
From > 1 predictor variables	Multiple regression	
Categorical data:		
2 or more variables	Chi-square[4]	Chi-square[4]
Better for low sample size	Fisher's exact test	Fisher's exact test

[1]Parametric statistics are good for continuous data that are normally distributed. If the assumption of normal distributed data (among others) is violated, the use of a parametric statistic is unreliable, and a nonparametric equivalent should be used. Nonparametric tests are also good for categorical data where appropriate.
[2]If multiple dependent variables are being compared, a Bonferroni correction on the *P* value (.05/k, where k is the number of comparisons being made) is appropriate.
[3]If measurements are recorded in the same subjects/patients on multiple occasions, a repeated measures ANOVA is appropriate. If multiple, related dependent variables are being analyzed in three or more groups, a multivariate analysis of variance (MANOVA) is appropriate. If there is a need to correct for a covariate or other confounding factor, an analysis of covariance (ANCOVA) is appropriate.
[4]Because these tests are appropriate for categorical data, they may be considered parametric or nonparametric.

- Further, nonparametric statistical tests are also appropriate for categorical data and for data sets with very small sample sizes (few subjects or specimens).

Tests to Compare Two Groups of Continuous Data

- The principles underlying the t-test were developed by an employee of a beer brewing company. Because of proprietary interest regarding the use of advanced mathematics and statistics for brewing quality control, publications on the development were written under the pseudonym "Student" (Student, 1908). This explains the term Student's t-test.
- Variations of *Student's t-test* can be used to compare paired or independent data, although references to the test typically refer to the independent samples t-test.
- The *paired samples t-test* is used to compare data recorded (1) in the same patient or subject on two occasions, (2) in two tests of the same specimen, or (3) from two subjects/samples that have been matched or paired. This is also called the *dependent samples t-test.* For example, this test would be used to compare outcomes reported by patients on a visual analogue scale before and after they undergo surgical intervention.
- The *Wilxocon signed rank sum test* is the nonparametric equivalent of the dependent samples t-test.
- *The independent samples t-test* is used to compare data collected from two different groups. For example, this test would be used to compare vertical jump heights (continuous data) in patients who underwent ACL reconstructions with either patellar tendon autograft (group 1) or hamstring autograft (group 2).
- The *Mann-Whitney U test* is the nonparametric equivalent of the independent samples t-test.
- The *Bonferroni correction* is an adjustment to the *P* value (probability value; see later section) threshold that will indicate statistical significance. There is a possibility for error when multiple t-tests are performed to compare multiple outcomes (dependent variables) between the two groups. Therefore a more conservative *P* value is appropriate.
    - For example, assume that a comparison is operationally defined as being "statistically significant" when the *P* value is less than .05. When scores from three different outcome measures, the correction factor would be $P = (.05/3) = .017$, where 3 is the number of t-tests (or nonparametric equivalents) being performed in the analysis. Therefore, with a Bonferroni correction, a particular test will be "statistically significant" only if the *P* value is less than .017. Because ANOVA models (see later) account for this type of error, Bonferroni corrections are not necessary.

Tests to Compare Three or More Independent Groups

- The *analysis of variance (ANOVA or F-test)* is appropriate for comparing data from three or more independent groups. For example, to compare outcome scores among hypothetical treatment groups A, B, and C, the ANOVA test will be able to describe whether there are ($P < .05$) or are not ($P > .05$) any differences among the treatment groups but will NOT be able to describe where the specific differences are located; therefore, post hoc tests are necessary (see next section).
- *Post hoc* (Latin, "after the fact") testing: Specific tests (similar to t-tests) are used after a statistically significant ($P < .05$, for example) ANOVA test in order to determine the exact location of the group differences. In the hypothetical example just described, post hoc tests would be used to compare outcomes as follows: (1) between treatment groups A and B, (2) between treatment groups A and C, and (3) between treatment groups B and C. It is necessary to locate the exact location of statistically significant differences, because each comparison may or may not be different with a "significant" ANOVA test. Examples of common post hoc tests are Tukey's, Sidak, Bonferroni (not the same as the *P* value correction), Dunnet's, Scheffe, and Neuman-Keuls tests.
- *Multivariate analysis of variance (MANOVA) tests* are appropriate when there are multiple, related dependent variables. For example if it is necessary to compare age, height, weight, and range of motion among four different treatment groups, a MANOVA test is appropriate. Post hoc testing follows as described previously, in order to determine the exact location of the differences.
- *Analysis of covariance (ANCOVA) tests* are appropriate when there are confounding factors that must be accounted for in the statistical analysis. For example, if the comparison of an outcome score after surgery is confounded by preoperative (baseline) values, the ANOVA can be adjusted in order to account for baseline scores while comparing outcomes between treatment groups. Post hoc testing follows as described previously in order to determine the exact location of differences.
- *Repeated measures ANOVA tests* are appropriate for serial testing at multiple (more than two) time points: before surgery, 3 months following surgery, 6 months following surgery, and so on. Post hoc testing follows as described previously in order to determine the exact location of differences.
- The *Kruskal-Wallis test* is the nonparametric equivalent of the analysis of variance test and is appropriate when data are not normally distributed or are categorical.

Factorial Designs

- Multiple independent variables are common in research designs. For example, both gender and intervention may be grouping variables in a single research design.
- Multiple independent variables can be described in factorial designs. For example a 2×3 factorial design whereby gender and intervention are independent (grouping) variables, the integer, 2, represents the first independent variable, "gender," which has two levels, male and female. The second integer, 3, represents the second independent variable, "intervention," which has three levels, treatment groups A, B, and C.
- Normally distributed data from factorial designs can be compared with that from ANOVAs (one dependent variable), MANOVAs (if there are two or more related dependent variables), ANCOVA (if adjustment for a covariate is necessary), or a repeated measures ANOVA (if one of the independent variables involved repeated measurements of the same subject/sample).

Tests for Categorical Data

- *The chi-square (χ^2) test* is an appropriate test for two or more groups of categorical data; for example, to compare whether or not revision surgery was required for patients who underwent reconstruction using hypothetical device A or device B. In this example, the differences in the frequency of revision surgery (outcome of interest) between patients undergoing reconstruction using device A or B would be tested using the chi-square test. A "statistically significant" result would be interpreted as a relationship between device use and revision surgery. Specific trends can be identified by examining data frequency tables.
- *Fisher's exact test* is similar to the chi-square test but can be a more useful statistical test for small sample sizes or for data sets in which one or more categories contains very few or no data points. For example in the comparison of hypothetical devices A and B, if no patient who required revision surgery underwent reconstructions using device B, Fisher's exact test may be preferred.

Measures of Association

- *Correlations* describe the strength of a relationship between two variables. A *Pearson product-moment correlation coefficient (r)* is the test for correlating two arrays of continuous, normally distributed data (bivariate correlation). The value of the *r* coefficient can range from –1 to 0 to +1.
  - Values closer to +1 or 1 indicate stronger relationships.
  - Values closer to 0 indicate weaker relationships
- Correlation coefficients that are *positive* indicate *direct relationships*. In a correlation of two values collected on the same patient, positive correlations indicate a relationship in which patients who score high on one scale tend to also score high on the other scale. For example, height and weight are positively correlated, because taller people tend to be heavier. Likewise, correlation coefficients that are *negative* indicate *indirect relationships*, in which patients who score high on one scale tend to score low on another scale. For example, athletes who have higher body fat content tend to have slower sprint speeds.
- Correlation coefficients that are less than 0.33 are considered "weak"; those less than 0.66 are considered "moderate"; and those greater than 0.66 are considered "strong" (Fig. 10–3).
- *Spearman rank correlation coefficient (ρ, rho)* is the nonparametric equivalent to the Pearson correlation coefficient. It is appropriately used for non-normally distributed or categorical data.
- *Regression* describes the ability of one (*simple linear regression*) or more (*multiple regression*) variables to predict a specific outcome variable. The more variance explained, the better predictive value of the variables(s) on the outcome of interest. In simple linear regression, one set of numerical data is analyzed to determine predictive ability for an outcome of interest. In multiple regression, two or more predictor variables are used.
- The *coefficient of determination* (R^2) is the product of regression analysis that describes the proportion (%) of variance in the outcome that has been explained by the predictor variable.
  - For example, if the coefficient of determination from simple linear regression (dependent variable = sprint speed; independent variable = body weight) is

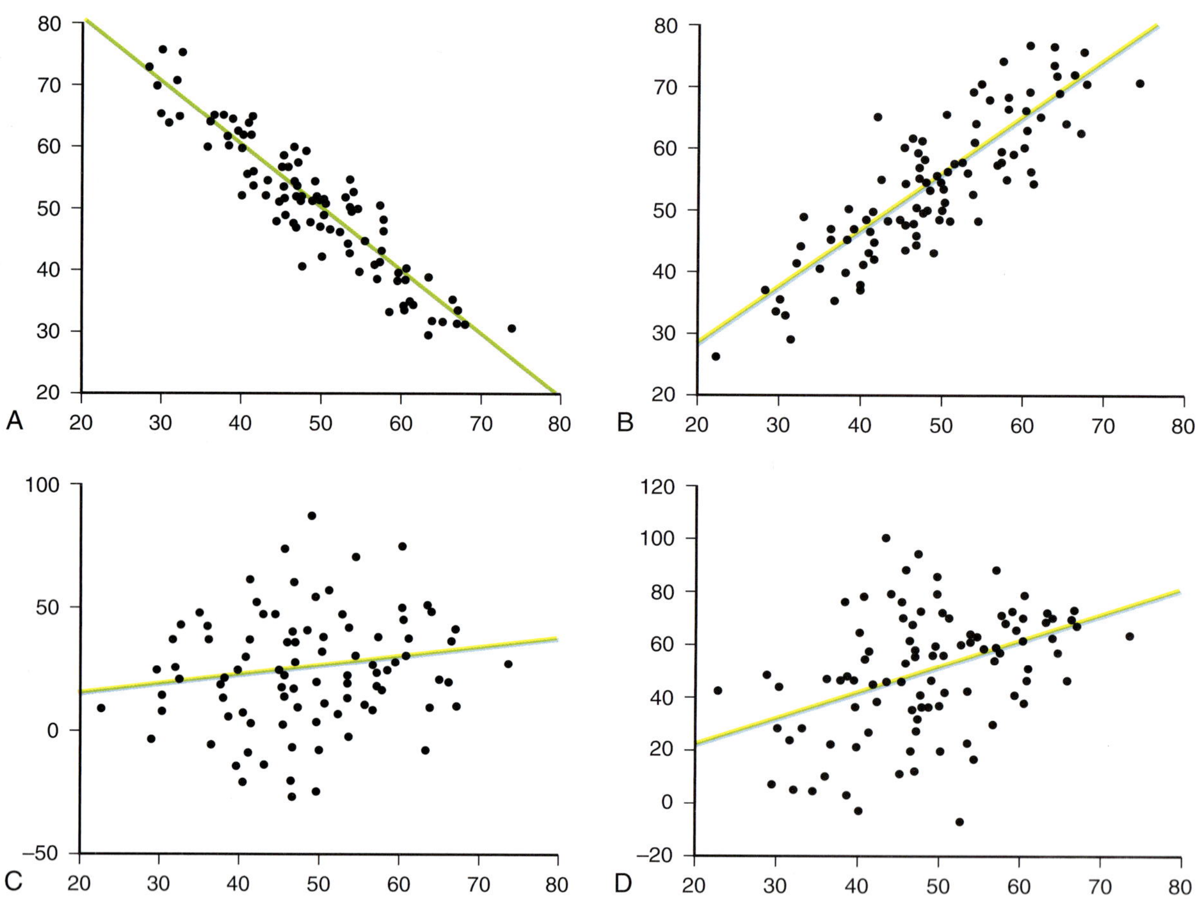

Figure 10–3 Scatterplots showing bivariate (2-variable) relationships. **A**, $r = -0.94$: strong negative correlation. **B**, $r = 0.85$: strong positive correlation. **C**, $r = 0.17$: weak positive correlation. **D**, $r = 0.42$: moderate positive correlation.

Table 10–5 Type I and Type II Statistical Error*

		Reality	
		There is a statistically significant difference between groups (+)	**There is NO difference between groups (–)**
Statistical Test Result	There is a statistically significant difference between groups (+)	Correct test result	*Type I error (alpha)*[†]
	Any observed differences are due to chance alone (–)	***Type II error (beta)***	Correct test result

*In statistical hypothesis testing, the *P* value is used to help make a decision about whether to reject or fail to reject your null hypothesis. Simply, if the *P* value is less than .5, the test is statistically significant (likely not due to chance). These tests, like other tests, are subject to false positives and false negatives.
[†]The likelihood of making this type of error is represented by the *P* value (probability) associated with a given statistical test result. Researchers are typically willing to make this error 5% of the time (5 out of 100); therefore if a *P* value is less than or equal to .05, a test is considered "statistically significant."

$R^2 = 0.81$, then we can interpret the predictive value of body weigh on sprint speed as follows: Approximately 81% of the variance in sprint speed can be explained by subjects' body weight; and 19% is explained by other variables (or error) that have not been included in the simple linear regression analysis.

- *Multiple regression* is used to determine the simultaneous predictive value of two or more independent (*predictor*) variables on the dependent (*outcome*) variable.
- *Logistic regression* is used when the outcome variable is categorical (typically dichotomous) and the predictor variables are categorical or continuous but not normally distributed.

Other Statistical Issues

- *Probability values* (*P* values) are associated with inferential statistical tests and are used to determine whether a test statistic (t-test, chi-square, ANOVA, F-test, etc.) is statistically significant. Traditionally, if a *P* value is less than or equal to .05, then a test result is interpreted as statistically significant. (This value is typically selected but it is arbitrary.) *P value* refers to the probability that a test result is due purely to chance alone. In other words, when you are comparing outcomes between two treatment groups and the t-test result is associated with a *P* value that is less than a certain threshold, the test statistic is said to be statistically significant. Therefore the appropriate conclusion is that the observed differences between the treatment groups are most likely NOT due to chance and more likely due to the intervention that separated the groups. If the *P* value is above the acceptable threshold, we conclude that the observed differences (or associations) were most likely due to chance alone, and not to any of the interventions or other grouping variables. A *P* value of.05 represents the *type I error rate (alpha)* and is interpreted as the number of times out of 100 that we are willing to be wrong when we conclude that a test result was statistically significant (Table 10–5).
- *Statistical power* is the ability to detect a group difference or correlation when it actually exists (see Table 10–5).
  - *Type II errors (beta)* occur when a statistical test indicates that a test comparing two treatment groups (t-test, for example) is not statistically significant, indicating no difference between groups, but there was actually a real difference that was missed by the statistical test. This is typically acceptable up to 20% of the time.
  - Similarly, acceptable statistical power should be greater than or equal to 0.80—that is, a statistical test should be able to detect actual relationships or group differences when they actually exist at least 80% of the time.
  - Statistical power is increased by higher sample sizes (more subjects), by decreased variability among data sets (lower standard deviations), and by designing studies in which there are greater group differences or treatment effects.
- *Power analyses* can be performed before a study, either on the basis of preliminary or pilot data or by using surrogate data, in order to determine how many subjects would be needed in the study (per group or intervention) so as to provide the greatest likelihood of finding a statistically significant result while accepting a maximum type I error

rate of 5% ($P = .05$) and with statistical power (1-beta) exceeding 80%.

- Clinical importance is NOT implied if a *P* value indicates a statistically significant test result. It is the responsibility of the scientist or clinician to determine whether the magnitude of the differences or the strength of associations is important or meaningful to clinical populations.
- *Confidence intervals (CIs)* quantify the precision of the mean calculated from a study sample data. CIs are calculated from study data means and standard deviations and describe an estimated range of values within which a population parameter will fall. Data sets with higher variability and higher standard deviations have larger confidence interval ranges. A *95% confidence interval* describes a range of data values for which we are 95% certain that the actual value representative of the entire population lies somewhere within the calculated upper and lower limits of the CI (see Fig. 10–2). CI calculations are appropriate for normally distributed data.
- *Effect sizes* measure the magnitude of a treatment effect. These statistics not only describe the mean difference between treatment groups but also account for data variability. If data are highly variable, then the estimated effect size will weaken.
  - Effect sizes range in values from 0 to infinity; values closer to 0 indicate no treatment effect, higher values are interpreted as being stronger.
  - Effect sizes less than 0.2 are considered small, those less than 0.5 are considered medium, and those 0.8 and higher are considered large. Effect sizes can be useful when one is considering the clinical importance of research findings.

Review Questions

1. You are reviewing continuous data from an outcomes study and notice that most of the subjective outcomes scores cluster around values from 80% to 90%. Two of the values are 12% and 14%. These values will cause your data distribution to be:
A. Positively skewed.
B. Negatively skewed.
C. Excessively kurtotic.
D. Normally distributed.

2. An experiment is designed to determine the ability to predict work status (working vs. not working) from maximum lift capacity during a strength test. The appropriate statistical test is:
A. Pearson *r* correlation coefficient.
B. Logistic regression.
C. Multiple linear regression.
D. Spearman rho correlation coefficient.

3. When prospectively comparing patients who were randomly allocated to treatment group A or treatment group B, researchers observed that 25 of 50 patients with treatment A had a complication. Only 6 of 50 patients with treatment B had a complication. If you want to determine the likelihood of a complication between the 2 treatment groups, which statistic would be most appropriate?
A. Independent samples t-test.
B. ANOVA
C. Relative risk.
D. Odds ratio.

4. Your study is designed to compare subjective knee function ratings, using a percentage from 0 to 100, between patients who received microfracture and those who received osteochondral plug transfer and an abrasion chondroplasty. Preliminary analysis indicates that the data are excessively skewed and kurtotic. What is the best test for these data?
A. Independent samples t-test with a Bonferroni correction.
B. Repeated measures ANOVA.
C. Kruskall-Wallis test.
D. Mann-Whitney U test.

5. The results from your ANOVA test reveals a *P* value of .02 and is interpreted as statistically significant. What is the appropriate action?
A. Post-hoc tests to determine the exact location differences.
B. Evaluate confidence intervals and effect sizes for additional information.
C. The differences between groups are clinically important.
D. No additional interpretation is necessary.

6. A range of values is calculated from a large data set collected in a multiple-site clinical trial that provide 95% certainty that the population parameter lies somewhere within those values. You notice that the range is larger for data that have a higher standard deviation. What measure is being described?
A. Effect size.
B. Sensitivity.
C. Positive predictive value.
D. Confidence interval.

7. What statistic describes the ability of a clinical test to detect true-positive test results relative to all patients who actually have a given disease or injury?
A. Sensitivity.
B. Specificity.
C. Positive predictive value.
D. Negative predictive value.

8. In a prospective clinical trial, the relative risk for infection following surgery in patients who

have been randomly assigned to group A and group B (control) is 3.1. How is this value interpreted?
A. Treatment group A has a reduced risk for infection.
B. The odds ratio would have been the preferred method for calculating risk.
C. Patients in treatment group A are 3.1 times more likely to have an infection following surgery.
D. There is a 310% higher risk for infection in group A.

9. A clinical diagnostic test for SLAP tears is found to have very high specificity. During an examination, you perform this test and the result is positive, indicating the patient has a SLAP tear. Which of the following can you most reasonably conclude about this test?
A. There is high certainty that the patient has a SLAP tear.
B. You can rule out SLAP tear with a positive test result.
C. This test would be best suited as a screening test.
D. This test must have a very low false-negative rate.

10. A study is designed to longitudinally compare preoperative and postoperative outcomes in patients who had knee joint injections for painful osteoarthritis with those in matched patients who did not have injections. What type of study design is most appropriate?
A. Retrospective cohort.
B. Prospective case-control.
C. Prospective case series.
D. Cross-sectional.

References and Resources

De Muth, J.E., 2008. Preparing for the first meeting with a statistician. Am. J. Health Syst. Pharm. 65, 2358–2366.

Greenfield, M.L., Kuhn, J.E., Wojtys, E.M., 1996. A statistics primer. Am. J. Sports Med. 24, 393–395.

Greenfield, M.L., Kuhn, J.E., Wojtys, E.M., 1996. A statistics primer. P values: Probability and clinical significance. Am. J. Sports Med. 24, 863–865.

Greenfield, M.L., Kuhn, J.E., Wojtys, E.M., 1997. A statistics primer: Power analysis and sample size determination. Am. J. Sports Med. 25, 138–140.

Greenfield, M.L., Kuhn, J.E., Wojtys, E.M., 1997. Current concepts: A statistic primer: Descriptive measures for continuous data. Am. J. Sports Med. 25, 720–723.

Greenfield, M.L., Wojtys, E.M., Kuhn, J.E., 1997. A statistics primer: Tests for continuous data. Am. J. Sports Med. 25, 882–884.

Greenfield, M.L., Kuhn, J.E., Wojtys, E.M., 1998. A statistics primer: Confidence intervals. Am. J. Sports Med. 26, 145–149.

Greenfield, M.L., Kuhn, J.E., Wojtys, E.M., 1998. A statistics primer: Correlation and regression analysis. Am. J. Sports Med. 26, 338–343.

Greenfield, M.L., Kuhn, J.E., Wojtys, E.M., 1998. A statistics primer: Validity and reliability. Am. J. Sports Med. 26, 483–485.

Kocher, M.S., Zurakowski, D., 2004. Clinical epidemiology and biostatistics: A primer for orthopaedic surgeons. J. Bone Joint Surg. Am. 86A, 607–620.

Kuhn, J.E., Greenfield, M.L., Wojtys, E.M., 1996. A statistics primer: Hypothesis testing. Am. J. Sports Med. 24, 702–703.

Kuhn, J.E., Greenfield, M.L., Wojtys, E.M., 1997. A statistics primer: Prevalence, incidence, relative risks, and odds ratios: Some epidemiologic concepts in the sports medicine literature. Am. J. Sports Med. 25, 414–416.

Kuhn, J.E., Greenfield, M.L., Wojtys, E.M., 1997. A statistics primer: Statistical tests for discrete data. Am. J. Sports Med. 25, 585–586.

Kuhn, J.E., Greenfield, M.L., Wojtys, E.M., 1997. A statistics primer: Types of studies in the medical literature. Am. J. Sports Med. 25, 272–274.

McKeon, P.O., Medina, J.M., Hertel, J., 2006. Hierarchy of research design in evidence-based sports medicine. Athletic Therapy Today 11, 42–45.

Medina, J.M., McKeon, P.O., Hertel, J., 2006. Rating the levels of evidence in sports medicine research. Athletic Therapy Today 11, 38–41.

Overholser, B.R., Sowinski, K.M., 2007. Biostatistics primer: Part I. Nutr. Clin. Pract. 22, 629–635.

Overholser, B.R., Sowinski, K.M., 2008. Biostatistics primer: Part 2. Nutr. Clin. Pract. 23, 76–84.

Sprent, P., 2003. Statistics in medical research. Swiss Med. Wkly. 133, 522–529.

Wang, D., Bakhai, A., Maffulli, N., 2003. A primer for statistical analysis of clinical trials. Arthroscopy 19, 874–881.

Wojtys, E.M., Greenfield, M.L., Kuhn, J.E., 1996. A statistics primer: Statistical terminology—part 2. Am. J. Sports Med. 24, 564–565.

Answer Key

CHAPTER 1

Team Physician Responsibilities Questions

1. E
2. C
3. D
4. D

Pre-participation Physical Examination Questions

1. D
2. A

Return-to-Play Questions

1. B
2. A
3. E

Legal and Ethical Considerations Questions

1. B
2. D

CHAPTER 2

Cardiovascular Issues Questions

1. D
2. D
3. E

Pulmonary Issues Questions

1. D
2. B

Environmental Illness Questions

1. C
2. C
3. D

Infection Questions

1. C
2. D

Dermatology Questions

1. D
2. D

Nonmusculoskeletal Injury Questions

1. B
2. D

Supplement Questions

1. B
2. E

Nutrition and Eating Disorders Questions

1. A
2. B

The Female Athlete Questions

1. C
2. A

Special Populations Questions

1. E
2. C

CHAPTER 3

Anatomy and Biomechanics Questions

1. A
2. E
3. A
4. B

Diagnosis Questions

1. D
2. C
3. C
4. D

Arthroscopy Questions

1. E
2. C
3. C

Instability Questions

1. E
2. C
3. E

Rotator Cuff Disease Questions

1. B
2. C
3. D
4. E

Superior Labrum/Biceps Pathology Questions

1. E
2. E
3. C
4. B

Clavicle Disorders Questions

1. A
2. C
3. B
4. C

Glenohumeral Arthrosis Questions

1. B
2. A
3. D
4. D

The Thrower's Shoulder Questions

1. E
2. A

CHAPTER 4

Anatomy and Functional Biomechanics Questions

1. A
2. B
3. E

History, Physical Examination, and Imaging Questions

1. C
2. A

Medial-Sided Elbow Pain Questions

1. B
2. E

CHAPTER 5

Bone and Joint Questions

1. B
2. B
3. C
4. D

Tendon/Muscle Questions

1. B
2. B
3. E
4. E

Neurovascular Questions

1. A
2. B

History and Physical Examination Questions

1. E
2. C
3. E
4. B

Tendon Injury Questions

1. C
2. D
3. B

Ligament Injury Questions

1. A
2. C
3. B
4. B

Fracture Questions

1. C
2. E
3. D

CHAPTER 6

Anatomy and Biomechanics Questions

1. B
2. A
3. C
4. B

History, Physical Examination, and Imaging Questions

1. D
2. D
3. B
4. E

Arthroscopy Questions

1. C
2. E
3. C

Meniscus Questions

1. D
2. C
3. C

Ligament Injury Questions

1. E
2. A
3. D

Osteochondral Lesions Questions

1. B
2. D
3. E

Synovial Lesions Questions

1. D
2. C
3. B

Patellofemoral Disorders Questions

1. B
2. E
3. B

Pediatric Sports Knee Disorders Questions

1. D
2. E
3. C

CHAPTER 7

Anatomy Questions

1. C
2. B
3. E
4. D
5. C

Bursitis and Contusions Question

1. B

Syndromes Questions

1. A
2. B
3. B
4. B
5. C
6. A
7. C
8. C

Fracture Questions

1. A
2. B
3. B
4. D
5. D
6. A2, B5, C4, D1, E3

Dislocation, Avascular Necrosis, and Nerve Entrapment Questions

1. E
2. B
3. B
4. C
5. D
6. B
7. Answer: posterior labral tearing, chondral shear of the femoral head, anterior labral tearing (with reduction).

Arthroscopy Questions

1. A
2. B
3. A
4. C
5. A
6. B
7. D
8. B
9. True.
10. Flexion, internal rotation and axial compression.
11. False. Abnormalities also include labral degeneration/tearing and chondral damage to the anterior superior acetabulum.

CHAPTER 8

Anatomy and Biomechanics Questions

1. B
2. D
3. C

History, Physical Examination, and Imaging Questions

1. C
2. B
3. A

Arthroscopy Questions

1. B
2. C
3. D

Acute Sprains Questions

1. D
2. B
3. C

Ankle Instability Questions

1. D
2. B
3. C

Osteochondral Lesion Questions

1. C
2. B
3. C

Peroneal Subluxation Questions

1. B
2. B
3. D

Achilles Tendon Rupture Questions

1. B
2. D
3. C

Stress Fracture Questions

1. C
2. D
3. C

Turf Toe Questions

1. C
2. D
3. A

CHAPTER 9

Head Injuries Questions

1. D
2. D

Cervical Spine Questions

1. B
2. C
3. E

Lumbar Spine Questions

1. E
2. E
3. A
4. E

CHAPTER 10

Review Questions

1. B
2. B
3. C
4. C
5. A
6. D
7. A
8. C
9. A
10. B

Index

Note: Page numbers followed by *f* indicate figures and followed by *t* indicate tables.